A CONSUMER'S GUIDE TO
EES

DOES YOUR DOCTOR CHARGE TOO MUCH?

JAMES DAVIS

Davis, James B.
 Does Your Doctor Charge Too Much? : a consumer's guide to physician fees / James Davis.
  p.   cm.
 Includes index.
 ISBN 1-885987-02-1
  1. Medical fees--United States. 2. Consumer education.
I. Title.
R728.5.D379   1997   97-5172
362.1'029'6--dc21

ISBN 1-885987-02-1

Health Information Press
A Division of PMIC
4727 Wilshire Blvd, Suite 300
Los Angeles, California 90010
1-800-MED-SHOP

http://www.medicalbookstore.com

Printed in the United States of America

Copyright© 1997 under the Uniform Copyright Convention. All rights reserved. This book is protected by copyright. No part of it may be reproduced, stored in a retrieval system, or transmitted in any form or by any means, electronic, mechanical, photocopying, recording, or otherwise, without written permission from the publisher.

FOREWORD

Today's consumers are far more sophisticated in their general knowledge of medical services. However, they are still mostly in the dark about what medical, surgical and diagnostic procedures should or will cost...until they get the doctor's bill or a copy of the health insurance plan's explanation of benefits. This lack of understanding often results in the consumer paying hundreds or thousands of dollars out of his or her own pocket for medical care they thought was covered by their health insurance plan.

Many consumers believe that their health insurance plan covers everything. But the reality is that all health insurance benefits are limited to some degree by the coverage contract between the insurance company and the insured. If your doctor charges you more than the contract allows, you may have to pay the difference, which could be substantial.

You may believe that you can depend on your doctor, whose income and livelihood depend on a clear understanding of these issues, to know everything about this and automatically do it right on your behalf. The truth is that most doctors would prefer to just practice medicine and ignore the subjects of billing and insurance. Unfortunately, many do exactly that, with serious consequences for themselves and their patients. Improper handling of health insurance claims costs doctors and their patients millions of dollars a year in lost insurance benefits.

Finding ways to reduce payments to doctors and control medical billing fraud continues to be the focus of health care reform proposals by politicians. Yet did you know that virtually all medical practices are operated as discount businesses? Or that for every doctor who is committing billing fraud there are many more who aren't charging enough for their services?

How do you find out if your doctor's fees are fair, based upon those charged by other doctors in your community? How do you know if your health insurance plan or HMO is paying a fair amount to your doctor? How do you challenge a "too high" fee by your doctor or a "too low" payment by your health insurance plan? How can you "shop" for elective medical procedures and even negotiate a lower fee? This book answers these questions and more. It may save you some money and will definitely help you make informed decisions about your health insurance coverage and the cost of your medical care.

DISCLAIMER

This publication is designed to offer basic information regarding medical billing, health insurance claims and doctors' fees. The information presented is based on the analysis of a database of medical fees and the experience and interpretations of the author. Though all of the information has been carefully researched and checked for accuracy and completeness, neither the author nor the publisher accept any responsibility or liability with regard to errors, omissions, misuse or misinterpretation.

CONTENTS

FOREWORD & ACKNOWLEDGMENTS i

INTRODUCTION AND OVERVIEW 1

INSURANCE TERMINOLOGY 5

HEALTH INSURANCE 15

    Key Points Regarding Health Insurance 15
    Who's Who in Health Insurance 15
    Types of Insurance Carriers 17
    Limitations of Insurance Coverage 21
    Determining Eligibility and Verifying Benefits ... 24
    Should Your Doctor Bill Your Insurance? 25
    How Health Insurance Pays Your Doctor 26
    Health Insurance Fraud 30

DOCTOR BILLING 33

    Key Points Regarding Doctor Billing 33
    Billing and Payment Policies 34
    Forms and Documents 35
    Medical Coding Systems 36

DOCTOR FEES 39

    Key Points Regarding Doctor Fees 39
    Doctors Have Difficulty Obtaining Fees 40
    Traditional Methods of Adjusting Fees 40
    Doctors Are Running Discount Businesses 41
    Your Right to Know Fees in Advance 42

HOW TO COMPARE FEES 45

    The Superbill 45
    The Health Insurance Claim Form 45
    Why Health Insurance Claims Are Rejected 47
    The Explanation of Benefits 49

DOES YOUR DOCTOR CHARGE TOO MUCH?

How to Challenge the Doctor's Fee	52
How to Challenge the Insurance Payment	53
Source of the Fee Data	54
Format of the Fee Data	55
A Short Course in Statistics	57
Geographic Variability and Adjustment	58
How to Adjust Fees for Your Location	59
Specialty Differentials	60

DOCTOR VISITS ... 61

Office or Other Outpatient Services	62
Hospital Observation Services	62
Hospital Inpatient Services	62
Consultations	62
Emergency Department Services	63
Critical Care Services	63
Neonatal Intensive Care Services	63
Nursing Facility Services	63
Rest Home or Custodial Care Services	64
Home Services	64
Prolonged Services	64
Case Management Services	64
Care Plan Oversight Services	65
Preventive Medicine Services	65
Newborn Care	65

MEDICINE SERVICES ... 67

Immunization Injections	67
Infusion Therapy	68
Therapeutic Injections	68
Psychiatric Services	68
Biofeedback	69
Kidney Dialysis Services	69
Gastroenterology Services	70
Ophthalmology Services	70
Ear, Nose and Throat Services	72
Cardiovascular Services	74
Non-invasive Diagnostic Studies	78
Pulmonary Services	79
Allergy and Immunology Services	80
Neurology Procedures	81

Central Nervous System Assessments 82
Chemotherapy Administration 83
Dermatology Procedures 83
Physical Therapy and Rehabilitation 83
Osteopathic Manipulation Treatment 85
Chiropractic Manipulation Treatment 85
Special Services and Reports 85

SURGERY SERVICES 87

Integumentary System 87
Musculoskeletal System Surgery 97
Respiratory System Surgery 134
Cardiovascular System Surgery 141
Spleen and Lymphatic System Surgery 154
Mediastinum and Diaphragm Surgery 155
Digestive System Surgery 156
Urinary System Surgery 174
Male Genital System Surgery 181
Laparoscopy and Hysteroscopy 185
Female Genital System Surgery 186
Maternity Care and Delivery 190
Endocrine System Surgery 192
Nervous System Surgery 193
Eye and Ocular Adnexa Surgery 204
Auditory System Surgery 211

RADIOLOGY SERVICES 215

Diagnostic Radiology 215
Diagnostic Ultrasound 225
Radiation Oncology 227
Nuclear Medicine 229

LABORATORY SERVICES 233

Automated Laboratory Panels 233
Organ or Disease Oriented Panels 234
Drug Testing 234
Therapeutic Drug Assays 234
Evocative/Suppression Testing 235
Consultation (Clinical Pathology) 236

Urinalysis 236
Chemistry 236
Hematology and Coagulation 245
Immunology 248
Transfusion Medicine 252
Microbiology 253
Anatomic Pathology 255
Surgical Pathology 256
Other Laboratory Procedures 257

APPENDIX 259

Geographic Variability and Adjustment 259
How to Adjust Fees for Your Location 260
Geographic Adjustment Factors by State 261

THE AUTHOR 270

INDEX 271

INTRODUCTION & OVERVIEW

Does your doctor charge too much? The answer could be *yes*, *no*, *maybe*, *sometimes*, or *probably not*...depending on the doctor, the service, or even where you live. A doctor may charge too much for some services and not enough for others. The doctor's charge may be reasonable, but your health insurance plan may not pay the doctor enough, leaving you to pay the difference.

So why is this important to you and me? Because it costs us money—a lot of money. Directly or indirectly, we all pay for our own health care. We pay it directly by paying the doctor in full or by paying the difference between what the doctor charges and what our health insurance plan pays. We pay it directly by paying all or a portion of our health insurance premiums. We pay it indirectly with our taxes, which support Medicare, Medicaid and a variety of other government health programs, from which we may or may not personally benefit.

Finding ways to reduce payments to doctors and control supposedly rampant billing fraud continues to be the focus of health care reform proposals. Yet, in spite of the national furor over the high cost of medical care, virtually all medical practices are run as discount businesses. When a doctor accepts what your health insurance pays as full payment, or when he/she gives up as much as fifty percent for bad debt collection, or when he/she accepts capitation or discounted payments from managed care organizations, or when he/she provides services to Medicare or Medicaid patients, the doctor is running a discount business.

Working with physicians over the past three decades has given me a unique perspective that politicians don't have. Of course there is some billing fraud, committed by a few dishonest people. But for every doctor that anyone can find who is committing fraud, I can find nine more who are not charging enough for their services.

The problem is not billing fraud. The problem is the combined result of improper coding and billing of medical services, poor handling of health insurance claims by the doctor's staff, and the adversarial relationship between doctors and health insurance companies.

The relationship between doctors and health insurance plans has traditionally been an adversarial one. Part of the reason is that doctors resent the control over their practice and the amount of time required to complete health insurance claim forms—only to have to wait for their payment, which is often reduced.

Another reason for this adversarial relationship is that the doctors and the health insurance plans have different economic missions. The doctor's economic mission is to provide his services and be paid as soon as possible. To many doctors, the mission of private health insurance plans often seems to be to pay the doctor less, pay him later, or pay him nothing. The reason for this is simple.

Most for-profit health insurance plans are publicly held companies or subsidiaries of publicly held companies. Their main economic mission is to make a profit and provide a profitable return on investment for their shareholders. However, taking away the profit motive doesn't necessarily improve the relationship.

For the most part, Medicare and Medicaid health insurance carriers are bottomless pits of bureaucratic inefficiency drowning in a sea of constantly changing rules and regulations. For example, your doctor's telephone call regarding a specific coding or billing problem to six different provider relations representatives of the same Medicare carrier may result in six different answers to the same question!

Many non-profit health plans, such as Blue Cross, are known as slow payers. However, in a non-profit environment, if there is no money to pay claims or to hire staff to process claims, what other choice do they have? Rumors abound of insurance claims examiners tossing handfuls of claims into wastebaskets to eliminate backlogs.

It is possible for you and your doctor to win this adversarial game, but the doctor has to know the rules, and you have to help him. So what can you do to help?

- You can learn more about the business side of medicine.

- You can learn more about the benefits and limitations of your own health insurance plan.

- You can make sure the doctor's office has current information about your health insurance plan.

- You can ask the doctor's staff questions about charges, billing policies, payment options and health insurance.

- You can negotiate lower fees for some medical services and elective surgical procedures.

- You can question the doctor's office about fees that appear to be too high.

- You can question your health insurance plan about delays in payments, denial of benefits, and low payments to your doctor.

- You can help your doctor get paid by your health insurance plan by getting more involved in the process when necessary.

SUPPORT FROM ORGANIZED MEDICINE

The American Medical Association (AMA), which represents about 40 percent of all doctors licensed to practice medicine in the United States, supports the distribution of fees and prices for medical services and procedures to consumers. In the AMA's *Policy Compendium*, 1995 Edition, the AMA refined its Health Access America program and made the following recommendations:

- *Physicians should retain the right to charge their patients their usual fee that is fair, irrespective of insurance/coverage arrangements between the patient and the insurers. (This right may be limited by contractual agreement). An accompanying responsibility of the physician is to provide the patient adequate fee information prior to the provision of the service. In circumstances where it is not feasible to provide fee information ahead of time, fairness in application of market-based principles demands such fees be subject, upon complaint, to expedited professional review as to appropriateness.*

- *In order to facilitate cost-conscious, informed market-based decision making in health care, physicians, hospitals, pharmacies, durable medical equipment suppliers, and other health care providers would be required to make information readily available to consumers on fees/prices charged for frequently provided services, procedures and products, prior to the provision of such services, procedures and products.*

DOES YOUR DOCTOR CHARGE TOO MUCH?

INSURANCE TERMINOLOGY

Doctors are trained during medical school to speak a foreign language called medical terminology. This language allows medical professionals to communicate clearly and precisely with each other, but unfortunately it usually inhibits their ability to communicate effectively with patients and the patient's family.

Doctors also use special terminology on patient bills, health insurance claim forms, managed care contracts and in dealing with insurance companies. The complexity of this foreign language is further complicated by various federal and state government agencies charged with the responsibility of managing Medicare, Medicaid, CHAMPUS and other health care programs.

In order to understand doctors' bills, doctors' fees, and your own health insurance benefits, you need to have a basic knowledge of the words, phrases and acronyms that doctors, government agencies and health insurance plans use to describe services, regulations, benefits and payment policies.

Accident and health insurance: Health insurance under which benefits are payable in case of disease, accidental injury or accidental death.

Allowed charge: The amount that your health insurance plan allows for services and procedures billed by your doctor. The allowed charge may be exactly what the doctor charged or may be a lower amount.

Anniversary: The beginning of a benefit year for a subscriber group.

Assignment of benefits: When the health insurance subscriber authorizes the health insurance plan to pay the doctor directly for any allowable benefits.

Balance billing: When the doctor bills the beneficiary for the difference between what the doctor charged and the amount paid by your health insurance plan.

Beneficiary: A person eligible to receive benefits under a health insurance plan.

Benefit package: Services covered by a health insurance plan and the financial terms of such coverage, including cost sharing and limitations on amounts of services.

Blue Cross: (Mostly) nonprofit, community service organizations, providing in-hospital health care services to their subscribers. Some Blue Cross plans have converted to for-profit status recently.

Blue Shield: Nonprofit voluntary organization which provides subscribers with coverage for expenses (other than hospital costs). May also process health insurance claims for programs like Medicare.

Bundling: The use of a single payment for a group of related procedures or services.

Capitation: A census-driven payment system wherein a health insurance plan provides medical services for a fixed monthly fee. Doctors contracting with the plan may be paid in the same manner.

Carrier: The insurance company which writes and administers the health insurance policy.

Case management: Monitoring and coordinating the delivery of health services for individual patients to enhance care and manage costs. Often used for patients with specific diagnoses or who require high-cost or extensive health care services.

CHAMPUS: Civilian Health and Medical Program of the Uniformed Services. A federally funded comprehensive health benefits program designed to provide eligible beneficiaries a supplement to medical care in military and Public Health Service facilities.

Claim: A demand to the health insurance company, by the insured person, for payment of benefits under a policy.

Claim form: A form used to present health insurance claim information in an organized manner to the health insurance company.

Claims examiner: An employee of a health insurance company who is responsible for handling health insurance claims received from patients, hospitals and doctor's offices.

INSURANCE TERMINOLOGY

Coding: A logical system for identifying and defining medical procedures, services, supplies, materials and diagnoses.

Coinsurance: A provision of a health insurance plan which requires the beneficiary to share in the cost of certain covered expenses on a percentage basis. Also known as copayment.

Comprehensive medical insurance: A health insurance policy designed to give the protection offered by both a basic and a major medical health insurance policy.

Conversion privilege: The right of an individual insured under a group plan to convert to an individual plan if the individual leaves the group.

Copayment: See COINSURANCE.

Coordination of benefits: A provision in a health insurance plan that states that when a patient is covered under more than one group insurance plan, the benefits paid by all plans will be limited to 100 percent of the actual charge.

Cost sharing: The portion of payment for health expenses that the beneficiary must pay, including the deductibles, copayments, coinsurance, and extra bill.

Coverage decision: A decision by a health plan or insurer whether to pay for or provide a medical service or technology for particular clinical indications.

CPT: Current Procedural Terminology. A logical system of medical procedure codes and descriptions published annually by the American Medical Association. This procedure coding system is accepted by virtually all commercial health insurance plans and is required by Medicare and Medicaid.

Cross-over patient: A patient who has both Medicare and Medicaid coverage.

Customary charge: The doctor's standard charge for a given service. Typically calculated by health insurance plans as the doctor's median charge for the service over a prior 12 month period.

Deductible: A specific amount which a subscriber must pay toward the cost of medical treatment before the benefits of the program go into effect. Deductibles may be individual or family.

Deductible carryover: A feature whereby covered charges in the last three months of the calendar year may be carried over to be counted toward the next year's deductible.

Dependents: The spouse and children of the insured as defined in the health insurance contract.

Down coding: A process used by health insurance claims examiners to reduce the value of services billed by doctors by changing the codes submitted.

Dual choice: A health insurance benefit offered by an employer which permits eligible employees a choice of health insurance plans.

Enrollee: See INSURED.

EOB: See EXPLANATION OF BENEFITS.

Exclusions: Specific services or conditions which the health insurance plan will not cover or which are covered at a limited rate.

Explanation of benefits: A form included with a check from the health insurance plan which explains the benefits that were paid and/or charges that were rejected.

Fee for service: Refers to paying medical doctors for individual services rendered.

Fee schedule: A list of pre-determined payments for medical services.

Gatekeeper: A primary care doctor in an HMO who reviews and evaluates patients for referral to specialists. The gatekeeper's mission is to reduce unnecessary services and costs.

Geographic adjustment factor: An adjustment made to a doctor's charges to Medicare based upon where the doctor practices. The adjustment is based upon the work performed and the average practice expenses and malpractice costs in the area where the services are provided.

Global service: A group of related medical services that are treated as a single unit for the purpose of coding, billing and payment.

INSURANCE TERMINOLOGY

Group contract: A contract between an HMO and a subscribing group of beneficiaries which specifies rates, performance, relationships, schedule of benefits, and other conditions, usually for a 12 month period.

HCFA: Health Care Financing Administration. The U.S. Government agency with responsibility for the Medicare and Medicaid programs.

HCFA1500: A universal health insurance claim form that is required for Medicare billing and generally accepted by all health insurance plans.

Health Insurance Company: A company engaged in the business of selling health insurance plans to individuals or groups.

Health Insurance Plan: An organization that acts as an insurer for an enrolled population. May be structured as a fee-for-service or managed care plan.

Health Insurance Policy: An agreement between the health insurance company and the beneficiary which defines the limitations of coverage and specific benefits. A health insurance company may sell hundreds of different health insurance plans.

Health Maintenance Organization: See HMO

HMO: An organization that provides comprehensive health services to its members in return for a fixed prepaid fee. There are four types of HMOs: group, staff, independent practice association, and network.

ICD-9-CM: International Classification of Diseases. A standardized system of describing diagnoses by code numbers developed and maintained by the World Health Organization.

Indemnity schedule: See SCHEDULE OF ALLOWANCES.

Independent Practice Association: An HMO that contracts with individual doctors to provide services to HMO members in a negotiated per capita or fee-for-service rate. Doctors maintain their own offices and can contract with other HMO's and see other fee-for-service patients.

Insurance clerk: One of the doctor's employees who has been assigned the very important job of filing and managing health insurance claims in the medical office.

Insured: The person who represents the family unit in relation to the insurance program. Usually the employee whose employment makes this coverage possible.

Insurer: See CARRIER.

International classification of diseases: See ICD-9-CM.

IPA: See Independent Practice Association

Limited License Practitioner: A professional licensed to perform certain health services in independent practice; for example, podiatrists, dentists, optometrists and chiropractors.

Major medical insurance: Health insurance to finance the expense of major illnesses and injuries. Major medical policies usually include a substantial deductible clause. Above the initial deductible, major medical insurance is characterized by large benefit maximums.

Managed care: Any system of health service payment or delivery arrangements where the health plan attempts to control or coordinate use of health services by its enrolled members in order to contain health expenditures, improve quality, or both. Arrangements often involve a defined delivery system of doctors with some form of contractual arrangement with the plan.

Maximum fee schedule: A compensation arrangement in which a participating doctor agrees to accept the a pre-defined amount from a list supplied by the health insurance plan as the total fee for covered services.

Maximums: The maximum amount a health insurance plan will pay for a specific benefit or policy during a specified time period.

Medicaid: A state/federal government sponsored medical assistance program to enable eligible recipients to obtain essential medical care and services.

Medicare: A federal health insurance program for people 65 or over and for disabled persons with chronic renal disorders.

Medicare Fee Schedule: A schedule of fees for medical, surgical and diagnostic procedures which must be used to bill services to Medicare.

INSURANCE TERMINOLOGY

Medicare Part A: The Medicare Hospital Insurance program which covers hospital and related post-hospital services. As an entitlement program, it is available without payment of a premium. Beneficiaries are responsible for an initial deductible per spell of illness and coinsurance for some services.

Medicare Part B: The Medicare Supplementary Medical Insurance program which covers the costs of doctor services, outpatient lab, x-ray, DME and certain other services. As a voluntary program, Part B requires payment of a monthly premium. Beneficiaries are responsible for a deductible and coinsurance payment for most covered services.

Medigap insurance: Private health insurance policies designed to supplement Medicare coverage. Benefits may include payment of Medicare deductibles, coinsurance, and balance bills, and payment for services not covered by Medicare.

Participating physician: A doctor who signs a participation agreement, agreeing to accept assignment on all Medicare claims for a period of one year.

Policy holder: See INSURED.

PPO: Preferred Provider Organization

Pre-authorization: The process of obtaining permission to perform a service from the health insurance plan before the service is performed. Sometimes referred to as pre-certification.

Precertification: See PRE-AUTHORIZATION.

Pre-determination: The process of obtaining an estimate of what the health insurance plan will pay for a specific service or procedure before the service is rendered.

Preferred Provider Organization: A managed care health plan that contracts with networks or panels of doctors to furnish services and be paid on a negotiated fee schedule. Enrollees are offered a financial incentive to use doctors on the preferred list, but may use non-network doctors as well.

Premium: An amount paid periodically to purchase health insurance benefits.

Primary carrier: The health insurance company which has first responsibility to pay for medical services under Coordination of Benefits.

PRO: See Peer Review Organization

Proof of eligibility: Evidence of eligibility for insurance benefits.

Provider: The person who provides covered medical services, procedures and supplies to the beneficiary covered by a health insurance plan.

Reasonable charge: For any service covered by a health insurance plan, the lower of the customary charge by a particular doctor for that service and the customary charge by doctors in the same geographic area for the same service.

Relative value scale: An index that assigns specific numeric values to medical services. Multiplying the relative value by a conversion factor results in a fee.

Release of information: The patient's signature indicating consent to the release of information necessary for settlement of his or her health insurance claim.

Schedule of allowances: A list of specific amounts which the health insurance plan will pay toward the cost of medical services provided.

Secondary carrier: The health insurance plan which is second in responsibility to pay for medical services under Coordination of Benefits.

Site-of-service differential: The difference in the amount paid by your health insurance plan when the same service is performed in different places. For example, an outpatient visit in the doctor's office or a hospital clinic.

Specialty differential: A difference in the amount paid for the same service when performed by doctors in different specialties. For example, an office visit by a general practitioner or a neurosurgeon.

Subscriber: See INSURED.

Superbill: A form used by doctors to record office visits and services. May be used under some circumstances by patients who wish to file their own health insurance claim forms.

Supplemental health services: Benefits offered by an HMO that exceed their basic health service requirements.

Supplier: Providers, other than doctors, of health care services. These include independent laboratories, durable medical equipment suppliers, ambulance services, orthotists, prosthetists, and portable X-ray providers.

INSURANCE TERMINOLOGY

Table of allowances: See SCHEDULE OF ALLOWANCES.

Third party administrator: An administrative organization other than the insurance company or health care provider that collects health insurance premiums, pays health insurance claims and provides administrative services.

Unbundling: The process of coding, billing and requesting payment for services that are generally included in a global charge by listing the services and fees separately.

Upcoding: The process of selecting a medical procedure code for a service that is more intense, extensive, or has a higher charge, than the service actually provided.

Underwriter: See CARRIER.

Usual, customary, and reasonable: A method of determining benefits by comparing your doctor's charges to those of his or her peers in the same community and specialty.

Utilization review: The process of reviewing services provided to determine if those services were medically necessary and appropriate.

Workers' compensation: State laws which provide coverage of medical expenses for employees who are injured during performance of their work.

HEALTH INSURANCE

Most doctors would prefer to practice medicine and leave the subject of insurance to their staff. But health insurance, with its rules, regulations, forms and terminology is here to stay. Nearly 200 million Americans, 88 percent of the population, are now covered in one way or another by health insurance. Health insurance plans currently pay about 70 percent of all health care costs in the United States. Depending upon your doctor's specialty, from 60 to 90 percent of his practice income will be from health insurance plans.

KEY POINTS REGARDING HEALTH INSURANCE

- All health insurance plans have limitations of coverage.

- Depending on deductibles and copayments, you may have to pay a significant portion of a doctor's charges out of your own pocket.

- The relationship between doctors and health insurance plans is frequently adversarial.

- Your doctor's staff may not bill your health insurance plan properly.

- Your health insurance plan may not pay your doctor properly, leaving you to pay more than your fair share of the bill.

Following is a comprehensive overview of what health insurance is; the relationships betweenf doctors, beneficiaries and health insurance plans; insurance claims processing; and some useful tips to maximizing your health insurance benefits.

WHO'S WHO IN HEALTH INSURANCE

Before we get into a detailed description of how health insurance works, it is appropriate that we identify the major participants.

THE CARRIER

The insurance company which writes and administers your health insurance policy is commonly referred to as the CARRIER. It is also known as the insurer, underwriter, insurance company or administrative agent. Health insurance carriers are responsible for providing coverage as outlined in the contract between the carrier and the insured (you) or contracting group (your employer, union, association). The health insurance carrier cannot be expected to provide payment for which coverage has not been purchased.

Each health insurance carrier offers many different health insurance plans. Also, most government health care programs are administered by health insurance carriers, with the notable exception of most Medicaid programs which are managed by data processing companies. Thus, a single health insurance carrier may sell individual policies and group plans, and also administer a government program such as Medicare. Health insurance plans fall into three basic groups:

Group Policies

Group policies are often benefits of employment that are provided by the employer with little or no cost to the insured. "Coordination of Benefits" is a clause in most group policies which limits the amount that will be paid to a patient who has coverage under more than one group policy.

Individual Policies

Individual policies are those purchased by individuals. There are also health care benefits provided under the individual's other insurance policies, such as home owners and auto insurance. There is no coordination of benefits under individual policies.

Government Programs

Government programs are designed to provide benefits and health care for individuals who would not otherwise be able to afford them.

THE PROVIDER

The provider is the person who provides covered services, procedures and supplies to the beneficiaries. The provider may be a doctor, chiropractor, physical therapist or other health care professional who treats the patient.

The provider may also be the pharmacist who fills the prescription, the outside laboratory that conducts tests, or the medical supply house that rents or sells the patient equipment such as a wheelchair or walker. In the medical office, when the nurse or in-house laboratory provides services under the doctor's supervision, the doctor is still considered the provider.

THE INSURED

The insured is the person who represents the family unit in relation to the health insurance plan. This may be the employee, whose employment makes this coverage possible. This person may also be known as the enrollee, certificate holder, policy holder, or subscriber.

THE BENEFICIARIES

The beneficiary is the person eligible to receive benefits under a health insurance policy. This refers to you and any family members (dependents) covered by your health insurance plan. Dependents include the spouse (husband or wife) and children of the insured as defined in the contract.

TYPES OF INSURANCE CARRIERS

There are currently over 600 health insurance carriers and over 900 HMOs in the United States, and three or four times as many health insurance plans. The different types of health insurance carriers fall into seven categories: commercial carriers, Blue Cross and Blue Shield, Medicare, CHAMPUS, Medicaid, worker's compensation, and health maintenance organizations (HMOs).

COMMERCIAL CARRIERS

Commercial health insurance carriers offer contracts to individuals and groups under which payments are made to the beneficiary (or to the providers if they have accepted assignment of benefits) according to an indemnity table or schedule of benefits for specified medical services. In general most plans conform to one of three basic types:

Basic Medical Plans

Basic medical plans pay total costs up to a maximum, usually around $5,000, for all but a few exclusions such as cosmetic surgery and mental disorders. There may or may not be a deductible, which is an amount the beneficiary must pay. The costs may be incurred in the hospital, home or office.

Major Medical Plans

Major medical plans are designed for catastrophic situations only, and there is no payment under such plans for minor health problems. They usually take up where basic plans leave off, and almost always have a large deductible and copayment.

Comprehensive Medical Plans

Comprehensive medical plans consist of combinations of basic medical plans and major medical plans. These plans provide the best coverage of the three types of commercial insurance plans.

BLUE CROSS AND BLUE SHIELD

The Blue Cross and Blue Shield organization is not a single company, but rather a confederation of 62 independent, community-based Blue Cross and Blue Shield plans. About one in four Americans are covered by a Blue Cross or Blue Shield plan. Blue Cross and Blue Shield plans also contract with the government to pay Medicare health insurance claims. Currently, 85 percent of all Medicare Part A (hospital) health insurance claims and 68 percent of all Medicare Part B (doctor) health insurance claims are processed by Blue Cross and Blue Shield plans.

Blue Cross

Blue Cross plans are mostly nonprofit, community service organizations providing health care services to their subscribers. They are called pre-payment plans because individuals pay in advance for the health services they may need. Blue Cross was initially founded for the purpose of covering hospital stays and remains as such in some states. In many states, the Blue Cross and Blue Shield plans have effectively merged to provide comprehensive coverage for hospital and non-hospital services. Some Blue Cross plans have converted to for-profit status in order to compete more successfully.

Blue Shield

Blue Shield plans are nonprofit voluntary associations originally established so that subscribers may pay in advance for expenses incurred for surgery, in-hospital medical care, and in some plans, outpatient emergency services. As subscribers pay a premium in advance to receive these benefits, Blue Shield plans are also pre-payment plans.

Blue Shield is not a commercial health insurance company. A person becomes a member by entering into a contract with his or her local Blue Shield Plan, and by paying regular dues. He or she becomes a subscriber, not a policyholder, and retains a certificate, not a policy, which tells him or her what to expect when medical services are required.

Under a contract in which the patient has both Blue Shield and Blue Cross coverage, the Blue Cross plan typically pays for hospital services and the Blue Shield plan typically pays for professional services. Blue Cross and Blue Shield also administer Medicare, Medicaid, and CHAMPUS programs in many states. In addition, Blue Cross and Blue Shield plans across the country are developing joint ventures, merged care programs, prepaid group practices and health maintenance organizations (HMOs).

MEDICARE

Medicare is a government health insurance program administered by the Health Care Financing Administration (HCFA), a department of the Social Security Administration. Medicare Part A is hospital insurance, including skilled nursing facilities and home health care in certain cases, for almost everyone over the age of 65, the permanently disabled, and those with chronic renal disease. Coverage under Part A Medicare is automatic.

Medicare Part B, also known as Supplementary Medical Insurance (SMI) covers doctor services, laboratory tests and x-rays. Although a voluntary program, almost all who are eligible sign up. Those who are receiving social security benefits and some others have the premium for Part B coverage deducted from their monthly checks, while the rest pay their premium directly to the Social Security Administration.

Medicare Part B has an annual deductible and a 20 percent copayment. Many Medicare patients also maintain supplemental health insurance coverage, known as MEDI-GAP, which provides coverage for all or part of the difference between what Medicare pays and the total charges.

CHAMPUS

CHAMPUS, which stands for Civilian Health and Medical Program of the Uniformed Services, is a program that makes health care benefits available to dependents of active military personnel, as well as retired military personnel and their families. Under the CHAMPUS program, beneficiaries can go to non-military doctors for medical care and have part of the cost of care paid by the federal government. At age 65, all CHAMPUS beneficiaries are transferred to the Medicare program.

WORKER'S COMPENSATION

Worker's compensation covers medical expenses and disability benefits for workers whose injuries or illnesses are the result of doing their jobs. Anyone who employs more than a specific number of workers is required by law to carry worker's compensation insurance with a carrier of the employer's choice.

With the exception of emergencies, treatment for worker's compensation cases must be authorized in advance. There is a lot of second opinion review involved in some cases where it is not exactly clear that the injury or illness was indeed work related, or if there is a dispute about the level of disability. In addition, there are a variety of additional reports and forms which must completed by the doctor and filed with the worker's compensation insurance carrier.

The premiums for worker's compensation insurance are paid by employers. This gives the employer some rights with regard to receiving regular reports from your doctor, sending you to another doctor for a second opinion, and questioning or challenging your disability or inability to work.

MEDICAID

Medicaid is a health care assistance program administered jointly by the federal and state governments. Each state sets up and operates its own program within the general guidelines set down by the federal government. Some states offer only the minimum services required by the program while other states offer expanded services financed by a combination of federal and state funds.

Medicaid is the most difficult health insurance carrier for doctors to deal with. Regulations limit the diagnostic procedures performed, the type of treatment given, and the medications that can be prescribed. Decisions regarding hospitalization are restricted. Health insurance claims are frequently rejected or denied outright. Payment to doctors is typically 30%-33% of billed charges and in many cases does not cover the cost of doing the paperwork, much less the cost of providing the service. Because of the very low payments, many doctors no longer accept Medicaid patients.

HEALTH MAINTENANCE ORGANIZATIONS (HMOs)

Health maintenance organizations, more commonly known as HMOs, are pre-paid group practice plans where the patient or the patient's employer pays monthly premiums. When medical services are rendered, the patient either does not pay any additional payment or pays small co-payments and any deductibles required by the plan. Health maintenance organizations are the most popular of all the pre-paid health plans.

LIMITATIONS OF INSURANCE COVERAGE

When health insurance coverage is purchased, the benefits are spelled out clearly in the terms of the contract. However, few people bother to read it. The limits of coverage under a given contract are a business agreement based on economic reasoning. Health insurance plans with more limits and less coverage cost less than plans with fewer limits and more coverage. The benefits to which a patient is entitled are determined by the terms of the contract. The health insurance carrier is obligated to provide coverage only for those services specified in the contract.

EXCLUSIONS AND PRE-EXISTING CONDITIONS

All health insurance plans include one or more exclusion clauses covering listed exclusions and pre-existing conditions. Specific exclusions in terms of services, procedures and/or supplies may be listed. Anything listed as an exclusion is not covered under the terms of the policy, which means that no benefits will be paid for these conditions. Examples of typical listed exclusions include:

- Routine physicals

- Routine PAP smears

- Well-baby care

- Newborn problems within first 24 hours of birth

Depending upon the terms of the policy, coverage for treatment of pre-existing conditions may also be excluded or limited. This is a particular problem if you have a pre-existing condition and are covered by an employer paid group-health plan. If you change jobs, you will probably have to convert to your new employer's health plan. If you have a pre-existing condition, the new employer's health plan may decide not to provide coverage at all, or may provide coverage for everything but your pre-existing condition.

Many of the health care reform proposals being considered by Congress include both mobility of health insurance coverage—meaning you can take it with you when you switch jobs—and a requirement that all group health insurance plans cover all members of the group without exclusion.

MAXIMUM COVERAGE AMOUNTS

Most health insurance policies have specific maximum dollar amounts that they will pay. These may be annual maximums, lifetime maximums, or maximums for a specific illness. The typical illnesses and injuries that you and your family will experience as part of ordinary life will not generally deplete your health insurance benefits. However, a heart transplant, a liver transplant, many forms of cancer treatment, or a case of AIDS could put you in a position of literally running out of health insurance benefits.

Under an *annual maximum* insurance policy, benefits become available again at the beginning of the next benefit year or calendar year depending upon the terms of the policy. Under a *lifetime maximum* insurance policy, some conditions are not totally excluded. However, coverage is discontinued after a specific limitation has been reached.

MENTAL AND ADDICTIVE DISORDERS

The most common limitation is a separate schedule of benefits that covers mental, psychoneurotic and personality disorders, and the treatment of drug and alcohol addiction. These may be excluded completely, or subject to limitations.

BENEFIT PERIOD LIMITATION

The term *benefit period* may be used to describe maximums allowed for a specific illness. This limitation most often applies to hospitalization. However, there are similar limitations on payment for outpatient treatment of alcoholism, drug addiction and mental illness.

DEDUCTIBLES

A deductible is a specified amount that the covered person must pay toward the cost of medical treatment before the benefits of the health insurance policy go into effect. Most health insurance policies contain deductible clauses.

However, the amount and type of deductible depends upon the specific plan. The amount of the deductible is generally related to the premium. The insured may choose a higher deductible in exchange for lower premiums, or the insured may choose no deductible in exchange for seeking care only from specified providers.

Individual/family Deductible

Under some policies, the deductible must be met on each individual family member. Others are written so that the first family expenses meeting the specified dollar value will satisfy the deductible for the year.

Deductible carryover

This means that the insured may apply some or all of the deductible for health care expenses incurred in the last three months of the year to deductibles for the following year.

Coinsurance or copayment

Also referred to as copayment, coinsurance is a provision of an insurance plan which requires the insured to share the cost of certain covered services on a percentage basis. The majority of health insurance policies include some form of coinsurance.

DUAL COVERAGE

A patient may have coverage under more than one health insurance policy. This is known as dual coverage. With respect to dual coverage, it is important to consider the three basic types of health insurance policies as they each have different ways of dealing with dual coverage.

Individual Plans

Individual plans are required by law to pay full benefits as specified by the health insurance policy regardless of any other health insurance coverage the patient may have. There is no coordination of benefits under individual health insurance policies.

Group Plans

Group health insurance plans most often include a coordination of benefits clause. Also known as non-duplication of benefits, it is a provision of a group health insurance plan that specifies that when a patient is covered by more than one group health insurance plan, total benefits paid by all policies are limited to 100 percent of the actual charges. No group plan pays more than it would without the coordination of benefits clause.

It is now law in some states that when a dependent is covered under multiple group insurance plans, the insured's date of birth is to be used to determine which insurance coverage is primary. In other words, in these states, if a child is covered as a dependent under insurance plans where the mother is the insured on one and the father the insured on the other, the insurance plan of the older parent is to be considered the primary carrier.

Government Plans

If a patient has dual coverage that includes a government health care plan, such as Medicaid, the government plan is always considered supplementary to private or group health insurance plans. Medicare is the major exception to this rule as many of its insureds also have supplemental health insurance policies, known as MEDI-GAP plans, to help with uncovered expenses.

DETERMINING ELIGIBILITY AND VERIFYING BENEFITS

Most doctors' offices have you fill out patient registration forms on your first visit. This form usually includes information about your health insurance. If you do not have health insurance, you will probably be asked to pay by check or credit card at the end of the visit.

The doctor has a right to expect to be paid for his services. Therefore, it is very important that the doctor's office determine that a patient is eligible for health insurance benefits before providing non-emergency services or treatment. Most doctors' offices are willing to make reasonable financial arrangements with patients.

PRE-AUTHORIZATION

Pre-authorization refers to the process of getting advance permission from the health insurance carrier before providing certain services to the beneficiary. In general, the process involves informing the health insurance carrier of the doctor's plans and the health insurance carrier granting permission for the procedure if covered under the patient's plan.

Many health insurance carriers require pre-authorization, as a condition of their policies, before they will agree to pay for certain hospital admissions, inpatient or outpatient surgeries, and elective procedures. The purpose of pre-authorization is to reduce health care costs by reducing or eliminating unnecessary services.

Most Medicaid programs have rigid pre-authorization programs for all non-emergency hospitalization and surgeries. Many commercial health insurance plans now require pre-authorization for non-emergency hospitalization and/or specific surgical procedures such as total abdominal hysterectomy.

An important point is to note that pre-authorization is usually required for non-emergency hospitalizations, some elective surgeries, and certain diagnostic procedures. Pre-authorization may also result in a demand or request for a second opinion by the carrier prior to granting permission for the procedure. Many health insurance carriers now offer reduced premiums in return for revised plans which include some pre-authorization.

PRE-DETERMINATION

In addition to verifying your health insurance coverage, the doctor may want to find out if his fees for a specific service or procedure will be covered. This process is called pre-determination. The purpose of pre-determination is for the doctor and the patient or insured to be fully informed of what portion of the doctor's charges will be paid by the health insurance carrier.

Pre-determination is helpful to the doctor because it provides him assurance that all or a portion of his fees will be paid by the insurance carrier. In addition, pre-determination allows the doctor's office and the insured to make arrangements for the payment of any difference between the doctor's fees and the amount paid by the health insurance carrier before the service is rendered.

SHOULD YOUR DOCTOR BILL YOUR INSURANCE?

Absolutely. Ten or fifteen years ago, doctors' offices routinely gave their patients itemized statements of the services rendered, instructed patients to file their own health insurance claims, and billed the patient directly. Patients typically waited until the health insurance plan paid them or the doctor before paying any balance due.

Many doctors have learned that completing and filing health insurance claims for their patients helps the doctor get paid faster. If the doctor accepts assignment of benefits on health insurance claims, the health insurance carrier will pay the doctor directly. In addition, it relieves the patient of the anxiety and frustration of completing forms to help the doctor get paid.

HOW HEALTH INSURANCE PAYS YOUR DOCTOR

There are three basic methods of payment used by health insurance plans to pay your doctor. As many health insurance companies offer a variety of plans that create different relationships between the company, the doctor, and the patient, the doctor may be paid by different methods for different plans of the same health insurance company.

FEE-FOR-SERVICE/DISCOUNTED FEE-FOR-SERVICE

Doctors using *fee-for-service* submit itemized health insurance claim forms which include all services and procedures rendered. This is the most common method of billing by most doctors in the United States. Approximately 46% of all payments by health insurance plans to the average doctor are based on fee-for-service or discounted fee-for-service, according to a study done by The InterStudy Competitive Edge: HMO Industry Report 6.2, Minneapolis 1996.

Unless there are special circumstances, the doctor submits his usual charge for each item billed. The health insurance carrier processes the doctor's fee-for-service claim using one of the following methods:

Usual, Customary and Reasonable Charge

Payment based upon usual, customary and reasonable charges, commonly referred to as *UCR*, is the payment system used by most private health insurance plans. The *usual* fee is what your doctor charges most of the time for a specific service or procedure for the majority of his patients. The *customary* fee is determined by health insurance carrier profiles. The typical customary fee is based on the 90th percentile of all fees charged by doctors with the same specialty in the same geographic location for a specific procedure or service. The *reasonable* fee is the lesser of the usual fee, the customary fee, or is justifiable due to special circumstances of the particular case.

How UCR Works

As explained above, the health insurance carriers determine the customary fees for doctors within the same grouping and geographic area. Unless justified by special circumstances, the health insurance carrier will never allow more than

HEALTH INSURANCE

the customary fee for a specific procedure or service. The coinsurance clause affects the amount which the health insurance plan actually pays.

The following examples illustrate how UCR and coinsurance would work for a hypothetical medical procedure billed by four different doctors in the same geographic area. Let's presume that the customary fee for the procedure, as determined by the health insurance carrier, is $ 225.00.

- Dr. Katz submits a claim for his usual fee of $ 220.00. As this is his usual fee, and lower than the customary fee, the carrier "allows" the $220.00 fee.

- Dr. McKellar submits a claim for her usual fee of $ 250.00. As this is her usual fee, but higher than the customary fee, the carrier "allows" $225.00.

- Dr. Williams submits a claim for his fee of $ 250.00 which is higher than his usual fee but is considered reasonable by the carrier because of special circumstances. After a review of the claim, the carrier "allows" $250.00.

- Dr. Davis submits a claim for her usual fee of $175.00. As this is her usual fee, and lower than the customary fee, the carrier "allows" the $175.00 fee.

If the health insurance plan had no coinsurance clause, each provider would be paid the allowed amount. However, if the plan had a 20 percent coinsurance clause: Dr. Katz would be paid $176.00, Dr. McKellar would be paid $180.00, Dr. Williams would be paid $200.00 and Dr. Davis would be paid $140.00—all for exactly the same service.

You may be required to pay the difference between what the doctor charges and what your health insurance plan pays, unless the doctor is accepting health insurance benefits as payment in full. The following chart more clearly indicates the difference in payment amounts to the doctor and the potential amounts you might have to pay out of your own pocket.

DOCTOR	**FEE**	**ALLOWED**	**PAID**	**YOU PAY**
Dr. Katz	$220	$220	$176	$44
Dr. McKeller	$250	$225	$180	$70
Dr. Williams	$250	$250	$200	$50
Dr. Davis	$175	$175	$150	$25

In this example, Dr. Mckellar's fee is more than the health insurance carrier's statistical customary fee for the service. Any doctor's fee that is significantly higher than the health insurance carrier's customary fee, without explanation, should be questioned. You should not have to pay more out of pocket because a doctor charges significantly more than other doctors in the same area.

Schedule of Benefits

A schedule of benefits is a list of specified amounts which the health insurance carrier will pay toward the cost of medical services provided. It is also known as Table of Allowances, Table of Benefits, Indemnity Schedule or Schedule of Allowances. The dollar amounts listed on the Schedule of Benefits represents the total obligation of the health insurance carrier with respect to payment for a specific procedure, service or supply. It does not in any way relate to the doctor's actual charge.

Most health insurance plans which use a Schedule of Benefits to determine payments also include a coinsurance clause. The insured is responsible for the coinsurance amount (typically 20 percent), plus the difference, if any, between the actual charge and the amount allowed by the schedule.

Maximum Fee Schedule

A maximum fee schedule is a payment plan in which the participating doctor agrees to accept the maximum fee schedule amount for a given procedure, service or supply as his or her total payment for a covered service. The payment is not based upon what the doctor charges. The fee schedule may be developed from UCR databases, relative value scales or some combination of the two. Government programs, such as Medicare and Medicaid, are the most common examples of this type of payment plan. Since January 1992, payments for Medicare services have been based on a maximum fee schedule.

CAPITATION

A capitation plan is a pre-paid health insurance plan wherein the health insurance carrier pays the contracting doctor a specified amount, usually on a monthly basis, for each of the health insurance carrier's beneficiaries who have selected the doctor for their health care. This type of payment system is being seen more often as doctors in private practice are subcontracted by HMOs to provide services to their subscribers. Under a capitation system you should not be billed for any service or procedure, unless it is not covered by your health insurance plan. According to the study cited above, approximately 29 percent of all payments by health insurance plans to average doctors are based on capitation.

RELATIVE VALUE SCALE

A *relative value scale* (RVS) is a system of assigning a numeric value to specific medical services and procedures. The numeric value assigned to a specific service is relative to similar or related services. In order to use RVS to calculate a fee, a multiplier known as a *conversion factor* is used. The conversion factor is a dollar amount. To calculate a fee using RVS, the doctor simply multiplies the relative value by the conversion factor. Most relative value scales have different conversion factors for medicine procedures, surgery procedures, radiology procedures and laboratory procedures.

The California Medical Association (CMA) pioneered the use of relative values in 1954 with the *California Relative Value Study* (CRVS). This system was used for setting fees by doctors in California and many other states for almost 20 years, until the federal government decided that it was a form of price fixing and forced the CMA to stop publishing the relative values. CRVS set the precedent and foundations for both the current procedure coding system used nationwide and for the Medicare Fee Schedule implemented in 1992.

Early relative value scales were based upon a statistical analysis of doctor charges and had no relationship to the work involved in providing the service or procedure. Later studies by government agencies, health insurance carriers and others calculated relative values by including the following factors:

- The time involved in performing the service or procedure.

- The skill required to perform the service or procedure.

- The severity of the patient's condition.

- The risk of the service or procedure to the patient.

- The risk of the service or procedure to the doctor (malpractice).

- The cost of operating a medical practice.

Many health insurance carriers use a relative value scale combined with their own conversion factors to determine payment for medical services and procedures. Some health insurance carriers use a combination of UCR and a relative value scale to determine payments to doctors. Approximately 25 percent of all payments by health insurance plans to the average doctor are based on relative value scales, according to The InterStudy report.

The Medicare Fee Schedule

In 1986, Congress created the Physician Payment Review Committee (PPRC) to advise it on reforms of the methods used to pay doctors and other providers under the Medicare program. The PPRC commissioned a two-year study to determine the correct relative values of medical services and procedures based upon the actual work involved. The study was performed by researchers at Harvard University and was financed by the Health Care Financing Administration.

The study found that the current charges for medical services and procedures were not closely related to the costs of providing the services and procedures. The study also found that most non-technical services, such as office visits and general medical services, were under-valued (under-priced) and that most technical services, such as surgeries, radiology services, and complex diagnostic procedures, were over-valued (over-priced).

This study became the foundation for the Medicare Fee Schedule, established by the Omnibus Budget Reconciliation Act of 1989 (OBRA89). After much study and debate, but little effective opposition from organized groups of doctors, the Medicare Fee Schedule became a requirement for billing the Medicare program on January 1, 1992.

Traditionally in the area of medical billing, the policies and procedures mandated by Medicare are implemented a short time later by Medicaid, followed by private health insurance carriers. This being no exception, a significant number of Blue Cross, Blue Shield and other health plans have converted to a payment system similar to the Medicare Fee Schedule.

HEALTH INSURANCE FRAUD

Due to the rapidly escalating costs of health care, and the underlying assumption that doctors are responsible for the major portion of this escalation, there is increased activity on the part of Medicare, Medicaid and private health insurance carriers to detect cases of fraud and abuse.

We stated in the Introduction that for every single case of billing fraud by doctors that anyone can find, we can find many more doctors who are not charging enough. However, due to the publicity value and the possible deterrent affects on others, the emphasis by government and private insurance fraud investigators is to vigorously detect, pursue, punish and publish all cases of fraud and abuse.

HEALTH INSURANCE

FRAUD BY DOCTORS AND OTHER HEALTH CARE PROVIDERS

The following examples, taken from the *Medicare Carrier's Manual*, published by the Health Care Financing Administration for health insurance carriers who process Medicare health insurance claims, provide specific situations that are considered fraudulent. While these examples apply specifically to the Medicare program, private health insurance carriers generally take the same position when investigating fraud.

- Billing for services or supplies that were not provided.

- Altering health insurance claim forms to obtain a higher payment amount.

- Doctor's deliberate application for duplicate payment. (This would include billing Medicare and the beneficiary for the same service or billing both Medicare and another insurance carrier to attempt to be paid twice.)

- Soliciting, offering, or receiving a kickback, bribe or rebate.

- False representation with respect to the nature of the services rendered, charges for the services rendered, identity of the person receiving the services, dates of service, etc.

- Claims for non-covered services billed as covered services. (For example, routine foot care billed as a more involved form of foot care to obtain payment.)

- Claims involving collusion between a doctor and a beneficiary, resulting in higher costs to the Medicare program.

- Use of another person's Medicare card to obtain medical care.

- Alteration of claims history records to generate fraudulent payments.

FRAUD BY HEALTH INSURANCE CARRIERS

It should be clearly understood that doctors are not the only ones committing health insurance fraud. Health insurance carriers also commit fraudulent acts which cost tax payers millions of dollars every year. Following are some recent cases that made national headlines.

In a case that raises new questions about a state's ability to monitor medical care for millions of Medicaid enrollees who are being steered into HMOs, a San Diego physician recently alleged that ProCare, Inc., a managed care company, falsified medical records to pass a state inspection.

In April 1996, Blue Shield of California agreed to plead guilty to federal criminal charges that it engaged in a years-long conspiracy to falsify government audit reports on the health insurer's processing of billions of dollars worth of Medicare claims. Blue Shield agreed to pay a $1.5 million fine to settle the criminal charges.

In May 1996, the Justice Department claimed that Foundation Health Plan, commonly known as FHP, may have overcharged as much as $15 million on its health benefit contracts for federal employees over a five-year period.

FRAUD BY PATIENTS

Consumers also commit health insurance fraud. The fraud you usually hear about includes faking work-related injuries, faking injuries after an automobile accident or faking injuries after falling in a store or other public place. This fraud costs consumers billions of dollars a year. In addition, there are other forms of fraud committed by patients, including:

- The use of another person's health identification card to obtain medical care.

- Collusion between a doctor and a beneficiary, resulting in higher costs to the health insurance carrier.

DOCTOR BILLING

Getting paid by your health insurance plan is not a simple task for your doctor's office. In order to report and bill medical services, procedures and diagnostic tests to your health insurance plan, your doctor and his staff must learn and manage a variety of administrative tasks related to filing health insurance claims.

The doctor's office must have written policies and procedures which support the billing, coding and collections processes. They must use forms and documents which are current, accurate and conform to legal requirements. They must use current medical coding systems, required by law, to report all services and procedures to your health insurance plan. They must understand how health insurance carriers work and develop effective strategies and systems that allow maximum payment with minimal effort. And even if they do all of this properly they still may not get paid.

KEY POINTS REGARDING DOCTOR BILLING

- Many of the documents your doctor's office may ask you to complete and sign are required by law. Billing forms and documents provide the fundamental information needed for your doctor's office to bill your health insurance plan.

- Accurate and complete billing forms and documents can make a significant difference in how much, or even if, your doctor gets paid by your health insurance plan. It also can affect how much you may have to pay.

- Doctors must use several complex coding systems to report services and procedures to health insurance carriers. The doctor's payment, and the amount you may have to pay, depends on the accurate use of these coding systems.

- The doctor's billing staff must keep track of hundreds of constantly changing rules, regulations and policies for billing Medicare, Medicaid, worker's compensation, managed care plans, and private health insurance plans.

- Helping your doctor with this information is the best way to make sure you receive the maximum allowed benefits from your health insurance plan.

BILLING AND PAYMENT POLICIES

When you visit your doctor, or are scheduled for a surgical or diagnostic procedure, you should be informed in advance of what the service will cost. Unfortunately, many doctor's offices do not do this automatically and many patients never ask because they mistakenly believe that their health insurance policy will pay for everything.

If the doctor's office staff does not inform you regarding billing and payment, you should take the initiative and ask. Some questions related to billing and payment policies that you need answers to include:

- What are the estimated costs and are you expected to pay at the time of service?

- If you are expected to pay, what are your payment options: check, cash, credit cards?

- Will the doctor's office bill you, and if they will is there a finance or service charge for unpaid balances?

- Does the doctor's office file health insurance claims for all patients for all services?

- Does the doctor accept assignment of benefits?

- What about any balance remaining after my health insurance plan has paid?

- Does the doctor's office participate in Medicare?

- How does the doctor's office handle deductibles and coinsurance?

- What about my secondary insurance?

FORMS AND DOCUMENTS

When you visit your doctor's office, or are seen by a doctor in the hospital, you usually have to fill out a variety of forms. This is particularly true on the first visit to a new doctor. While you may consider this a burden, the accuracy and completeness of the information you provide on these forms can significantly affect the benefits paid by your health insurance plan.

In order to collect the information required for creating accounts, posting charges, and billing patients and health insurance carriers properly, the doctor's office must develop, maintain and use proper billing forms and documents. Many of these forms are required by various federal, state and local laws.

The best time for the doctor's office to collect billing information is when the patient is first seen. However, collecting this information is sometimes difficult when you receive services at a location other than the doctor's office. Hospital consultations, emergency room services, inpatient surgeries without pre-operative office visits are all examples of situations where the patient is not seen in the doctor's office prior to provision of services and may not be seen in the office after provision of services.

Under these circumstances the doctor providing the service should try to collect information and signatures required to bill your health insurance plan. But many doctors are uncomfortable discussing billing issues and others consider the collection of information beneath their dignity. So more likely, you will get a phone call or a letter from the doctor's billing staff asking for the information and signatures.

Another example is the independent laboratory. Frequently your doctor will send a blood sample or other specimen to an independent laboratory for analysis. The laboratory, which is another form of medical practice supervised by doctors, performs the test, sends the results to your doctor, and then sends you or your health insurance company a bill without ever seeing you.

It is to your benefit to make sure that any doctor or other provider who provides services to you or your family has accurate and complete information needed to bill your health insurance plan.

- Carry your health insurance identification card with you. All health insurance carriers issue cards to their beneficiaries and many of the cards have valuable information such as special telephone numbers or even an explanation of basic coverage provided in addition to patient identification.

- Notify your doctor's office during your next visit of any changes of employment or other status which may affect your health insurance coverage. Most group health insurance plans have a waiting period of at least 30 days and frequently 60 or 90 days before the employee is eligible for coverage.

MEDICAL CODING SYSTEMS

When a doctor provides a service or performs a procedure he makes an entry in your medical record. In addition, he or his staff must code the service or procedure for billing purposes. Coding is a uniform method of identifying and defining services, procedures, and medical supplies and equipment for billing and payment purposes.

Prior to 1983 there were over 120 different medical coding systems in use in the United States. In order to bill health insurance claims properly, the doctor's office had to keep track of numerous codes and coding systems, as well as special claim forms required by different health insurance plans.

Today, doctors use only three nationally recognized coding systems to report services and procedures. The purpose of this simplification of coding systems was to provide a uniform language that accurately described medical, surgical, and diagnostic services, and provided an effective means for reliable nationwide communication between and among doctors and health insurance plans.

Two of the coding systems, CPT and HCPCS, are used to report services and procedures—or "what" the doctor did. The third coding system, ICD-9-CM, is used to report the patient's condition, diagnosis or symptoms—or "why" the doctor provided the service or procedure. These coding systems are required by federal and state laws for government health insurance programs and are required or accepted by virtually all other health insurance plans.

PROCEDURE CODING

Procedure coding is used to define the service, procedure or supply that is provided. The first of the two procedure coding systems is *Physicians' Current Procedural Terminology*, more commonly known as CPT. CPT is revised and published annually by the American Medical Association.

IMPORTANT FORMS AND DOCUMENTS

Selection of the proper CPT code has a significant impact on if, and how much, the doctor is paid for his/her services. Likewise, it may have a significant impact on how much you have to pay out of your own pocket. The CPT coding system includes codes, descriptions and guidelines for over 7,000 medical and surgical services and diagnostic procedures. The codes listed in the fee section of this book are CPT codes. Following are examples of CPT codes for well-known medical services and procedures:

10060	Incision and drainage of abscess
81000	Urinalysis
44950	Appendectomy
71020	Chest x-ray, two views
90704	Immunization; influenza virus vaccine
99201	Office or other outpatient visit, new patient

The second procedure coding system used by doctors is the <u>H</u>CFA <u>C</u>ommon <u>P</u>rocedure <u>C</u>oding <u>S</u>ystem, more commonly known as HCPCS. HCPCS is revised and published annually by the Health Care Financing Administration. The HCPCS coding system is used by doctors and other health care providers to bill Medicare for supplies, materials, durable medical equipment and injections which are not listed or not clearly defined in CPT. HCPCS codes must be used when billing Medicare. Some private health insurance carriers also allow or mandate the use of HCPCS codes, mostly carriers that also process Medicare claims. There are over 2,400 HCPCS codes covering supplies, materials, injections and services. Following are examples of HCPCS codes for medical services and procedures:

A4206	Syringe with needle; sterile 1cc
E0112	Crutches, underarm, wood; pair
G0085	Individual psychotherapy, inpatient hospital, 45-50 minutes
H5300	Occupational therapy
J2510	Injection, penicillin g procaine, up to 600,000 units
Q0084	Chemotherapy administration by infusion technique only, per visit

There are no HCPCS codes or associated fees listed in this book. This information is provided in the event that you are a Medicare beneficiary and find codes of this type on your doctor's bill or explanation of benefits.

DIAGNOSIS CODING

Diagnosis coding is used to explain why the doctor performed specific services or procedures. Diagnosis codes are used to report illnesses, injuries,

37

signs, symptoms and ill-defined conditions. The diagnosis coding system used in the United States is the *International Classification of Diseases, 9th Revision*, more commonly known as ICD-9, which was originally published by the World Health Organization. The ICD-9 includes codes, descriptions and guidelines for over 14,000 illnesses, injuries, and symptoms.

As with procedure codes, selection of the proper diagnosis code has a significant impact on if, and how much, the doctor is paid by your health insurance carrier. Likewise, it may have a significant impact on how much you have to pay out of your own pocket. The Medicare program includes severe monetary penalties and even the possibility for exclusion from the Medicare program for failure to use diagnosis codes properly. Following are examples of ICD-9 diagnosis codes:

042	Human immunodeficiency virus [HIV] disease
174	Malignant neoplasm of female breast
410.21	Acute myocardial infarction of inferolateral wall
540.0	Acute appendicitis with generalized peritonitis
V01.5	Contact with or exposure to rabies
E910.0	Accidental drowning and submersion while water skiing

CODING ERRORS BY THE DOCTOR'S OFFICE

Doctors do not always use the correct procedure or diagnosis codes when billing services and procedures. This is usually due to a lack of proper training and/or the lack of current coding resources. But it can also result from an attempt to simplify the billing process by using just a few codes repeatedly. This failure to code properly could cost you a lot of money if the doctor bills you for the unpaid balance after your health insurance plan has paid the doctor.

CODING CHANGES BY HEALTH INSURANCE CARRIERS

One of the ways that a health insurance plan can pay your doctor less is by changing the procedure codes that your doctor submits. Insurance claims examiners are trained to identify opportunities to reduce the value of procedure codes billed by your doctor whenever possible. This process, known as down-coding, costs doctors and their patients millions of dollars annually.

Down-coding allows the health insurance carrier to reduce payment, delay payment while the doctor's office provides supporting documentation, or even deny payment. Frequently, the doctor's office accepts the reduced payment without complaint or appeal, and bills the patient for the unpaid balance.

DOCTOR FEES

In today's more competitive market environment, fees have become an important part of the doctor's marketing strategy. So how do doctors decide what to charge for a service or procedure? Is it like product pricing where they figure out the cost of a service then add a reasonable profit margin? Do they all get together as a group and decide what the charge for a specific service will be? Is there a single national guideline or database or list of medical fees? The answer to all of the above questions is *no*.

KEY POINTS REGARDING DOCTORS' FEES

- Doctors are typically reluctant to discuss fees with each other due to competition or the possibility of legal action based on collusion.

- It is difficult for doctors to obtain fee information, profiles, relative values, or conversion factors from most private health insurance carriers. In addition, medical associations are prevented by federal antitrust legislation from disclosing the results of fee surveys.

- Traditional methods of setting or adjusting fees may result in the doctor charging too much, or too little, and may result in you paying more than you should out of your own pocket.

- The Medicare Fee Schedule, required by law for billing the Medicare program, will most likely become the method used for payment by all health insurance plans.

- If your doctor charges a fee that is more than your health insurance plan will pay, you may have to pay the difference.

- Almost all fees charged by doctors are reduced or discounted either voluntarily or involuntarily.

- It is important to ask questions about fees, billing policies, and payment options before services are rendered.

DOCTORS HAVE DIFFICULTY OBTAINING FEES

It is difficult for doctors to acquire accurate information about medical fees. Under Federal Trade Commission (FTC) rules, doctors are prohibited from discussing medical fees with each other. They can discuss anything else about patients, but they can't discuss what they charge for specific services or procedures.

Many medical associations and medical specialty societies regularly perform surveys of their members' fees for services and procedures. However, under the same FTC ruling, these associations and societies are not allowed to publish the results of their fee surveys.

Fee schedules published by health insurance plans for doctors who agree to see patients enrolled in the plan are always discounted and are not a reliable source for current charges. Likewise, the Medicare Fee Schedule, required by federal law for billing the Medicare program, lists fees that are discounted as much as 50 to 60 percent below non-Medicare fees for the same service.

Private health insurance plans generally do not publish or inform doctors about the maximum allowance, better known as the customary fee, for specific services and procedures. If they did, then every doctor would simply charge the maximum amount, which would increase the amounts paid by the health insurance plan. So the doctor's staff has to use a combination of resources to develop fees that are reasonable, fair, and competitive.

TRADITIONAL METHODS OF ADJUSTING FEES

The consensus among health care management consultants is that most doctors do not have a logical basis for setting or raising their fees. Prior to 1992, doctors used a variety of methods to review and adjust their fees.

One of the most common methods was to increase all fees annually by a certain percentage, say 5 or 10 percent. A variation of this method was to review and increase the fees for selective procedures, usually those that were high volume services. Other doctors would try to figure out what the *going rate* was for popular services and procedures and then simply make sure their fees were the same. All of these methods were simple to calculate and easy to implement.

Some doctors ignored the issue of raising fees until they had a cash flow problem or needed to increase profits for some reason. Then they would discover that their fees were much lower than the going rates and implement large fee increases. This was known as the *catch-up* method. Sometimes the doctor's cash flow would actually decrease as a result of using this method because angry patients would leave the practice.

Other doctors used the Relative Value System described previously to set and increase fees. The concept was very simple. Each medical service or procedure was assigned a numeric value related to similar services and procedures. Each doctor used a conversion factor to calculate fees. For example, if a given procedure was valued at 10 units and the conversion factor was $10.00, the fee would be set at $100.00.

INFLATION AND INCREASED OPERATING COSTS

While the national economy has been relatively stable for several years, the cost of living has continued to increase between 3 to 6 percent annually based upon the Consumer Price Index (CPI). This means that it costs us 3 to 6 percent more each year to purchase the basic goods and services we need. It also means we need to increase our net income (what we have left to spend after taxes and other deductions) by 3 to 6 percent per year just to stay even.

During the same period the cost of running a doctor's office has increased by about 9 percent per year. So the typical doctor's office must increase net income by at least 9 percent per year to stay even with increased operating costs. As a result, most doctors have had to increase the volume of patients they see or find other ways to generate income. Some have quit private practice and joined with clinics or larger medical groups. Others have simply taken early retirement.

DOCTORS ARE RUNNING DISCOUNT BUSINESSES

In spite of the continuous national furor over medical fees, the truth is that, with very few exceptions, all medical practices are operated as discount businesses. Some of the more typical types of discounts includes:

- Giving a discount for cash payment at the time of service.

- Discounting services as a professional courtesy.

- Accepting insurance payment from a private carrier as payment in full.

- Accepting payments on accounts without interest charges.

- Referring accounts to a collection agency.

- Writing off an account as a bad debt.

- Accepting a capitation payment or discounted payment from a managed care organization such as an HMO, IPA or PPO.

- Participating in Medicare.

- Providing services to Medicaid patients.

YOUR RIGHT TO KNOW FEES IN ADVANCE

Many doctors' offices discuss fees in advance with patients who call to make an appointment. This lets the patient know what the charges will be, if the doctor accepts health insurance, and what payment options the patient has. Numerous studies have confirmed that when patients are about to undergo major medical procedures, their first concern is outcome, and their second concern is how much it is going to cost and how they are going to pay for it. Unfortunately, most patients never express this concern voluntarily.

Most doctors readily discuss their findings, treatment plans and the probable outcome(s) with their patients, but many totally neglect any discussion of fees or payment methods. Doctors are reluctant to discuss fees in part because they don't think of themselves as business people. They typically delegate this responsibility to their office manager or billing manager.

In addition to appreciating the information, discussing the potential cost gives patients the ability to make an informed decision regarding the service. In order to gain a little perspective on this issue, ask yourself the following questions:

- Would you order a meal in an expensive restaurant from a menu without prices?

- Would you allow a mechanic to perform major service on your car without an estimate of what it was going to cost?

- Would you allow a contractor to begin construction on your new kitchen or bathroom without a bid?

While I'm sure you answered *no* to each of the previous questions, many patients have diagnostic procedures, surgical procedures or begin long-term medical treatments having absolutely no idea what it will cost, or if their health insurance will pay for it.

Restaurants, automobile mechanics and contractors know better than to provide service without an agreement regarding payment. Yet many doctors' offices expect the patient to agree to expensive medical services and procedures without any advance knowledge of their cost. If the doctor or his staff does not discuss fees with you, then you have to take the initiative as an informed consumer.

DOES YOUR DOCTOR CHARGE TOO MUCH?

HOW TO COMPARE FEES

To compare a doctor's fee to the nationwide fees listed in this book, you need the procedure code (CPT) and the amount charged. You can find this information on a copy of your doctor's Superbill, a copy of your health insurance claim form, or from the explanation of benefits sent to you by your health insurance plan.

THE SUPERBILL

When you visit your doctor's office or are seen by a doctor in a hospital or other facility, the doctor must record what services were provided for billing and statistical purposes. Most doctors use a document called a *Superbill* for this purpose. The document may also be called a visit slip, encounter form, or charge slip.

The Superbill includes a list of procedure codes and descriptions for the most common services or procedures that the doctor performs, along with other information. The doctor records the services or procedures by making check marks on the Superbill. The doctor's billing staff then uses the Superbill to bill your health insurance plan.

An example of a typical Superbill is found on the following page. You can use the Superbill to review the doctor's charges immediately. You don't have to wait until your health insurance plan has been billed. To compare what your doctor charged with the fees listed in this book you need the CPT procedure code for each service or procedure, and the amount charged.

THE HEALTH INSURANCE CLAIM FORM

The *HCFA1500* is the most commonly used health insurance claim form. The form is required by Medicare and accepted by virtually all private health insurance carriers. An example of a typical HCFA1500 is found in the next pages. Most doctors bill your health insurance plan directly using the HCFA1500 claim form.

DOES YOUR DOCTOR CHARGE TOO MUCH?

INTERNAL MEDICINE GROUP — 4186
8330 West Third Street
Los Angeles, CA 90048
(708) 920-0700
LICENSE: P12345
FEIN: 95-4210732

DATE OF SERVICE: 03,15,97
ACCOUNT NUMBER: 6,9,4,3,1
ACCOUNT NAME (LAST, FIRST): DAVIS, JAMES
TIME: 60"

☒ NEW PATIENT ☐ ASSIGNED?
DX #1 786.50 **DX #2** **DX #3** **DX #4**

OFFICE VISITS NEW PATIENT
CODE	DESCRIPTION	DX	FEE
99201	Brief		
99202	Limited		
99203	Intermediate		
99204	Extended		
X 99205	Comprehensive		275

OFFICE VISITS ESTABLISHED PATIENT
99211	Minimal		
99212	Brief		
99213	Intermediate		
99214	Extended		
99215	Comprehensive		

CONSULTATIONS INITIAL OFFICE
99242	Intermediate		
99243	Extended		
99245	Comprehensive		

PROCEDURES
10000*	Drain Skin Lesion		
20550*	Injection, Tendon Sheath		
36415*	Routine Venipuncture		
45330	Sigmoidoscopy		
X 93000	EKG Complete		75
93040	Rhythm EKG with Report		
94010	Spirometry Complete		

INJECTIONS AND IMMUNIZATIONS
90702	Immunization; DT		
90703	Immunization; Tetanus Toxoid		
90724	Immunization; Influenza		
90782	Injection, IM/SQ		
90784	Injection, IV		
90788	Injection, Antibiotic		

RADIOLOGY
| 71010 | X-Ray Exam Chest | | |
| X 71020 | X-Ray Exam Chest | | 95 |

LABORATORY
80019	Lab Panel 19+ Tests		
80052	Premarital Profile		
80060	Hypertension Panel		
80061	Lipid Profile		
80070	Thyroid Panel		
80072	Arthritis Panel		
81000	Urinalysis		
82270	Stool for Occult Blood		
82310	Calcium		
82465	Serum Cholesterol		
82565	Blood Creatinine		
82643	Ria for Digoxin		
82951	Glucose Tolerance Test		
83718	Blood Lipoprotein		
84075	Alkaline Phosphatase		

LABORATORY (Cont'd)
84295	Blood Sodium		
84450	SGOT		
84460	SGPT		
84478	Blood Triglycerides		
85014	Hematocrit		
85022	Automated Hemogram		
85031	Manual Hemogram		
85048	White Blood Cell Count		
85580	Blood Platelet Count		
85610	Prothrombin Time		
85651	RBC Sedimentation Rate		
86580	Skin Test, TB		
87060	Culture, Throat or Nose		

SUPPLIES
| 99070 | Supplies & Materials | | |

MISCELLANEOUS
98900	Med Conference, 30 Min		
98902	Med Conference, 60 Min		
98920	Telephone Call, Brief		
98921	Telephone Call, Intermediate		
99000	Specimen Handling		
99080	Special Reports		

DIAGNOSIS ICD-9 CM
Abnormal loss weight 783.2 · B.hypertensive hrt dis 402.1 · Diabetes w/comp NOS 250.00 · Herpes zoster 053.9 · Mixed hyperlipid 272.2 · Phlebitis unsp 451.9
Acute bronchitis 466.0 · B.neoplasm lg bowel 211.3 · Diaphragmatic hernia 553.3 · Hypercholesterolemia 272.0 · Myalgia unsp 729.1 · Pleurisy unsp 511.9
Acute URI NOS 465.9 · Bronchitis NOS 490 · Diverticula colon 562.1 · Hyperlipidemia 272.4 · Myeloma multiple 203.0 · Pneumonia, org NOS 486
Allergic rhinitis 477.9 · Bronchitis obstr chr 491.2 · Diverticulitis colon 562.11 · Hypertension benign 401.1 · MI unsp 410.90 · Polycythemia vera 283.4
Alzheimer's disease 331.0 · Calculus kidney 595.0 · Diverticulosis colon 562.10 · Hypertension essential 401.0 · MI old 412 · Polymyalgia rheum 725
Anemia iron def unsp 280.9 · Cardiomyopathies 425.4 · Dizziness & giddiness 780.4 · Hypertension NOS 401.9 · Nasopharyngitis acute 460 · Preop chest xray/EKG V99.99
Anemia unsp 285.9 · Cataract NOS 366.9 · Duodenal ulcer unsp 532.9 · Hyperten heart dis NOS · Neuralgia, neuritis 729.2 · Prostate hyperplasia 600
Anemia protein def 281.9 · Cerebrovasc dis other 437.0 · Dyspepsia 536.8 402.90 · Obesity 278.0 · Pul heart dis unsp 416.9
Angina pectoris unsp 413.9 · Cerebral thrombosis 434.0 · Edema 782.3 · Hypopotassemia 276.8 · Osteoarthritis unsp 715.90 · Pyrexia unk origin 780.6
Anxiety state NOS 300.00 · Cerebrovasc dis NOS 437.9 · Emphysema other 492.8 · Hypothyroidism unsp 244.9 · Osteoporosis NOS 733.00 · Renal failure 586
Aortic valve disord 424.1 · ✓Chest pain NEC 786.59 · Esophagitis 530.1 · Impacted cerumen 380.4 · Osteoarthrosis gen 715.0 · Rheumatoid arthritis 714.0
Aortocoronary bypass · ✓Chest pain unsp 786.50 · Gastritis unsp 535.5 · Intermed cor syndrome 411.1 · Other abn blood chem 790.6 · Rhythm disord, other 427.89
V45.81 · Chr airway obstr NEC496 · Gen osteoarthrosis 715.09 · Intest obstruction NOS 560.9 · Other comp med care999.9 · Senile dementia 290.0
Apoplexia 436 · Chr isch heart dis NEC 414.8 · Gout NOS 274.9 · Intracereb hemorr 431 · Other bursitis 727.3 · Sx: abd pain, cramps 789.0
Arrhythmia 427.9 · Chr renal failure 585 · Gouty arthritis 274.0 · Irritable colon 564.1 · Other cellulitis unsp 682.9 · Sx: nausea & vomiting 787.0
Arthropathy unsp 716.9 · Cirrhosis liver 471.5 · Heart dis isch NEC 411.8 · Isch heart dis unsp chr 414.9 · Pain in limb 729.5 · Sx: headache face pain 784.0
ASCVD 429.2 · Constipation 564.0 · Heart fail congestive 428.0 · Isch heart dis chronic 414.0 · Painful respiration 786.52 · Sx: shortness breath 786.09
Asthma w/o status 493.90 · Contact dermatitis 692.9 · Heart failure NOS 428.9 · Kidney disord unsp 593.9 · Palpitations 785.1 · Syncope & collapse 780.2
Atherosclerosis gen 440.9 · Convulsions, seizures 780.3 · Hematuria benign ess 599.7 · Lumbago 724.2 · Parkinson disease 332.0 · Systemic lupus eryth 710.0
Atrial fibrillation 427.31 · Cough 786.2 · Hemiplegia 342.9 · Lymphomas NEC 202.8 · Peptic ulcer unsp 533.9 · Thyrotoxicosis NOS 242.9
Atrial flutter 427.32 · Cystitis unsp 595.9 · Hemorr GI tract unsp 578.9 · Malaise & fatigue 780.7 · Periph vasc dis unsp 443.9 · Trans cereb isch unsp 435.9
Backache unsp 724.5 · Dehydration 276.5 · Hemorr rectum & anus 569.3 · Melena blood in stool 587.1 · Pernicious anemia 281.0 · Unsp septicemia 038.9
· Depress disord NEC 311 · Hemorrhoids unsp 455.6 · Mitral valve disord 424.0 · Pharyngitis acute 462 · Unsp sinusitis chr 473.9

RELEASE & ASSIGNMENT
I authorize release of any information necessary to process my insurance claim and assign and request payment directly to my physicians.
SIGNED _____ DATE _____

RECALL & RETURN
RETURN ☐ DAYS ☐ WEEKS ☐ MONTHS
NEXT APPOINTMENT _____ DATE _____ TIME _____ AM/PM

ACCOUNTING INFORMATION
PRIOR BALANCE	0
TODAY'S CHARGES	445
TOTAL DUE	
AMOUNT PAID	445
NEW BALANCE	0

© PMIC REV. 1/97

SAMPLE SUPERBILL SHOWING SERVICES, DIAGNOSES AND FEES

Unless you are filing your own health insurance claim, you will not usually receive a copy of the HCFA1500. If you file your own health insurance claims, or you ask the doctor's office for a copy of your health insurance claim form, you can use the information on the form to review fees in this book.

To compare what your doctor charged with the fees listed in this book, you need the CPT procedure code for each service or procedure and the amount charged. This information is found in BOX 24 of the HCFA1500.

COLUMN D   PROCEDURES, SERVICES OR SUPPLIES

Under the heading CPT/HCPCS you will find a five-digit code that defines what the doctor is billing for. This code is used by the doctor's office or hospital to report the procedure or service performed and may also be used to bill for supplies.

The health insurance company uses this code to determine the benefits payable to the doctor or hospital. The code listed in this column is what you need in order to compare the charges on your health insurance claim form to the range of charges listed in this book.

COLUMN F   CHARGES

The amount listed in this column is what the doctor or hospital is charging your health insurance plan for the procedures or services rendered. The fact that a certain amount is listed does not mean that this is what the doctor will be paid. The amount listed in this column is what you use to compare your doctor or hospital charges to the range of charges listed in this book.

WHY HEALTH INSURANCE CLAIMS ARE REJECTED

You would think that filling in a health insurance claim form would a be relatively simple and error free process for the doctor's staff. After all they do them all the time. But many claim forms, especially those that are typed instead of computer generated, include simple errors which frequently result in the health insurance claims being delayed or denied. The most common reasons for health insurance claim rejection are:

- The patient's or insured's subscriber number and/or group number is incorrect or missing (BOX 1A).

DOES YOUR DOCTOR CHARGE TOO MUCH?

HEALTH INSURANCE CLAIM FORM

CARRIER: EMPLOYERS HEALTH INSURANCE, 987 ROXBURY DRIVE, GREEN BAY, WI 69123

1. Program	OTHER (X)
1a. Insured's I.D. Number	999-99-9999
2. Patient's Name	DAVIS, JAMES B
3. Patient's Birth Date / Sex	09 09 59 / M (X)
4. Insured's Name	SAME
5. Patient's Address	867 S VICTORIA AVE
City / State	LOS ANGELES, CA
Zip Code	90005
6. Patient Relationship to Insured	Self (X)
8. Patient Status	Single (X) / Employed (X)
11. Insured's Policy Group or FECA Number	8369-W
14. Date of Current Illness/Injury	03 15 97
21. Diagnosis	1. 786 50

24. Services

Date of Service	Place	Type	Procedure (CPT)	Diagnosis	Charges
03 15 97	11		99205	1	275 00
03 15 97	11		93000	1	75 00
03 15 97	11		71020	1	95 00

25. Federal Tax I.D. Number	95-123456
26. Patient's Account No.	00069431
27. Accept Assignment	YES (X)
28. Total Charge	$445 00
29. Amount Paid	$ 00
30. Balance Due	$445 00
33. Physician's Billing Name & Address	INTERNAL MEDICINE GROUP, 8330 WEST THIRD STREET, LOS ANGELES, CA 90048

(APPROVED BY AMA COUNCIL ON MEDICAL SERVICE 8.88) **PLEASE PRINT OR TYPE**
APPROVED OMB-0938-0008 FORM HCFA-1500 (12-90). FORM RRB-1500.
APPROVED OMB-1215-0055 FORM OWCP-1500. APPROVED OMB-0720-0001 (CHAMPUS)

HCFA1500 HEALTH INSURANCE CLAIM FORM

- The doctor's signature (or facsimile) is missing (BOX 31).

- Dates are obviously incorrect (BOX 24 A). For example, surgery is dated prior to pre-operative exam, or discharge date is before admission date, or date(s) are missing entirely.

- The ICD-9 diagnosis does not correspond with or support the services or procedures (BOX 21).

- The ICD-9 diagnosis is missing or incomplete (BOX 21).

- Reasons for multiple visits made the same day are not listed on the claim.

- The charges are not itemized (BOX 24).

- Necessary information about prescription drugs or durable medical equipment prescribed by the doctor is not included (BOX 24).

- The procedure codes are missing or incorrect (BOX 24 D).

- The patient identification is incomplete (BOX 2-BOX 11).

- The fee column is left blank (BOX 24 F). Many health insurance carriers will not process a claim which has blank fees.

- The claim is difficult to read due to smudges or handwriting. Believe it or not, some doctor's offices actually submit handwritten health insurance claims!

If your doctor prepares a health insurance claim form and gives it to you to file with your health insurance plan, take the time to review the claim form before you mail it to your health insurance carrier. This will give you the opportunity to catch and correct any obvious errors before the claim is mailed. This minor investment in your time will pay off in fewer delays, denials and development letters from your health insurance carrier.

THE EXPLANATION OF BENEFITS

With the exception of most managed care plans, you will receive an *Explanation Of Benefits* (EOB) from your health insurance carrier for services billed by your doctor(s). You can use the EOB to make sure that all of the services were billed properly and that the health insurance carrier is paying reasonable benefits.

- Are all charges listed on the health insurance claim also listed on the EOB?

- Is there an explanation for any unpaid or unprocessed charges?

- Are all of the codes on the EOB exactly the same as those on the health insurance claim?

- Does the payment for each procedure meet with your expectation or agree with your pre-authorization form?

If your answer to any of these questions is no, you need to carefully review the health insurance claim or Superbill and file an immediate appeal with the health insurance carrier.

The sample EOB on the following page is typical of the type of form you will receive from your health insurance plan. Note that the information is similar to what is on the HCFA1500 health insurance claim form. This particular form includes the procedure code, a brief generic description of the service, the date of service, and the amount charged by the doctor. The form includes a column for services not covered, a column listing the discount or penalty, codes and explanations for the reductions and finally a calculation of the eligible expenses and the amount paid. The sample EOB also illustrates many of the reasons that your doctor's charges may be reduced, delayed or denied due to deductibles, limitation of benefits, or error by the doctor's office. By reviewing the sample EOB, we can determine that several of the charges were applied to the deductible, that the deductible has now been met, that there is a benefit limitation on one of the charges, and that the doctor's office made a coding error on two services.

DEDUCTIBLE AND COPAYMENT

- This charge was applied to the plan deductible, and the balance is owed by the insured.

- The deductible is now satisfied, and the balance is paid at the indicated percent.

- The copayment amount for the visit is the insured's responsibility.

- The insured is only liable for the amount in the insured's responsibility field.

DOCTOR FEES

EMPLOYERS HEALTH
1100 EMPLOYERS BLVD. GREEN BAY, WI 54344
TOLL FREE 800-558-4444

PAGE 1 OF 1
017365
600857274

If you have questions, call 1-800-558-4444

DATE 01/22/1996

PATIENT	DOCUMENT NO.	EMPLOYEE/INSURED	GROUP NO.	INSURED NO.
JAMES B DAVIS	P08725361	JAMES B DAVIS	8020517	999-99-9999

JAMES B DAVIS
867 S VICTORIA AVE
LOS ANGELES   CA   90005

SUMMARY OF PAYMENT

PROVIDER
WEISS MICHAEL H MD INC

TOTAL AMOUNT CHARGED	PAID BY OTHER PLAN	PAID BY YOUR PLAN	INSURED'S RESPONSIBILITY
755.00		230.40	437.08

PROC CODE	SERVICE	DATE OF SERVICE	TOTAL CHARGE	NOT COVERED	DISCOUNT OR PENALTY	REMARKS SEE BELOW	ELIGIBLE EXPENSE	DEDUCTIBLE APPLIED	PAID AT %	BENEFITS
82270	DIAGNOSTIC LAB	12/05/1995	15.00		3.37	310	11.63		100	11.63
99215	EXAMINATION	12/05/1995	125.00		31.01	310 B06	10.00			
							83.99		100	83.99
71020	DIAG XRAY	12/05/1995	65.00		8.80	310	56.20		100	56.20
93015	DIAG XRAY	12/05/1995	250.00		33.10	310 B33	59.81		100	
						B01	157.09	157.09		59.81
93016	DIAG XRAY	12/05/1995	100.00	100.00		90N				
93000	DIAG XRAY	12/05/1995	75.00	75.00		90N				
85024	DIAGNOSTIC LAB	12/05/1995	20.00		4.88	310 B01	15.12	15.12		
85651	DIAGNOSTIC LAB	12/05/1995	15.00		3.24	310 B01	11.76	11.76		
84439	DIAGNOSTIC LAB	12/05/1995	30.00		3.12	310 B01	26.88	26.88		
84443	DIAGNOSTIC LAB	12/05/1995	60.00			310 B02	39.15	39.15		
							20.85		90	18.77
	TOTALS		755.00	175.00	87.52		492.48	250.00		230.40

B01   THIS CHARGE WAS APPLIED TO THE PLAN DEDUCTIBLE, BALANCE OWED BY INSURED
B02   THE DEDUCTIBLE IS NOW SATISFIED, BALANCE PAID AT THE INDICATED PERCENT
B06   THE CO-PAYMENT AMOUNT FOR THE VISIT IS THE INSURED'S RESPONSIBILITY
B33   THIS SERVICE HAS A LIMITED BENEFIT, PLEASE REFER TO THE PLAN/CERTIFICATE
310   INSURED IS ONLY LIABLE FOR AMOUNT IN THE INSURED'S RESPONSIBILITY FIELD
90N   CODING ERRORS HAVE BEEN DETECTED. THIS CODE IS EXCLUDED AS IT IS PART OF A MORE GLOBAL CODE.

AMOUNT	CHECKS ISSUED TO:	ANNUAL ACCUMULATION FOR:	
230.40	WEISS MICHAEL H MD INC	INDIVIDUAL DEDUCTIBLE	250.00
		FAMILY DEDUCTIBLE	250.00

SAVE FOR FUTURE REFERENCE. DUPLICATES ARE NOT AVAILABLE. PLEASE SAVE FOR ADDITIONAL INFORMATION

SAMPLE HEALTH INSURANCE EXPLANATION OF BENEFITS

LIMITATION OF BENEFITS

- This service has a limited benefit, please refer to the plan/certificate.

CODING ERRORS

- Coding errors have been detected. This code is excluded since it is part of a more global code.

Of particular concern in this example are the coding errors made by the doctor's office. If these errors are not questioned by either the doctor or the insured and then re-billed properly to the health insurance plan, the insured has to pay $175.00 out of his/her own pocket.

HOW TO CHALLENGE THE DOCTOR'S FEE

Unlike most goods and services that we purchase, there is no warranty on medical services. If you see the doctor and feel better, you pay the bill. If you don't feel better, you still have to pay the bill. If you have surgery and it fixes the problem, you pay the bill. If the surgery doesn't fix the problem, you still have to pay the bill.

However, you do have a right to question the doctor's fees if they are significantly higher than the customary fees in the community or if the doctor's office makes coding errors on the health insurance claim form—especially if you are responsible for the balance remaining after your health insurance plan has paid the doctor. If you have compared the doctor's fees with the fees in this book, applied the geographic adjustment factor from the appendix, and find some or all of them to be significantly higher than the 90th percentile, or if your health insurance plan did not pay for some services because of coding errors, you should take the following steps:

- Call the doctor's office and ask for an explanation of the charges. Explain clearly that you believe that the doctor's fees are too high or that a coding error was made on the health insurance claim form. Listen carefully to what you are told by the doctor's office staff and make notes.

- If you are not satisfied with the explanation of the fees or coding error, ask for an immediate reduction of the charges. Don't be surprised if the doctor's billing staff either refuses to honor your request or says they will have to ask the doctor and get back to you.

- If you do not receive a response within two or three days, write the doctor a letter explaining clearly that you believe that his fees are too high, or that a coding error was made, and that you want him to reduce his fees so that you will only have to pay your fair share.

- If you do not receive a response to your phone call or letter within a reasonable time, call your health insurance company and file a complaint. Explain the steps you have taken and offer to send copies of your letter, your explanation of benefits, and copies of the pages of this book which include the services in question. Ask them to contact the doctor on your behalf.

- You may wish to file a complaint with the local Better Business Bureau.

- Be prepared to change doctors. Most doctors, like most other businesses, know that it costs more to get a new customer than to keep an existing one. Therefore, unless they strongly disagree with your position, they will usually honor your request. If they don't, find a new doctor.

- If the doctor refuses to negotiate the fee, and if the amount you have to pay due to over-charging or coding errors is hundreds or thousands of dollars, you should consult your attorney. Many doctors are aware that a significant percentage of medical malpractice cases start out as disputes over a doctor's fees. A phone call or letter from an attorney will usually resolve the matter.

HOW TO CHALLENGE THE INSURANCE PAYMENT

As we have explained, most health insurance plans will delay, reduce or deny payment whenever possible. You are generally responsible for the doctor's bill whether your health insurance plan pays or not. If your health insurance plan pays less than it should, and the doctor's fees are reasonable, and no coding errors were made, you may have to pay a significant portion of the doctor's bill out of your own pocket.

If you have compared the doctor's fees with the fees in this book and find them to be at or below the 90th percentile, but your health insurance plan either down-coded the service or allowed less than the customary fee, and you have to pay the difference, you should take the following steps:

- Call the doctor's office and explain the situation. In most cases, they will have already appealed the denial or reduction to your health insurance plan. If they haven't submitted an appeal, ask them to do so immediately.

- If you are a member of a group health insurance plan, call your health plan manager and ask them to help you obtain the benefits you are entitled to. Health insurance carriers are usually far more responsive to someone who is responsible for thousands of beneficiaries than they are to an individual.

- If you do not receive a response within two or three days, write the health insurance carrier a letter explaining clearly that you believe that they are not paying enough on your claim. Include copies of the pages of this book which include the services in question. Ask for an immediate review.

- If you do not receive a response to your letter within a reasonable time, write your state insurance commissioner and file a complaint. When requesting assistance from your state insurance commissioner, send a cover letter explaining clearly your complaint, along with copies of any correspondence sent to or received from the health insurance carrier. You should also include copies of the pages of this book which include the fees you are disputing.

  Health insurance carriers usually respond quickly to investigations started by the state insurance commissioner. This can be an effective tool, but should be used only after regular appeal processes have failed. In some states, the insurance commissioner will act only at the request of the consumer. In others, the insurance commissioner will also act on the request of the doctor as the consumer's advocate.

- If the health insurance carrier refuses to negotiate the fee, and if the amount you have to pay due to over-charging or coding errors is hundreds or thousands of dollars, you should consult your attorney. Don't expect your health insurance carrier to be as responsive to a call or letter from an attorney as your doctor would be.

SOURCE OF THE FEE DATA

The usual, customary and reasonable (UCR) fees listed in this book were developed over a period of several years. More than 100 million actual doctor charges, as well as a supplemental database derived from more than 600 million submitted charges, were analyzed to develop the fee database. The database is updated continuously to maintain current information.

In addition to this book for consumers, the database is used to publish *Physician Fees*, an annual professional publication used for fee schedule review and management by thousands of doctors, hospitals, other medical professionals, and health insurance carriers. The Medicare fees listed in this book are taken directly from the Medicare Fee Schedule published annually in the *Federal Register*.

FORMAT OF THE DATA

Each entry includes the procedure code, a short description or definition of the procedure, UCR fees at the 50th, 75th and 90th percentiles and the national average Medicare fee. The relatively few procedure codes without UCR and Medicare fees were omitted.

CODE

This is the five-digit code which defines the service or procedure. All codes listed in this book are CPT codes. CPT codes are used by doctors, hospitals and health insurance carriers nationwide to define medical services, procedures and diagnostic tests. CPT codes are revised and published annually by the American Medical Association. The CPT codes listed in this book were abstracted from the Medicare Fee Schedule published in the December 1996 *Federal Register*.

SHORT DESCRIPTION

This is a short or abbreviated description of the service or procedure. The short descriptions are from the Medicare Fee Schedule. Many of the short descriptions have been revised for consistency and readability. Wherever possible, lay descriptions have been used in place of medical terminology.

In reviewing the listing of codes and descriptions, you will find many listings where the descriptions are the same for different codes. For example:

99281 Emergency department visit
99282 Emergency department visit
99283 Emergency department visit
99284 Emergency department visit
99285 Emergency department visit

33405 Replace aortic valve
33406 Replace aortic valve
33411 Replace aortic valve
33412 Replace aortic valve
33413 Replace aortic valve

In the case of CPT visit codes from 99200-99499, the code with a higher number typically, but not always, represents a higher valued procedure and will have higher fees. For other CPT codes, and particularly the surgery codes from 20000-69999, the codes represent different techniques or variations of the same surgical procedure.

Your doctor's office can give you the full description for any service or procedure listed in the CPT book. The full descriptions for these procedures may also be found in *Physicians' Current Procedural Terminology* (CPT), 1997, published by the American Medical Association. CPT can be special ordered from your local bookstore or you may find a copy in your local library.

50TH

The 50th percentile fee for the service or procedure. The 50th percentile is that point where one-half (50%) of all fees for a given procedure are at or below the amount listed and one-half (50%) of all fees are higher than the amount listed.

75TH

The 75th percentile fee for the service or procedure. The 75th percentile is that point where three-fourths (75%) of all fees for a given procedure are at or below the amount listed and one-fourth (25%) percent of all fees are higher than the amount listed.

90TH

The 90th percentile fee for the service or procedure. The 90th percentile is that point where nine-tenths (90%) of all fees for a given procedure are at or below the amount listed and one-tenth (10%) of all fees are higher than the amount listed. The 90th percentile fee is also what many health insurance carriers use as the customary fee. Unless there are special circumstances, the health insurance carrier will usually not pay or allow the doctor more than the 90th percentile fee.

MC

The national average Medicare fee for the service or procedure. The Medicare fee is calculated from the Medicare Fee Schedule as published in the December 1996 *Federal Register*. You will note that the Medicare fees are significantly lower than the UCR fees. This is not an indicator of the financial worth of the service, but reflects the reduced fees paid to doctors by the Medicare program. Some fees listed do not have a fee in the Medicare (MC) column. This is either because the service is not covered by Medicare, or an appropriate Medicare fee has not yet been determined, or, as in the case of most laboratory services, a method other than the Medicare Fee Schedule is used to set fees.

A SHORT COURSE IN STATISTICS

The usual, customary and reasonable (UCR) fees in this book are presented as percentiles. The use of percentiles provides a better perspective than using averages or low-to-high fee ranges. The easiest way to understand percentile distribution is by showing it as a curve. The chart below illustrates the distribution curve for CPT code 99205, which is an office visit for a new patient, of about 60 minutes duration.

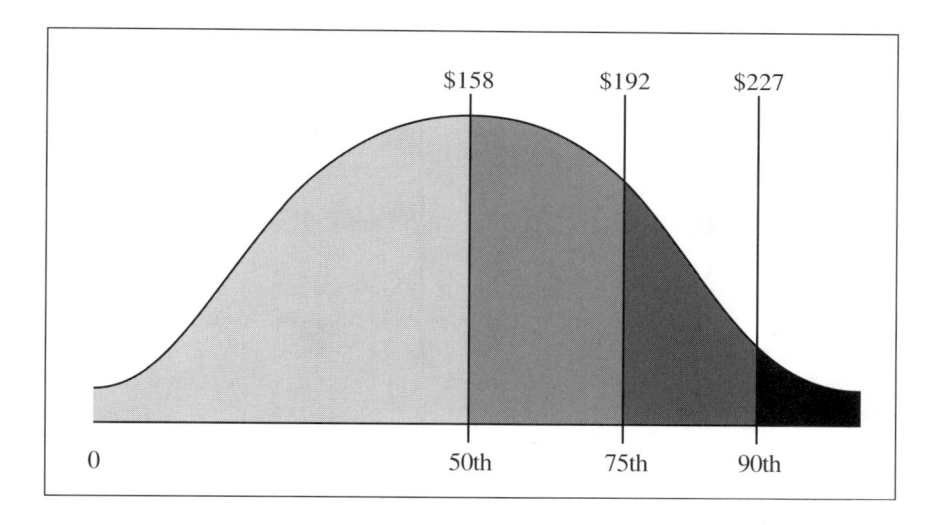

In this example, the 50th percentile fee for the service is $158. If you arranged all of the doctor's fees for this service in fee order, one-half of the fees would be at or below $158 and one-half would be above $158. If your doctor charged $125 for this service, his/her fee would be below the 50th percentile.

If your doctor charged $275 for this service, his/her fee would be above the 90th percentile. The 90th percentile is usually the maximum amount allowed by health insurance companies. So even though your doctor charged more, the health insurance company would allow only $227.

Depending upon the type of plan you have and whether you have to pay deductibles and/or coinsurance, you would have to pay the difference between what your health insurance paid and what the doctor charged.

On the sample HCFA1500 health insurance claim form you will see a listing for three charges. If you look up each of these codes in the fee reference section of this book, you will find the following:

Code	Short Description	50th	75th	90th	MC
99205	Office visit, new patient; 60 mins	158	192	227	121
93000	Electrocardiogram, complete	54	69	84	27
71020	Chest x-ray	74	93	110	32

In this example, the first and third procedures billed are below the 90th percentile. However, the second procedure is significantly higher than the 90th percentile and will probably be reduced by the health insurance plan. In this case, it is important to determine your financial responsibility in the event that the doctor's charges are higher than the ranges.

GEOGRAPHIC VARIABILITY AND ADJUSTMENT

The percentile fees presented in this book are based on national fee data. However, doctors' fees vary substantially by geographic area. In rural areas and smaller towns and cities, doctors' fees may be significantly lower than the percentiles presented in this book. Likewise, in larger cities, doctors' fees may be significantly higher than the fees presented. There are two primary reasons for the geographic variation in doctors' fees; namely, the cost of running a medical practice and the cost of medical malpractice insurance.

The cost of practice includes rent, employee costs, and other overhead costs, but not medical malpractice costs. According to the cost of practice indexes published in the Medicare Fee Schedule, New York City has the highest cost of practice and small cities in eastern Missouri have the lowest cost of practice. The cost of running a medical practice in New York City is almost 68% higher than running a medical practice in a small city in eastern Missouri.

The second reason for the geographic variation in doctors' fees is the cost of medical malpractice insurance. According to the malpractice expense indexes published in the Medicare Fee Schedule, New York City has the highest cost of medical malpractice insurance and South Dakota has the lowest cost of medical malpractice insurance. Medical malpractice insurance costs are about 248 percent higher in New York City than they are in South Dakota.

In order to more accurately determine the percentile of the doctors' fees in the area where you live, we have included an appendix of geographic adjustment factors. A *geographic adjustment factor* (GAF) is a multiplier used to determine the correct fee for a specific location of medical practice. The appendix includes a list of geographic adjustment factors for cities, counties, areas, regions and states which can be used to fine-tune the doctor fees listed in this book. The geographic adjustment factors listed in the appendix are based upon the Medicare Fee Schedule.

HOW TO ADJUST FEES FOR YOUR LOCATION

To use the geographic adjustment factor, first look up the CPT codes in the book that you want to compare to your doctor's fees or health insurance carrier allowances. Write down the 50th, 75th and 90th percentile fees for each CPT code. Then look up the geographic adjustment factor for your city, county, area, region or state in this appendix. Finally, multiply the percentile fees by the geographic adjustment factor to determine the adjusted fee.

In order to clearly illustrate, let's look at two medical services provided in Phoenix, New York City, and any city in South Dakota. We first look up and write down the percentile fees for each service. Then, looking up these locations in the appendix, we find that the GAF for Phoenix is 1.007, the GAF for New York City is 1.246 and the GAF for South Dakota is .866. Finally, we multiply the percentile fees by the GAF for each location to determine the adjusted fee.

Code	Short Description		50th	75th	90th	MC
99205	Office visit, new patient; 60 minutes		158	192	227	121
	Phoenix	(multiply by 1.007)	159	193	229	122
	New York City	(multiply by 1.246)	197	239	285	151
	South Dakota	(multiply by .866)	137	166	197	105
33513	CABG, vein, four		5644	7876	9664	2972
	Phoenix	(multiply by 1.007)	5684	7931	9732	2993
	New York City	(multiply by 1.246)	7032	9814	12041	3703
	South Dakota	(multiply by .866)	4888	6821	8369	2574

As these examples illustrate, medical fees in Phoenix are very close to the national average, medical fees in New York are almost 25 percent higher than the national average and medical fees in South Dakota are a little over 13 percent lower than the national average. As previously explained, these variations are due to the cost of practice and cost of medical malpractice insurance.

SPECIALTY DIFFERENTIALS

Traditional thinking is that a service performed by a medical specialist is worth more than the same service performed by a non-specialist. For example, a neurosurgeon might take the position that his office visit was worth more than an office visit by a general practitioner. In addition, there are physicians who justify higher fees based upon experience, reputation or technique.

Medicare does not recognize specialty differentials or allow higher charges based upon experience, reputation or technique. However, non-governmental health insurance plans may recognize and pay these higher charges. But if they don't, you may be required to pay the difference out of your own pocket.

DOCTOR VISITS

All doctors provide visit services. The office, hospital or emergency department visit is the first encounter with the doctor. During the visit the doctor takes a history, performs a physical examination, and orders appropriate diagnostic studies such as x-rays and laboratory tests. The doctor may also determine the diagnosis and order treatment during the visit.

The extent of the history and physical examination depends on the nature of the complaint and whether you are a new patient or an established patient. If you are a new patient with a significant complaint, the doctor will typically take a detailed history and perform a more thorough physical examination than if you are an established patient that the doctor knows from previous visits. A minor complaint from either a new or established patient may not require any past medical history or physical examination prior to treatment.

The visit code that the doctor chooses to bill your health insurance plan for the visit depends upon the location of the visit, whether you are a new or established patient, the extent of history obtained, the extent of the physical examination, the complexity of medical decision making, the nature of the presenting problem and the approximate amount of time. The amount of time involved in providing a visit service depends upon the location of the service.

For office visits and office consultations, *time* refers to the amount of time the doctor spends face-to-face with the patient while performing such tasks as taking the history, performing the physical examination, or counseling the patient. For inpatient hospital visits and hospital consultations, *time* refers to the total amount of time the doctor is reviewing medical records, examining the patient, writing in the medical record, ordering and reviewing test results, and communicating with other doctors and nurses as well as the patient's family. All times listed in this book are averages and may be higher or lower depending upon the actual clinical circumstances.

Diagnostic tests or studies ordered or performed, and therapeutic services such as immunizations or injections provided during the visit, are not considered to be included in the visit service. You should expect to be billed for any diagnostic tests or studies or therapeutic services in addition to the visit service.

MC = Medicare Fee

Code	Short Description	50th	75th	90th	MC

OFFICE OR OTHER OUTPATIENT SERVICES

New Patient

Code	Short Description	50th	75th	90th	MC
99201	Office visit; 10 mins	45	55	64	29
99202	Office visit; 20 mins	61	72	84	47
99203	Office visit; 30 mins	84	100	117	65
99204	Office visit; 45 mins	121	145	171	96
99205	Office visit; 60 mins	158	192	227	121

Established Patient

Code	Short Description	50th	75th	90th	MC
99211	Office visit; 5 mins	24	30	35	13
99212	Office visit; 10 mins	37	45	53	25
99213	Office visit; 15 mins	50	60	69	37
99214	Office visit; 25 mins	73	88	102	55
99215	Office visit; 40 mins	113	136	158	88

HOSPITAL OBSERVATION SERVICES

Code	Short Description	50th	75th	90th	MC
99217	Observation care discharge	77	95	114	59
99218	Observation care	88	107	127	65
99219	Observation care	135	162	191	105
99220	Observation care	171	205	241	134

HOSPITAL INPATIENT SERVICES

Code	Short Description	50th	75th	90th	MC
99221	Initial hospital care; 30 mins	100	123	146	64
99222	Initial hospital care; 50 mins	145	171	198	105
99223	Initial hospital care; 70 mins	183	216	251	134
99231	Subsequent hospital care; 15 mins	53	64	76	34
99232	Subsequent hospital care; 25 mins	74	89	106	49
99233	Subsequent hospital care; 35 mins	107	131	156	69
99238	Hospital discharge day; < 30 mins	79	95	111	58
99239	Hospital discharge day; > 30 mins	110	134	157	73

CONSULTATIONS

Code	Short Description	50th	75th	90th	MC
99241	Office consultation; 15 mins	77	95	113	44
99242	Office consultation; 30 mins	104	126	147	69

DOCTOR VISITS

Code	Short Description	50th	75th	90th	MC
99243	Office consultation; 40 mins	133	161	189	90
99244	Office consultation; 60 mins	177	212	246	125
99245	Office consultation; 80 mins	240	290	338	169
99251	Initial inpatient consult; 20 mins	89	111	133	46
99252	Initial inpatient consult; 40 mins	117	142	169	70
99253	Initial inpatient consult; 55 mins	147	178	210	92
99254	Initial inpatient consult; 80 mins	190	228	266	126
99255	Initial inpatient consult; 110 mins	241	289	338	171
99261	Follow-up inpatient consult; 10 mins	50	63	75	25
99262	Follow-up inpatient consult; 20 mins	73	90	108	43
99263	Follow-up inpatient consult; 30 mins	101	124	149	63
99271	Confirmatory consultation	69	88	107	36
99272	Confirmatory consultation	95	120	146	53
99273	Confirmatory consultation	122	155	188	75
99274	Confirmatory consultation	162	205	249	99
99275	Confirmatory consultation	211	267	325	136

EMERGENCY DEPARTMENT SERVICES

99281	Emergency department visit	48	60	70	21
99282	Emergency department visit	70	84	97	33
99283	Emergency department visit	106	128	147	60
99284	Emergency department visit	161	194	223	91
99285	Emergency department visit	236	284	325	144

CRITICAL CARE SERVICES

99288	Direct advanced life support	192	235	272	0
99291	Critical care services, first hour	257	319	384	176
99292	Critical care, additional 30 mins	122	153	185	85

NEONATAL INTENSIVE CARE SERVICES

99295	Initial neonatal critical care	915	1142	1380	721
99296	Subsequent neonatal critical care	481	600	725	358
99297	Subsequent neonatal critical care	245	306	370	179

NURSING FACILITY SERVICES

99301	Nursing facility care	72	87	103	59

MC = Medicare Fee

DOES YOUR DOCTOR CHARGE TOO MUCH?

Code	Short Description	50th	75th	90th	MC
99302	Nursing facility care	96	117	140	75
99303	Nursing facility care	135	160	187	107
99311	Nursing facility care, subsequent	45	53	63	34
99312	Nursing facility care, subsequent	65	76	88	51
99313	Nursing facility care, subsequent	92	109	128	67

REST HOME OR CUSTODIAL SERVICES

Code	Short Description	50th	75th	90th	MC
99321	Rest home visit, new patient	55	68	82	38
99322	Rest home visit, new patient	80	98	119	53
99323	Rest home visit, new patient	115	142	173	70
99331	Rest home visit, established patient	46	55	64	30
99332	Rest home visit, established patient	61	74	87	40
99333	Rest home visit, established patient	79	96	113	49

HOME SERVICES

Code	Short Description	50th	75th	90th	MC
99341	Home visit, new patient	67	76	87	57
99342	Home visit, new patient	83	96	110	75
99343	Home visit, new patient	113	131	150	98
99351	Home visit, established patient	56	67	78	45
99352	Home visit, established patient	74	88	103	57
99353	Home visit, established patient	97	116	135	72

PROLONGED SERVICES

Code	Short Description	50th	75th	90th	MC
99354	Prolonged service, office	110	146	188	88
99355	Prolonged service, office	63	85	111	88
99356	Prolonged service, inpatient	115	153	196	85
99357	Prolonged service, inpatient	75	102	132	85
99358	Prolonged service, no contact	95	129	168	0
99359	Prolonged service, no contact	49	66	86	0
99360	Physician standby services	103	140	182	0

CASE MANAGEMENT SERVICES

Code	Short Description	50th	75th	90th	MC
99361	Physician/team conference, 30 mins	75	101	132	0
99362	Physician/team conference, 60 mins	114	156	202	0
99371	Phone consultation	16	22	28	0
99372	Phone consultation, intermediate	38	52	68	0

DOCTOR VISITS

Code	Short Description	50th	75th	90th	MC
99373	Phone consultation, complex	56	77	100	0

CARE PLAN OVERSIGHT SERVICES

99375	Care plan oversight, 30-60 mins	98	126	159	76
99376	Care plan oversight, over 60 mins	131	178	231	0

PREVENTIVE MEDICINE SERVICES

99381	Preventive visit, new, infant	103	139	181	0
99382	Preventive visit, new, age 1-4	105	143	186	0
99383	Preventive visit, new, 5-11	101	137	179	0
99384	Preventive visit, new, 12-17	129	176	228	0
99385	Preventive visit, new, 18-39	120	163	212	0
99386	Preventive visit, new, 40-64	127	173	225	0
99387	Preventive visit, new, 65 & over	143	194	253	0
99391	Preventive visit, est, infant	80	109	141	0
99392	Preventive visit, est, age 1-4	90	122	158	0
99393	Preventive visit, est, 5-11	94	127	165	0
99394	Preventive visit, est, 12-17	108	147	191	0
99395	Preventive visit, est, 18-39	99	134	175	0
99396	Preventive visit, est, 40-64	108	146	190	0
99397	Preventive visit, est, 65 & over	87	116	148	0
99401	Preventive counseling, individual	40	48	58	0
99402	Preventive counseling, individual	74	91	109	0
99403	Preventive counseling, individual	105	129	154	0
99404	Preventive counseling, individual	143	176	209	0
99411	Preventive counseling, group	41	50	60	0
99412	Preventive counseling, group	72	88	105	0
99420	Health risk assessment test	76	93	111	0

NEWBORN CARE

99431	Initial care, normal newborn	135	166	198	80
99432	Newborn care not in hospital	110	135	161	86
99433	Normal newborn care, hospital	69	84	100	42
99435	Hospital newborn discharge day	157	193	230	108
99440	Newborn resuscitation	233	286	340	200

MC = Medicare Fee

DOES YOUR DOCTOR CHARGE TOO MUCH?

Code   Short Description   50th   75th   90th   MC

MEDICINE SERVICES

Medicine services include immunizations, injections, psychiatric services, dialysis and a variety of other diagnostic and therapeutic services and procedures. Many of these services are provided by specialists, such as gastroenterologists, ophthalmologists, cardiologists, dermatologists, pulmonologists, neurologists, oncologists and allergists. In addition, specific medicine services may be provided by physical therapists, osteopathic physicians and chiropractors.

These services may be rendered in the doctor's office, hospital or emergency department. Most of these services are provided during a visit, or as a result of a visit. Usually these services will be billed in addition to an office, hospital or emergency department visit. Any supplies or materials provided by the doctor, such as sterile trays or drugs, over and above those usually included with the office visit or other services rendered may also be billed.

Code	Short Description	50th	75th	90th	MC
IMMUNIZATION INJECTIONS					
90700	DTaP immunization	50	65	78	0
90701	DTP immunization	42	55	66	0
90702	DT immunization	20	26	32	0
90703	Tetanus immunization	18	24	28	0
90704	Mumps immunization	30	38	46	0
90705	Measles immunization	33	43	52	0
90706	Rubella immunization	34	44	52	0
90707	MMR virus immunization	55	72	86	0
90708	Measles-rubella immunization	41	54	64	0
90709	Rubella & mumps immunization	42	54	64	0
90710	Combined vaccine	60	78	93	0
90711	Combined vaccine	51	66	79	0
90712	Oral poliovirus immunization	37	48	58	0
90713	Poliomyelitis immunization	30	38	46	0
90714	Typhoid immunization	25	33	39	0
90716	Chicken pox vaccine	67	87	104	0
90717	Yellow fever immunization	24	31	37	0

MC = Medicare Fee

DOES YOUR DOCTOR CHARGE TOO MUCH?

Code	Short Description	50th	75th	90th	MC
90718	TD immunization	19	24	29	0
90719	Diphtheria immunization	22	29	35	0
90720	DTP/HIB vaccine	49	64	77	0
90721	Dtap/hib vaccine	69	89	107	0
90724	Influenza immunization	17	23	27	0
90725	Cholera immunization	22	28	34	0
90726	Rabies immunization	66	85	102	0
90727	Plague immunization	29	37	44	0
90728	BCG immunization	72	94	112	0
90730	Hepatitis A vaccine	55	71	85	0
90732	Pneumococcal immunization	25	32	37	0
90733	Meningococcal immunization	49	64	76	0
90735	Encephalitis virus vaccine	38	50	60	0
90737	Influenza B immunization	37	48	57	0
90741	Passive immunization, ISG	30	39	46	0
90742	Special passive immunization	51	66	80	0
90744	Hepatitis B vaccine, under 11	59	77	92	0
90745	Hepatitis B vaccine, 11-19	78	101	121	0
90746	Hepatitis B vaccine, over 20	85	110	132	0
90747	Hepatitis B vaccine, ill pat	78	101	121	0

INFUSION THERAPY

Code	Short Description	50th	75th	90th	MC
90780	IV infusion therapy, 1 hour	88	124	162	39
90781	IV infusion, additional hour	56	83	111	19

THERAPEUTIC INJECTIONS

Code	Short Description	50th	75th	90th	MC
90782	Injection (SC)/(IM)	13	19	26	4
90783	Injection (IA)	26	39	53	14
90784	Injection (IV)	36	53	71	17
90788	Injection of antibiotic	15	23	30	4

PSYCHIATRY SERVICES

Code	Short Description	50th	75th	90th	MC
90801	Psychiatric interview	147	191	235	113
90820	Diagnostic interview	121	156	193	108
90825	Evaluation of tests/records	88	114	142	0
90835	Special interview	140	181	223	107
90841	Psychotherapy	142	184	226	0

MEDICINE SERVICES

Code	Short Description	50th	75th	90th	MC
90842	Psychotherapy, 75-80 mins	201	254	308	138
90843	Psychotherapy, 20-30 mins	73	92	112	59
90844	Psychotherapy, 45-50 mins	116	147	178	83
90845	Medical psychoanalysis	93	121	149	71
90846	Special family therapy	96	124	153	80
90847	Special family therapy	116	148	181	91
90849	Special family therapy	103	134	164	28
90853	Special group therapy	58	77	96	28
90855	Individual psychotherapy	116	147	177	90
90857	Special group therapy	57	77	97	25
90862	Medication management	62	82	102	44
90870	Electroconvulsive therapy	147	190	234	80
90871	Electroconvulsive therapy	200	265	332	117
90875	Psychophysiological therapy	83	110	138	48
90876	Psychophysiological therapy	130	172	215	75
90880	Medical hypnotherapy	126	167	210	92
90882	Environmental manipulation	40	54	67	0
90887	Consultation with family	83	108	134	0
90889	Preparation of report	21	28	35	0

BIOFEEDBACK

90901	Biofeedback training	41	50	59	23
90911	Anorectal biofeedback	153	187	221	75

KIDNEY DIALYSIS SERVICES

90918	ESRD related services, month	813	1154	1516	450
90919	ESRD related services, month	662	941	1236	363
90920	ESRD related services, month	561	797	1046	322
90921	ESRD related services, month	339	482	633	230
90922	ESRD related services, day	32	43	56	15
90923	ESRD related services, day	25	36	47	12
90924	ESRD related services, day	21	30	39	11
90925	ESRD related services, day	15	21	28	8
90935	Hemodialysis, one evaluation	224	307	396	92
90937	Hemodialysis, repeated evaluations	408	553	706	161
90945	Dialysis, one evaluation	195	269	348	85
90947	Dialysis, repeated evaluations	308	437	574	143
90989	Dialysis training/complete	404	573	753	0

MC = Medicare Fee

Code	Short Description	50th	75th	90th	MC
90993	Dialysis training/incomplete	92	131	172	0
90997	Hemoperfusion	468	664	873	142

GASTROENTEROLOGY SERVICES

Code	Short Description	50th	75th	90th	MC
91000	Esophageal intubation	98	136	176	47
91010	Esophagus motility study	224	311	403	122
91011	Esophagus motility study	270	374	486	143
91012	Esophagus motility study	279	387	502	159
91020	Esophagogastric study	191	265	344	135
91030	Acid perfusion of esophagus	107	149	193	49
91032	Esophagus, acid reflux test	177	245	318	109
91033	Prolonged acid reflux test	270	373	485	149
91052	Gastric analysis test	136	188	244	55
91055	Gastric intubation for smear	111	153	199	58
91060	Gastric saline load test	74	103	133	40
91065	Breath hydrogen test	121	168	218	36
91100	Pass intestine bleeding tube	107	148	192	54
91105	Gastric intubation treatment	93	131	172	28
91122	Anal pressure record	224	310	403	146

OPHTHALMOLOGY SERVICES

Eye Examinations

Code	Short Description	50th	75th	90th	MC
92002	Eye exam, new patient	66	77	87	47
92004	Eye exam, new patient	95	109	124	76
92012	Eye exam, established patient	59	68	77	36
92014	Eye exam and treatment	80	92	105	53

Special Ophthalmological Services

Code	Short Description	50th	75th	90th	MC
92015	Refraction	19	25	32	0
92018	New eye exam and treatment	146	188	231	64
92019	Eye exam and treatment	97	125	153	58
92020	Special eye evaluation	46	58	71	22
92060	Special eye evaluation	51	66	82	35
92065	Orthoptic/pleoptic training	58	75	92	24
92070	Fitting of contact lens	142	183	225	64
92081	Visual field examination(s)	41	53	66	22

MEDICINE SERVICES

Code	Short Description	50th	75th	90th	MC
92082	Visual field examination(s)	64	82	101	31
92083	Visual field examination(s)	96	124	152	45
92100	Serial tonometry exam(s)	40	51	63	37
92120	Tonography and eye evaluation	44	57	70	36
92130	Water provocation tonography	54	70	86	42
92140	Glaucoma provocative tests	43	55	67	26
92225	Special eye exam, initial	62	83	105	28
92226	Special eye exam, subsequent	54	71	89	24
92230	Eye exam with photos	82	112	144	43
92235	Eye exam with photos	175	232	293	82
92240	Icg angiography	155	212	273	91
92250	Eye exam with photos	70	94	120	29
92260	Ophthalmoscopy/dynamometry	60	82	106	25
92265	Eye muscle evaluation	94	129	165	36
92270	Electro-oculography	93	127	164	50
92275	Electroretinography	139	191	245	63
92283	Color vision examination	43	59	76	15
92284	Dark adaptation eye exam	63	86	111	23
92285	Eye photography	40	55	71	16
92286	Internal eye photography	156	213	273	64
92287	Internal eye photography	121	166	214	79

Contact Lens Service

Code	Short Description	50th	75th	90th	MC
92310	Contact lens fitting	170	236	309	0
92311	Contact lens fitting	131	182	238	65
92312	Contact lens fitting	172	238	312	79
92313	Contact lens fitting	209	290	380	59
92314	Prescription of contact lens	134	186	244	0
92315	Prescription of contact lens	114	159	208	37
92316	Prescription of contact lens	148	205	269	55
92317	Prescription of contact lens	122	169	222	28
92325	Modification of contact lens	29	40	53	13
92326	Replacement of contact lens	77	108	141	55
92330	Fitting of artificial eye	177	246	322	75
92335	Fitting of artificial eye	147	204	267	84

Eye Glasses and Eye Prosthesis

Code	Short Description	50th	75th	90th	MC
92340	Fitting of eye glasses	38	53	70	0

MC = Medicare Fee

Code	Short Description	50th	75th	90th	MC
92341	Fitting of eye glasses	51	71	93	0
92342	Fitting of eye glasses	56	78	102	0
92352	Special eye glasses fitting	36	49	65	0
92353	Special eye glasses fitting	38	52	66	0
92354	Special eye glasses fitting	275	382	501	0
92355	Special eye glasses fitting	175	242	318	0
92358	Eye prosthesis service	62	86	112	0
92370	Repair and adjust eye glasses	36	50	66	0
92371	Repair and adjust eye glasses	35	49	64	0
92392	Supply of low vision aids	213	296	388	0
92393	Supply of artificial eye	761	1056	1384	0
92395	Supply of eye glasses	84	116	152	0
92396	Supply of contact lenses	129	180	236	0

EAR, NOSE AND THROAT SERVICES

Code	Short Description	50th	75th	90th	MC
92502	Ear and throat examination	168	223	280	89
92504	Ear microscopy examination	35	47	59	15
92506	Speech and hearing evaluation	79	105	132	46
92507	Speech/hearing therapy	54	72	90	28
92508	Speech/hearing therapy	31	41	51	15
92510	Rehab for ear implant	226	300	377	98
92511	Nasopharyngoscopy	134	178	223	70
92512	Nasal function studies	85	113	142	35
92516	Facial nerve function test	80	106	133	28
92520	Laryngeal function studies	162	215	270	43
92525	Oral function evaluation	199	265	333	85
92526	Oral function therapy	86	114	144	35

Vestibular Function Tests Without Electrical Recording

Code	Short Description	50th	75th	90th	MC
92531	Spontaneous nystagmus study	23	31	39	0
92532	Positional nystagmus study	34	45	57	0
92533	Caloric vestibular test	27	35	44	0
92534	Optokinetic nystagmus	10	14	17	0

Vestibular Function Tests With Electrical Recording

Code	Short Description	50th	75th	90th	MC
92541	Spontaneous nystagmus test	72	103	136	37
92542	Positional nystagmus test	68	96	127	33

MEDICINE SERVICES

Code	Short Description	50th	75th	90th	MC
92543	Caloric vestibular test	82	118	156	43
92544	Optokinetic nystagmus test	41	58	76	26
92545	Oscillating tracking test	43	61	80	22
92546	Sinusoidal rotational test	66	94	123	29
92547	Supplemental electrical test	38	55	72	20
92548	Posturography	140	199	263	85

Audiologic Function Tests With Medical Evaluation

Code	Short Description	50th	75th	90th	MC
92551	Pure tone hearing test, air	24	31	39	0
92552	Pure tone audiometry, air	28	36	44	16
92553	Audiometry, air and bone	41	51	62	24
92555	Speech threshold audiometry	23	30	37	14
92556	Speech audiometry, complete	37	47	57	20
92557	Comprehensive hearing test	75	94	114	43
92559	Group audiometric testing	33	43	53	0
92560	Bekesy audiometry, screen	22	28	35	0
92561	Bekesy audiometry, diagnosis	47	61	75	25
92562	Loudness balance test	24	31	38	15
92563	Tone decay hearing test	24	31	39	14
92564	Sisi hearing test	27	35	43	17
92565	Stenger test, pure tone	23	30	37	14
92567	Tympanometry	31	41	50	19
92568	Acoustic reflex testing	26	34	41	14
92569	Acoustic reflex decay test	26	34	41	15
92571	Filtered speech hearing test	24	32	39	14
92572	Staggered spondaic word test	11	15	18	3
92573	Lombard test	19	25	31	13
92575	Sensorineural acuity test	20	26	32	11
92576	Synthetic sentence test	25	33	40	16
92577	Stenger test, speech	38	50	61	26
92579	Visual audiometry (vra)	46	60	75	26
92582	Conditioning play audiometry	43	57	70	26
92583	Select picture audiometry	45	59	73	32
92584	Electrocochleography	164	213	263	88
92585	Auditory evoked potential	249	314	381	136
92587	Evoked auditory test	118	154	190	54
92588	Evoked auditory test	166	217	268	74
92589	Auditory function test(s)	41	54	66	19
92590	Hearing aid exam, one ear	111	145	179	0

MC = Medicare Fee

Code	Short Description	50th	75th	90th	MC
92591	Hearing aid exam, both ears	150	196	242	0
92592	Hearing aid check, one ear	35	46	57	0
92593	Hearing aid check, both ears	52	68	84	0
92594	Electro hearing aid test, one ear	35	45	56	0
92595	Electro hearing aid test, both ears	55	72	89	0
92596	Ear protector evaluation	43	57	70	21
92597	Oral speech device evaluation	139	181	223	80
92598	Modify oral speech device	92	120	148	55

CARDIOVASCULAR SERVICES

Therapeutic Services

92950	Heart/lung resuscitation (CPR)	347	447	543	201
92953	Temporary external pacing	218	283	345	35
92960	Heart electroconversion	312	400	485	139
92970	Cardioassist, internal	550	715	871	241
92971	Cardioassist, external	199	258	314	95
92975	Dissolve clot, heart vessel	1138	1478	1802	432
92977	Dissolve clot, heart vessel	527	685	835	278
92978	Intravascular ultrasound, heart	432	560	683	251
92979	Intravascular ultrasound, heart	266	346	422	154
92980	Insert intracoronary stent	2416	3138	3825	1057
92981	Insert intracoronary stent	916	1190	1451	328
92982	Coronary artery dilation	2568	3236	3874	858
92984	Coronary artery dilation	946	1229	1498	236
92986	Revision of aortic valve	2794	3628	4423	1069
92987	Revision of mitral valve	2432	3158	3850	1086
92990	Revision of pulmonary valve	2231	2897	3532	852
92992	Revision of heart chamber	3818	4959	6045	0
92993	Revision of heart chamber	4035	5240	6387	0
92995	Coronary atherectomy	2830	3676	4481	940
92996	Coronary atherectomy	758	984	1200	257

Cardiography

93000	Electrocardiogram, complete	54	69	84	27
93005	Electrocardiogram, tracing	42	55	68	16
93010	Electrocardiogram report	29	39	48	11
93012	Transmission of ECG	52	70	86	84

MEDICINE SERVICES

Code	Short Description	50th	75th	90th	MC
93014	Report on transmitted ECG	38	49	60	31
93015	Cardiovascular stress test	254	326	395	110
93016	Cardiovascular stress test	76	102	127	28
93017	Cardiovascular stress test	157	219	277	58
93018	Cardiovascular stress test	120	162	202	23
93024	Cardiac drug stress test	300	400	494	131
93040	Rhythm ECG with report	32	42	52	14
93041	Rhythm ECG, tracing	24	33	42	5
93042	Rhythm ECG, report	26	34	42	9
93224	ECG monitor/report, 24 hrs	323	409	492	160
93225	ECG monitor/record, 24 hrs	96	128	158	43
93226	ECG monitor/report, 24 hrs	137	179	219	76
93227	ECG monitor/review, 24 hrs	125	166	205	41
93230	ECG monitor/report, 24 hrs	321	405	484	169
93231	ECG monitor/record, 24 hrs	103	137	170	53
93232	ECG monitor/report, 24 hrs	185	247	305	75
93233	ECG monitor/review, 24 hrs	125	164	200	42
93235	ECG monitor/report, 24 hrs	260	347	428	126
93236	ECG monitor/report, 24 hrs	182	242	299	90
93237	ECG monitor/review, 24 hrs	114	152	188	35
93268	ECG record/review	212	283	349	158
93270	ECG recording	87	115	143	43
93271	ECG/monitoring and analysis	166	221	273	84
93272	ECG/review, interpret only	60	80	99	31
93278	ECG/signal-averaged	196	261	323	66

Echocardiography

Code	Short Description	50th	75th	90th	MC
93303	Echo transthoracic	362	481	595	211
93304	Echo transthoracic	198	263	325	115
93307	Echo exam of heart	373	483	587	199
93308	Echo exam of heart	213	289	362	109
93312	Echo transesophageal	511	694	868	251
93313	Echo transesophageal	182	247	309	54
93314	Echo transesophageal	451	612	766	197
93315	Echo transesophageal	460	625	782	269
93316	Echo transesophageal	94	128	160	54
93317	Echo transesophageal	365	496	620	215
93320	Doppler echo exam, heart	216	286	353	89
93321	Doppler echo exam, heart	131	179	223	51

MC = Medicare Fee

Code	Short Description	50th	75th	90th	MC
93325	Doppler color flow	182	238	291	105
93350	Echo transthoracic	573	770	956	155

Cardiac Catheterization

93501	Right heart catheterization	1525	2154	2816	813
93503	Insert/place heart catheter	483	663	852	183
93505	Biopsy of heart lining	718	1014	1326	318
93510	Left heart catheterization	2386	3371	4407	1527
93511	Left heart catheterization	2603	3677	4808	1499
93514	Left heart catheterization	3157	4459	5830	1976
93524	Left heart catheterization	3659	5169	6758	2014
93526	Right and left heart catheterization	3376	4769	6236	2058
93527	Right and left heart catheterization	4174	5896	7708	2114
93528	Right and left heart catheterization	4133	5838	7633	2070
93529	Right and left heart catheterization	4190	5918	7738	1885
93536	Insert circulation assist	1205	1702	2225	384
93539	Injection, cardiac catheterization	264	365	470	49
93540	Injection, cardiac catheterization	273	380	493	50
93541	Injection for lung angiogram	272	384	502	39
93542	Injection for heart x-rays	228	322	422	39
93543	Injection for heart x-rays	217	305	398	32
93544	Injection for aortography	236	332	434	31
93545	Injection for coronary x-rays	368	512	664	55
93555	Imaging, cardiac catheterization	669	945	1235	251
93556	Imaging, cardiac catheterization	936	1322	1729	382
93561	Cardiac output measurement	282	399	521	63
93562	Cardiac output measurement	151	213	278	34

Intracardiac Electrophysiologic Procedures

93600	Bundle of His recording	535	734	934	233
93602	Intra-atrial recording	398	545	694	169
93607	Right ventricular recording	519	712	906	234
93609	Mapping of tachycardia	1657	2272	2892	546
93610	Intra-atrial pacing	546	748	952	225
93612	Intraventricular pacing	526	721	917	235
93615	Esophageal recording	120	165	210	54
93616	Esophageal recording	245	336	428	106
93618	Heart rhythm pacing	1302	1784	2271	469

MEDICINE SERVICES

Code	Short Description	50th	75th	90th	MC
93619	Electrophysiology evaluation	2302	3156	4016	840
93620	Electrophysiology evaluation	3051	4183	5323	1159
93624	Electrophysiologic study	1000	1372	1746	326
93631	Heart pacing, mapping	1510	2071	2635	676
93640	Evaluation heart device	1261	1728	2199	536
93641	Electrophysiology evaluation	1910	2619	3333	690
93642	Electrophysiology evaluation	1792	2457	3127	632
93650	Ablate heart dysrhythm focus	2329	3192	4063	827
93651	Ablate heart dysrhythm focus	3195	4380	5575	1153
93652	Ablate heart dysrhythm focus	3476	4765	6065	1198
93660	Tilt table evaluation	402	552	702	0

Other Vascular Studies

Code	Short Description	50th	75th	90th	MC
93720	Total body plethysmography	88	114	137	39
93721	Plethysmography tracing	72	95	113	25
93722	Plethysmography report	55	72	85	14
93724	Analyze pacemaker system	1075	1404	1676	394
93731	Analyze pacemaker system	76	95	111	43
93732	Analyze pacemaker system	101	127	149	62
93733	Telephone analysis pacemaker	70	88	103	39
93734	Analyze pacemaker system	62	79	92	35
93735	Analyze pacemaker system	85	108	127	54
93736	Telephone analysis pacemaker	65	81	94	34
93737	Analyze cardio/defibrillator	78	100	117	41
93738	Analyze cardio/defibrillator	103	134	160	61
93740	Temperature gradient studies	76	99	119	22
93760	Cephalic thermogram	212	277	330	0
93762	Peripheral thermogram	284	371	443	0
93770	Measure venous pressure	25	33	39	12
93784	Ambulatory blood pressure monitoring	237	309	369	0
93786	Ambulatory blood pressure recording	104	136	162	0
93788	Ambulatory blood pressure analysis	98	128	152	0
93790	Review/report blood pressure recording	126	165	197	0
93797	Cardiac rehab	46	65	80	16
93798	Cardiac rehab/monitor	69	91	108	26

MC = Medicare Fee

Code	Short Description	50th	75th	90th	MC

NON-INVASIVE VASCULAR DIAGNOSTIC STUDIES

Cerebrovascular Arterial Studies

93875	Extracranial study	201	278	355	59
93880	Extracranial study	326	429	531	167
93882	Extracranial study	244	333	422	111
93886	Intracranial study	285	389	492	196
93888	Intracranial study	203	277	350	131

Extremity Arterial Studies

93922	Extremity study	197	268	339	61
93923	Extremity study	247	328	408	113
93924	Extremity study	256	349	442	125
93925	Lower extremity study	295	388	481	167
93926	Lower extremity study	197	269	340	112
93930	Upper extremity study	310	423	536	172
93931	Upper extremity study	216	295	373	114

Extremity Venous Studies

93965	Extremity study	195	267	339	68
93970	Extremity study	289	378	467	185
93971	Extremity study	204	278	352	123

Visceral and Penile Vascular Studies

93975	Vascular study	339	463	586	240
93976	Vascular study	248	338	428	161
93978	Vascular study	281	384	486	173
93979	Vascular study	210	286	362	116
93980	Penile vascular study	376	513	649	194
93981	Penile vascular study	267	364	461	144

Extremity Arterial-Venous Studies

93990	Doppler flow testing	228	311	394	105

MEDICINE SERVICES

Code	Short Description	50th	75th	90th	MC
PULMONARY SERVICES					
94010	Breathing capacity test	69	92	115	30
94060	Evaluation of wheezing	116	153	192	56
94070	Evaluation of wheezing	167	227	289	83
94150	Vital capacity test	24	34	44	0
94200	Lung function test (MBC/MVV)	43	58	75	17
94240	Residual lung capacity	79	105	132	40
94250	Expired gas collection	26	35	45	13
94260	Thoracic gas volume	72	98	126	29
94350	Lung nitrogen washout curve	71	96	123	34
94360	Measure airflow resistance	68	92	118	48
94370	Breath airway closing volume	49	66	85	23
94375	Respiratory flow volume loop	71	93	117	34
94400	CO_2 breathing response curve	105	144	184	45
94450	Hypoxia response curve	89	121	155	35
94620	Pulmonary stress testing	191	260	334	102
94640	Airway inhalation treatment	27	35	44	14
94642	Aerosol inhalation treatment	43	59	76	0
94650	Pressure breathing (IPPB)	33	45	58	14
94651	Pressure breathing (IPPB)	29	40	51	13
94652	Pressure breathing (IPPB)	41	56	72	17
94656	Initial ventilator management	196	272	352	80
94657	Continuous ventilator	99	131	165	48
94660	Positive airway pressure, CPAP	143	195	250	50
94662	Negative pressure ventilation, CNP	116	158	202	34
94664	Aerosol or vapor inhalations	40	53	67	18
94665	Aerosol or vapor inhalations	34	47	60	17
94667	Chest wall manipulation	41	54	67	20
94668	Chest wall manipulation	40	54	68	13
94680	Exhaled air analysis: O_2	133	182	233	39
94681	Exhaled air analysis: O_2, CO_2	182	248	318	65
94690	Exhaled air analysis	74	101	129	22
94720	Monoxide diffusing capacity	90	118	147	46
94725	Membrane diffusion capacity	113	155	198	75
94750	Pulmonary compliance study	71	97	124	37
94760	Measure blood oxygen level	30	42	56	9
94761	Measure blood oxygen level	51	69	87	24
94762	Measure blood oxygen level	75	103	132	40
94770	Exhaled carbon dioxide test	51	70	89	22

MC = Medicare Fee

Code	Short Description	50th	75th	90th	MC

ALLERGY AND IMMUNOLOGY SERVICES

Allergy Testing

Code	Description	50th	75th	90th	MC
95004	Allergy skin tests	4	5	7	3
95010	Sensitivity skin tests	11	14	17	9
95015	Sensitivity skin tests	11	14	18	9
95024	Allergy skin tests	6	8	10	5
95027	Skin end point titration	15	20	26	5
95028	Allergy skin tests	12	15	19	8
95044	Allergy patch tests	8	9	12	7
95052	Photo patch test	10	13	16	8
95056	Photosensitivity tests	8	11	14	6
95060	Eye allergy tests	18	24	30	12
95065	Nose allergy test	11	15	19	7
95070	Bronchial allergy tests	111	145	184	74
95071	Bronchial allergy tests	149	194	247	95
95075	Ingestion challenge test	122	159	202	97
95078	Provocative testing	20	26	33	9

Allergen Immunotherapy

Code	Description	50th	75th	90th	MC
95115	Immunotherapy, one injection	14	18	23	13
95117	Immunotherapy injections	21	29	36	17
95120	Immunotherapy, one injection	16	24	31	0
95125	Immunotherapy, many antigens	20	29	38	0
95130	Immunotherapy, insect venom	26	37	49	0
95131	Immunotherapy, insect venoms	35	51	66	0
95132	Immunotherapy, insect venoms	41	59	77	0
95133	Immunotherapy, insect venoms	49	70	91	0
95134	Immunotherapy, insect venoms	54	78	101	0
95144	Antigen therapy services	11	15	19	7
95145	Antigen therapy services	20	29	38	14
95146	Antigen therapy services	29	42	55	24
95147	Antigen therapy services	40	57	74	34
95148	Antigen therapy services	48	69	90	34
95149	Antigen therapy services	57	81	106	41
95165	Antigen therapy services	9	13	17	6
95170	Antigen therapy services	29	41	54	15
95180	Rapid desensitization	140	201	261	67

NEUROLOGY PROCEDURES

Code	Short Description	50th	75th	90th	MC
Sleep Testing					
95805	Multiple sleep latency test	470	635	809	260
95807	Sleep study	498	674	858	370
95808	Polysomnography, 1-3	632	855	1089	401
95810	Polysomnography, 4 or more	785	1062	1352	428
95812	Electroencephalogram (EEG)	244	330	420	101
95813	Electroencephalogram (EEG)	288	389	496	121
95816	Electroencephalogram (EEG)	195	264	336	90
95819	Electroencephalogram (EEG)	185	244	306	99
95822	Sleep electroencephalogram	205	278	354	117
95824	Electroencephalography	165	223	284	59
95827	Night electroencephalogram	252	340	433	145
Neuromuscular Testing					
95829	Surgery electrocorticogram	410	555	707	214
95830	Insert electrodes for EEG	191	258	329	82
95831	Limb muscle testing, manual	42	56	72	20
95832	Hand muscle testing, manual	43	58	74	18
95833	Body muscle testing, manual	84	114	145	29
95834	Body muscle testing, manual	88	118	151	41
95851	Range of motion measurements	39	54	70	14
95852	Range of motion measurements	36	48	62	9
95857	Tensilon test	81	110	140	35
95858	Tensilon test and myogram	164	222	282	86
95860	Muscle test, one limb	152	196	243	70
95861	Muscle test, two limbs	233	303	376	120
95863	Muscle test, 3 limbs	285	386	491	142
95864	Muscle test, 4 limbs	358	484	616	188
95867	Muscle test, head or neck	137	185	236	66
95868	Muscle test, head or neck	197	267	340	107
95869	Muscle test, limited	96	130	166	31
95872	Muscle test, one fiber	213	288	366	93
95875	Limb exercise test	105	141	180	65
95900	Motor nerve conduction test	79	105	133	36
95903	Motor nerve conduction test	95	128	163	40
95904	Sense nerve conduction test	78	105	133	31

MC = Medicare Fee

Code	Short Description	50th	75th	90th	MC
95920	Intraoperative nerve testing	308	417	530	163
95921	Autonomic nerve function test	66	89	114	39
95922	Autonomic nerve function test	69	94	119	41
95923	Autonomic nerve function test	66	89	114	39
95925	Somatosensory testing	227	301	379	72
95926	Somatosensory testing	224	298	376	72
95927	Somatosensory testing	190	257	328	72
95930	Visual evoked potential test	96	130	166	41
95933	Blink reflex test	116	157	200	64
95934	H reflex test	86	116	148	36
95936	H reflex test	91	123	156	37
95937	Neuromuscular junction test	99	127	155	49

Electroencephalographic Monitoring

Code	Short Description	50th	75th	90th	MC
95950	Ambulatory EEG monitoring	416	563	717	313
95951	EEG monitoring/videorecord	879	1189	1514	507
95953	EEG monitoring/computer	662	895	1139	361
95954	EEG monitoring/giving drugs	282	381	485	164
95955	EEG during surgery	267	362	460	140
95956	EEG monitoring/cable/radio	682	922	1174	371
95957	EEG digital analysis	289	390	497	144
95958	EEG monitoring/function test	571	772	983	315

Other Neurology Procedures

Code	Short Description	50th	75th	90th	MC
95961	Electrode stimulation, brain	331	448	571	189
95962	Electrode stimulation, brain	331	448	571	197

CENTRAL NERVOUS SYSTEM ASSESSMENTS/TESTS

Code	Short Description	50th	75th	90th	MC
96100	Psychological testing	197	266	339	64
96105	Assessment of aphasia	197	266	339	64
96110	Developmental test, limited	159	215	273	0
96111	Developmental test, extended	155	210	267	64
96115	Neurobehavior status exam	197	266	339	64
96117	Neuropsychological test battery	196	265	338	64

MEDICINE SERVICES

Code	Short Description	50th	75th	90th	MC
CHEMOTHERAPY ADMINISTRATION					
96400	Chemotherapy, (SC)/(IM)	26	39	51	5
96405	Intralesional chemotherapy	63	87	111	36
96406	Intralesional chemotherapy	98	136	174	55
96408	Chemotherapy, push technique	73	99	124	33
96410	Chemotherapy, infusion method	111	149	185	53
96412	Chemotherapy, infusion method	78	106	134	40
96414	Chemotherapy, infusion method	106	147	187	46
96420	Chemotherapy, push technique	78	108	138	43
96422	Chemotherapy, infusion method	109	152	194	43
96423	Chemotherapy, infusion method	46	64	81	17
96425	Chemotherapy, infusion method	76	105	134	49
96440	Chemotherapy, intracavitary	179	249	317	103
96445	Chemotherapy, intracavitary	199	276	351	104
96450	Chemotherapy, into CNS	154	214	273	90
96520	Pump refilling, maintenance	59	81	102	31
96530	Pump refilling, maintenance	68	93	116	37
96542	Chemotherapy injection	135	188	239	85
96545	Provide chemotherapy agent	59	82	104	0
96549	Chemotherapy, unspecified	32	47	62	0
DERMATOLOGY PROCEDURES					
96900	Ultraviolet light therapy	24	31	38	14
96910	Photochemotherapy with UV-B	32	41	50	20
96912	Photochemotherapy with UV-A	36	46	55	23
96913	Photochemotherapy, UV-A or B	89	116	140	47
PHYSICAL THERAPY AND REHABILITATION					
Modalities					
97010	Hot or cold packs therapy	24	32	39	0
97012	Mechanical traction therapy	28	36	43	15
97014	Electric stimulation therapy	26	34	41	13
97016	Vasopneumatic device therapy	28	37	45	15
97018	Paraffin bath therapy	29	38	46	11
97020	Microwave therapy	23	31	37	9
97022	Whirlpool therapy	28	36	43	12

MC = Medicare Fee

Code	Short Description	50th	75th	90th	MC
97024	Diathermy treatment	27	36	44	10
97026	Infrared therapy	25	33	40	9
97028	Ultraviolet therapy	23	31	37	9
97032	Electrical stimulation	28	37	45	13
97033	Electric current therapy	30	40	48	13
97034	Contrast bath therapy	24	31	38	10
97035	Ultrasound therapy	25	33	40	11
97036	Hydrotherapy	38	51	61	16

Therapeutic Procedures

Code	Short Description	50th	75th	90th	MC
97110	Therapeutic exercises	38	50	62	19
97112	Neuromuscular reeducation	34	45	55	19
97113	Aquatic therapy/exercises	43	58	72	21
97116	Gait training therapy	30	40	49	16
97122	Manual traction therapy	32	42	53	17
97124	Massage therapy	31	41	50	15
97150	Group therapeutic procedures	32	42	53	16
97250	Myofascial release	42	54	66	27
97260	Regional manipulation	33	43	54	13
97261	Supplemental manipulations	19	26	32	8
97265	Joint mobilization	51	68	85	27
97504	Orthotic training	35	46	58	19
97520	Prosthetic training	39	52	65	20
97530	Therapeutic activities	42	56	69	20
97535	Self care management training	43	58	72	20
97537	Community/work reintegration	43	58	72	20
97542	Wheelchair management training	38	51	63	14
97545	Work hardening	137	183	229	0
97546	Work hardening	66	89	111	0

Tests and Measurements

Code	Short Description	50th	75th	90th	MC
97703	Prosthetic checkout	39	52	65	15
97750	Physical performance test	50	66	83	23

Other Physical Medicine Procedures

Code	Short Description	50th	75th	90th	MC
97770	Cognitive skills development	53	71	89	24

MEDICINE SERVICES

Code	Short Description	50th	75th	90th	MC
OSTEOPATHIC MANIPULATIVE TREATMENT					
98925	Osteopathic manipulation, 1-2 regions	41	53	65	23
98926	Osteopathic manipulation, 3-4 regions	54	71	87	35
98927	Osteopathic manipulation, 5-6 regions	56	71	86	41
98928	Osteopathic manipulation, 7-8 regions	65	88	109	48
98929	Osteopathic manipulation, 9-10 regions	75	100	125	51
CHIROPRACTIC MANIPULATIVE TREATMENT					
98940	Chiropractic manipulation, 1-2 regions	42	57	71	24
98941	Chiropractic manipulation, 3-4 regions	54	72	90	30
98942	Chiropractic manipulation, 5 regions	66	89	111	37
98943	Chiropractic manipulation, extraspinal	48	64	80	0
SPECIAL SERVICES AND REPORTS					
99000	Specimen handling	15	21	27	0
99001	Specimen handling	14	19	26	0
99002	Device handling	27	39	51	0
99025	Initial surgical evaluation	44	63	83	0
99050	Medical services after hours	35	50	67	0
99052	Medical services at night	48	69	91	0
99054	Medical services at unusual hours	46	66	87	0
99056	Non-office medical services	31	44	58	0
99058	Office emergency care	37	53	70	0
99075	Medical testimony	280	399	528	0
99090	Computer data analysis	135	192	254	0
99100	Special anesthesia service	19	28	37	0
99116	Anesthesia with hypothermia	55	79	104	0
99135	Special anesthesia procedure	55	79	104	0
99140	Emergency anesthesia	21	30	39	0
99175	Induction of vomiting	77	109	141	48
99183	Hyperbaric oxygen therapy	184	258	331	133
99185	Regional hypothermia	46	65	84	22
99186	Total body hypothermia	136	192	248	75
99190	Special pump services	687	972	1254	0
99191	Special pump services	526	745	961	0
99192	Special pump services	360	509	657	0
99195	Phlebotomy	41	58	76	15

MC = Medicare Fee

DOES YOUR DOCTOR CHARGE TOO MUCH?

Code   **Short Description**   **50th**   **75th**   **90th**   **MC**

SURGERY SERVICES

Surgery services include the operation, local, metacarpal/digital block or topical anesthesia when used, and normal, uncomplicated follow-up care. This concept is referred to as a *package* for surgical procedures. When surgery services require the use of general anesthesia, the anesthesia service is billed separately by the anesthesiologist or the hospital.

Follow-up care for therapeutic surgical procedures includes only that care which is usually a part of the surgical service. Complications, exacerbations, recurrence or the presence of other diseases or injuries requiring additional services are reported separately from the surgery service. Follow-up care for diagnostic surgical procedures, such as endoscopy and injection procedures for radiography, includes only that care related to recovery from the diagnostic procedure itself. Care of the condition for which the diagnostic procedure was performed is not included and is reported separately.

Supplies and materials supplied by the doctor, such as sterile trays or drugs, which are considered over and above those usually included in the procedure may be reported separately. Visit services rendered by surgeons in the office, home or hospital, plus consultations and other medical services are reported using standard visit codes.

It is common for several surgical procedures to be performed at the same operative session. When multiple procedures are performed on the same day or at the same session, your health insurance plan will discount all procedures following the major procedure by 25-75 percent.

Code	Short Description	50th	75th	90th	MC

INTEGUMENTARY SYSTEM

Skin, Subcutaneous and Accessory Structures

Code	Short Description	50th	75th	90th	MC
10040	Acne surgery of skin abscess	59	77	95	58
10060	Drainage of skin abscess; simple	76	96	116	62

MC = Medicare Fee

Code	Short Description	50th	75th	90th	MC
10061	Drainage of skin abscess; complicated	163	211	263	113
10080	Drainage of pilonidal cyst; simple	97	126	157	53
10081	Drainage of pilonidal cyst; complicated	189	245	304	142
10120	Remove foreign body; simple	91	118	147	66
10121	Remove foreign body; complicated	232	301	375	145
10140	Drainage of hematoma/fluid	83	107	134	77
10160	Puncture drainage of lesion	72	91	111	61
10180	Complex drainage, wound	301	390	485	133
11000	Debride infected skin; up to 10%	69	88	110	41
11001	Debride infected skin; add 10%	59	81	105	23
11010	Debride skin, associated w/fracture	448	615	798	345
11011	Debride skin/muscle, w/fracture	534	733	952	411
11012	Debride skin/muscle/bone, w/fracture	742	1018	1323	571
11040	Debride skin partial	66	86	108	37
11041	Debride skin full	108	152	200	56
11042	Debride skin/tissue	188	268	356	72
11043	Debride tissue/muscle	364	518	688	157
11044	Debride tissue/muscle/bone	503	690	897	221
11050	Trim skin lesion	49	58	69	33
11051	Trim 2 to 4 skin lesions	63	74	86	47
11052	Trim over 4 skin lesions	73	90	108	51
11100	Biopsy of skin lesion	85	111	136	53
11101	Biopsy, each added lesion	54	72	90	28
11200	Remove skin tags	77	104	131	45
11201	Remove additional skin tags	39	53	68	18
11300	Shave skin lesion	77	100	126	43
11301	Shave skin lesion	109	140	175	62
11302	Shave skin lesion	141	179	221	80
11303	Shave skin lesion	152	199	251	109
11305	Shave skin lesion	90	117	146	49
11306	Shave skin lesion	142	186	234	69
11307	Shave skin lesion	133	174	219	85
11308	Shave skin lesion	199	261	328	117
11310	Shave skin lesion	103	133	166	58
11311	Shave skin lesion	133	170	212	78
11312	Shave skin lesion	161	210	264	95
11313	Shave skin lesion	224	292	368	128
11400	Remove benign skin lesion	91	119	150	56
11401	Remove benign skin lesion	116	150	187	78
11402	Remove benign skin lesion	150	196	247	99
11403	Remove benign skin lesion	197	257	324	123

SURGERY SERVICES

Code	Short Description	50th	75th	90th	MC
11404	Remove benign skin lesion	258	337	424	144
11406	Remove benign skin lesion	366	479	602	192
11420	Remove benign skin lesion	95	124	156	61
11421	Remove benign skin lesion	129	169	212	88
11422	Remove benign skin lesion	171	223	281	107
11423	Remove benign skin lesion	229	300	377	139
11424	Remove benign skin lesion	314	411	517	160
11426	Remove benign skin lesion	406	531	668	227
11440	Remove benign skin lesion	122	162	205	72
11441	Remove benign skin lesion	160	210	265	97
11442	Remove benign skin lesion	201	264	333	119
11443	Remove benign skin lesion	264	345	434	157
11444	Remove benign skin lesion	351	459	578	193
11446	Remove benign skin lesion	445	582	732	247
11450	Remove sweat gland lesion	461	603	759	225
11451	Remove sweat gland lesion	534	698	878	280
11462	Remove sweat gland lesion	454	594	747	202
11463	Remove sweat gland lesion	512	670	843	239
11470	Remove sweat gland lesion	507	663	834	249
11471	Remove sweat gland lesion	570	745	937	280
11600	Remove malignant skin lesion	160	208	255	101
11601	Remove malignant skin lesion	201	261	320	132
11602	Remove malignant skin lesion	250	317	384	158
11603	Remove malignant skin lesion	303	394	483	187
11604	Remove malignant skin lesion	378	491	602	212
11606	Remove malignant skin lesion	516	671	822	274
11620	Remove malignant skin lesion	187	243	297	108
11621	Remove malignant skin lesion	261	339	415	150
11622	Remove malignant skin lesion	332	432	529	184
11623	Remove malignant skin lesion	376	488	598	224
11624	Remove malignant skin lesion	474	616	755	272
11626	Remove malignant skin lesion	625	812	995	318
11640	Remove malignant skin lesion	253	329	403	129
11641	Remove malignant skin lesion	339	437	533	183
11642	Remove malignant skin lesion	419	543	664	223
11643	Remove malignant skin lesion	494	641	786	264
11644	Remove malignant skin lesion	587	763	935	326
11646	Remove malignant skin lesion	748	972	1191	421

MC = Medicare Fee

Code	Short Description	50th	75th	90th	MC

Nails

Code	Short Description	50th	75th	90th	MC
11720	Debride nail, 1-5	36	44	53	26
11721	Debride nail, 6 or more	60	75	90	44
11730	Remove nail plate	85	102	120	63
11731	Remove second nail plate	67	83	100	44
11732	Remove additional nail plate	51	64	77	32
11740	Drain blood from under nail	58	73	87	32
11750	Remove nail bed	268	337	407	156
11752	Remove nail bed/finger tip	372	463	556	219
11755	Biopsy nail unit	174	216	260	95
11760	Reconstruction of nail bed	246	306	367	99
11762	Reconstruction of nail bed	405	504	605	222
11765	Excision of nail fold, toe	108	134	161	47
11770	Remove pilonidal lesion	343	427	513	224
11771	Remove pilonidal lesion	737	917	1102	416
11772	Remove pilonidal lesion	894	1112	1336	478
11900	Injection into skin lesions	48	61	73	31
11901	Added skin lesions injection	68	85	102	48
11920	Correct skin color defects	393	487	587	118
11921	Correct skin color defects	540	670	807	141
11922	Correct skin color defects	205	254	306	36
11950	Therapy for contour defects	195	242	292	85
11951	Therapy for contour defects	294	365	440	98
11952	Therapy for contour defects	438	543	654	117
11954	Therapy for contour defects	513	636	766	123
11960	Insert tissue expander(s)	1293	1604	1931	678
11970	Replace tissue expander	1452	1802	2169	664
11971	Remove tissue expander(s)	333	413	497	185
11975	Insert contraceptive cap	177	219	264	0
11976	Remove contraceptive cap	210	260	313	109
11977	Remove/reinsert contraceptive cap	410	509	613	0

Wound Repair

Code	Short Description	50th	75th	90th	MC
12001	Repair superficial wound(s)	111	140	169	72
12002	Repair superficial wound(s)	146	182	220	85
12004	Repair superficial wound(s)	191	245	300	110
12005	Repair superficial wound(s)	243	312	381	142
12006	Repair superficial wound(s)	302	388	474	179

SURGERY SERVICES

Code	Short Description	50th	75th	90th	MC
12007	Repair superficial wound(s)	365	468	573	234
12011	Repair superficial wound(s)	137	171	206	80
12013	Repair superficial wound(s)	178	229	280	98
12014	Repair superficial wound(s)	217	278	340	118
12015	Repair superficial wound(s)	273	350	429	157
12016	Repair superficial wound(s)	340	436	534	203
12017	Repair superficial wound(s)	447	573	701	269
12018	Repair superficial wound(s)	571	732	896	436
12020	Closure of split wound	226	290	354	153
12021	Closure of split wound	188	241	295	97
12031	Layer closure of wound(s)	151	194	241	111
12032	Layer closure of wound(s)	199	257	319	138
12034	Layer closure of wound(s)	264	341	423	174
12035	Layer closure of wound(s)	323	416	517	215
12036	Layer closure of wound(s)	399	515	639	260
12037	Layer closure of wound(s)	480	618	768	320
12041	Layer closure of wound(s)	164	211	262	103
12042	Layer closure of wound(s)	204	263	327	127
12044	Layer closure of wound(s)	280	361	448	156
12045	Layer closure of wound(s)	344	443	551	191
12046	Layer closure of wound(s)	438	564	701	288
12047	Layer closure of wound(s)	493	636	790	298
12051	Layer closure of wound(s)	202	260	323	136
12052	Layer closure of wound(s)	262	338	420	168
12053	Layer closure of wound(s)	324	417	518	194
12054	Layer closure of wound(s)	418	538	669	245
12055	Layer closure of wound(s)	508	654	812	312
12056	Layer closure of wound(s)	627	808	1004	410
12057	Layer closure of wound(s)	716	923	1147	470
13100	Repair wound or lesion	223	292	355	167
13101	Repair wound or lesion	355	464	566	239
13120	Repair wound or lesion	287	376	458	184
13121	Repair wound or lesion	439	575	700	283
13131	Repair wound or lesion	362	474	578	231
13132	Repair wound or lesion	613	803	978	421
13150	Repair wound or lesion	345	452	550	223
13151	Repair wound or lesion	458	599	730	280
13152	Repair wound or lesion	748	979	1193	474
13160	Late closure of wound	675	884	1076	518
13300	Repair wound or lesion	971	1271	1548	461

MC = Medicare Fee

DOES YOUR DOCTOR CHARGE TOO MUCH?

Code	Short Description	50th	75th	90th	MC
14000	Skin tissue rearrangement	663	863	1044	359
14001	Skin tissue rearrangement	868	1130	1366	518
14020	Skin tissue rearrangement	792	1031	1247	449
14021	Skin tissue rearrangement	1093	1423	1720	645
14040	Skin tissue rearrangement	978	1274	1540	574
14041	Skin tissue rearrangement	1191	1550	1874	768
14060	Skin tissue rearrangement	1257	1628	1963	662
14061	Skin tissue rearrangement	1619	2108	2548	911
14300	Skin tissue rearrangement	1833	2387	2886	943
14350	Skin tissue rearrangement	1036	1349	1631	632
15000	Skin graft procedure	564	781	998	197
15050	Skin pinch graft procedure	393	544	695	232
15100	Skin split graft procedure	747	1033	1321	525
15101	Skin split graft procedure	412	571	729	143
15120	Skin split graft procedure	1205	1666	2130	630
15121	Skin split graft procedure	420	581	743	241
15200	Skin full graft procedure	661	914	1169	478
15201	Skin full graft procedure	246	340	435	139
15220	Skin full graft procedure	822	1137	1453	512
15221	Skin full graft procedure	313	433	553	130
15240	Skin full graft procedure	1073	1484	1897	604
15241	Skin full graft procedure	450	622	795	191
15260	Skin full graft procedure	1209	1672	2137	705
15261	Skin full graft procedure	563	779	995	225
15350	Skin homograft procedure	440	609	778	251
15400	Skin heterograft procedure	360	498	636	235
15570	Form skin pedicle flap	1006	1392	1779	626
15572	Form skin pedicle flap	1134	1569	2005	619
15574	Form skin pedicle flap	1302	1801	2302	626
15576	Form skin pedicle flap	1268	1754	2242	458
15580	Attach skin pedicle graft	977	1351	1727	562
15600	Skin graft procedure	475	657	840	203
15610	Skin graft procedure	511	706	903	231
15620	Skin graft procedure	631	874	1117	277
15625	Skin graft procedure	514	711	909	199
15630	Skin graft procedure	842	1165	1489	308
15650	Transfer skin pedicle flap	829	1147	1466	363
15732	Muscle-skin graft, head/neck	2455	3397	4342	1396
15734	Muscle-skin graft, trunk	2786	3854	4927	1532
15736	Muscle-skin graft, arm	2173	3006	3843	1361
15738	Muscle-skin graft, leg	2472	3419	4371	1283

SURGERY SERVICES

Code	Short Description	50th	75th	90th	MC
15740	Island pedicle flap graft	1430	1978	2528	847
15750	Neurovascular pedicle graft	1501	2077	2654	972
15756	Free muscle flap, microvascular	3671	5078	6491	2699
15757	Free skin flap, microvascular	3671	5078	6491	2699
15758	Free fascial flap, microvascular	3671	5078	6491	2699
15760	Composite skin graft	1100	1521	1944	655
15770	Derma-fat-fascia graft	1247	1725	2205	602
15775	Hair transplant punch grafts	268	370	473	290
15776	Hair transplant punch grafts	327	452	578	406
15780	Abrasion treatment of skin	959	1335	1729	321
15781	Abrasion treatment of skin	557	775	1004	346
15782	Abrasion treatment of skin	426	593	767	211
15783	Abrasion treatment of skin	329	458	593	240
15786	Abrasion treatment of lesion	97	136	176	102
15787	Abrasion treatment added lesions	65	91	118	23
15788	Chemical peel, face, epiderm	445	620	803	139
15789	Chemical peel, face, dermal	728	1014	1313	242
15792	Chemical peel, nonfacial	310	432	559	88
15793	Chemical peel, nonfacial	499	696	901	154
15810	Salabrasion	370	516	668	336
15811	Salabrasion	536	747	967	376
15819	Plastic surgery, neck	1546	2154	2788	697
15820	Revision of lower eyelid	1012	1410	1826	458
15821	Revision of lower eyelid	1059	1475	1909	511
15822	Revision of upper eyelid	914	1273	1648	407
15823	Revision of upper eyelid	1057	1472	1906	591
15824	Remove forehead wrinkles	1202	1674	2168	0
15825	Remove neck wrinkles	1171	1631	2112	0
15826	Remove brow wrinkles	909	1266	1639	0
15828	Remove face wrinkles	3264	4547	5886	0
15829	Remove skin wrinkles	3207	4468	5784	0
15831	Excise excessive skin tissue	2009	2799	3624	923
15832	Excise excessive skin tissue	1749	2436	3153	806
15833	Excise excessive skin tissue	1656	2307	2987	677
15834	Excise excessive skin tissue	1704	2373	3072	726
15835	Excise excessive skin tissue	1668	2323	3008	749
15836	Excise excessive skin tissue	1260	1755	2272	614
15837	Excise excessive skin tissue	1004	1399	1811	583
15838	Excise excessive skin tissue	953	1328	1719	525
15839	Excise excessive skin tissue	1220	1700	2200	454

MC = Medicare Fee

DOES YOUR DOCTOR CHARGE TOO MUCH?

Code	Short Description	50th	75th	90th	MC
15840	Graft for face nerve palsy	2375	3309	4283	1190
15841	Graft for face nerve palsy	2910	4053	5247	1613
15842	Graft for face nerve palsy	4067	5665	7334	2649
15845	Skin and muscle repair, face	2458	3424	4432	1166
15850	Remove sutures	149	208	269	0
15851	Remove sutures	98	137	177	38
15852	Dressing change, not for burn	118	165	213	44
15860	Test for blood flow in graft	249	346	449	139
15876	Suction assisted lipectomy	706	983	1273	0
15877	Suction assisted lipectomy	1245	1734	2245	0
15878	Suction assisted lipectomy	700	975	1262	0
15879	Suction assisted lipectomy	1206	1680	2175	0
15920	Remove tail bone ulcer	716	1009	1351	423
15922	Remove tail bone ulcer	1020	1436	1923	638
15931	Remove sacrum pressure sore	770	1084	1452	448
15933	Remove sacrum pressure sore	1223	1722	2307	704
15934	Remove sacrum pressure sore	1153	1624	2174	795
15935	Remove sacrum pressure sore	1570	2211	2961	1044
15936	Remove sacrum pressure sore	1153	1623	2173	929
15937	Remove sacrum pressure sore	1851	2606	3490	1149
15940	Remove pressure sore	865	1218	1631	483
15941	Remove pressure sore	1243	1750	2343	727
15944	Remove pressure sore	1156	1627	2179	836
15945	Remove pressure sore	1473	2074	2777	967
15946	Remove pressure sore	2291	3226	4320	1557
15950	Remove thigh pressure sore	548	771	1032	402
15951	Remove thigh pressure sore	984	1386	1856	738
15952	Remove thigh pressure sore	1086	1529	2047	731
15953	Remove thigh pressure sore	1268	1785	2390	876
15956	Remove thigh pressure sore	1631	2296	3074	1365
15958	Remove thigh pressure sore	1864	2624	3514	1404
16000	Initial treatment of burn(s)	62	87	116	40
16010	Treatment of burn(s)	108	152	203	39
16015	Treatment of burn(s)	358	504	675	187
16020	Treatment of burn(s)	62	87	116	37
16025	Treatment of burn(s)	122	172	230	90
16030	Treatment of burn(s)	191	269	361	103
16035	Incision of burn scab	495	697	934	261
16040	Burn wound excision	220	309	414	124
16041	Burn wound excision	419	590	790	253
16042	Burn wound excision	414	583	781	234

SURGERY SERVICES

Code	Short Description	50th	75th	90th	MC

Destruction of Lesions

Code	Short Description	50th	75th	90th	MC
17000	Destroy benign/premalignant lesion	71	89	110	39
17001	Destruction of additional lesions	34	45	58	16
17002	Destruction of additional lesions	20	26	33	12
17010	Destruction skin lesion(s)	135	177	224	59
17100	Destruction of skin lesion	55	70	87	36
17101	Destruction of 2nd lesion	31	42	54	12
17102	Destruction of additional lesions	18	26	34	8
17104	Destruction of skin lesions	187	245	310	79
17105	Destruction of skin lesions	131	172	218	42
17106	Destruction of skin lesions	409	537	679	257
17107	Destruction of skin lesions	840	1102	1394	508
17108	Destruction of skin lesions	1318	1730	2188	902
17110	Destruction of skin lesions	60	78	98	38
17200	Electrocautery of skin tags	66	86	109	41
17201	Electrocautery added lesions	37	49	62	21
17250	Chemical cautery, tissue	68	90	113	34
17260	Destruction of skin lesions	134	176	223	83
17261	Destruction of skin lesions	166	218	275	104
17262	Destruction of skin lesions	218	276	341	139
17263	Destruction of skin lesions	245	321	406	166
17264	Destruction of skin lesions	300	394	498	188
17266	Destruction of skin lesions	375	491	622	233
17270	Destruction of skin lesions	156	204	259	108
17271	Destruction of skin lesions	205	269	341	132
17272	Destruction of skin lesions	257	337	426	162
17273	Destruction of skin lesions	308	404	511	191
17274	Destruction of skin lesions	381	500	633	240
17276	Destruction of skin lesions	518	680	860	279
17280	Destruction of skin lesions	185	243	307	116
17281	Destruction of skin lesions	249	317	393	156
17282	Destruction of skin lesions	304	385	475	189
17283	Destruction of skin lesions	318	418	528	232
17284	Destruction of skin lesions	452	592	749	276
17286	Destruction of skin lesions	660	865	1094	366
17304	Chemosurgery of skin lesion	634	791	940	463
17305	2nd stage chemosurgery	342	439	530	207
17306	3rd stage chemosurgery	330	429	522	169
17307	Follow-up skin lesion therapy	322	418	509	172

MC = Medicare Fee

Code	Short Description	50th	75th	90th	MC
17310	Extensive skin chemosurgery	93	121	147	41
17340	Cryotherapy of skin	50	63	77	40
17360	Skin peel therapy	68	86	105	64
17380	Hair removal by electrolysis	66	83	102	0

Breast

Code	Short Description	50th	75th	90th	MC
19000	Drainage of breast lesion	94	132	177	50
19001	Drain added breast lesion	44	62	83	28
19020	Incision of breast lesion	327	458	613	195
19030	Injection for breast x-ray	109	153	205	65
19100	Biopsy of breast	157	207	259	79
19101	Biopsy of breast	435	572	717	232
19110	Nipple exploration	509	669	838	278
19112	Excise breast duct fistula	473	622	780	242
19120	Removal of breast lesion	635	827	1031	344
19125	Excision, breast lesion	724	929	1146	363
19126	Excision, additional breast lesion	367	482	604	182
19140	Remove breast tissue	908	1194	1496	395
19160	Remove breast tissue	861	1132	1419	421
19162	Remove breast tissue, nodes	1815	2385	2990	946
19180	Remove breast	1191	1565	1962	582
19182	Remove breast	1185	1557	1952	574
19200	Remove breast	2036	2676	3355	1041
19220	Remove breast	2488	3270	4098	1071
19240	Remove breast	1989	2614	3277	1021
19260	Remove chest wall lesion	1644	2161	2709	772
19271	Revision of chest wall	2761	3628	4548	1326
19272	Extensive chest wall surgery	3040	3995	5008	1352
19290	Place needle wire, breast	173	224	278	69
19291	Place needle wire, breast	89	117	146	36
19316	Suspension of breast	1641	2517	3431	1004
19318	Reduction of large breast	2277	3491	4760	1277
19324	Enlarge breast	732	1122	1530	371
19325	Enlarge breast with implant	1220	1871	2551	589
19328	Remove breast implant	614	942	1284	384
19330	Remove implant material	762	1168	1592	459
19340	Immediate breast prosthesis	1269	1946	2653	654
19342	Delayed breast prosthesis	1710	2621	3574	926
19350	Breast reconstruction	1012	1552	2116	667

SURGERY SERVICES

Code	Short Description	50th	75th	90th	MC
19355	Correct inverted nipple(s)	833	1278	1742	516
19357	Breast reconstruction	2642	4051	5523	1223
19361	Breast reconstruction	3456	5299	7223	1653
19364	Breast reconstruction	3394	5204	7094	1867
19366	Breast reconstruction	3398	5210	7103	1547
19367	Breast reconstruction	3377	5179	7060	1912
19368	Breast reconstruction	3997	6129	8355	2153
19369	Breast reconstruction	3643	5586	7615	2061
19370	Surgery of breast capsule	949	1455	1983	587
19371	Remove breast capsule	1128	1729	2357	719
19380	Revise breast reconstruction	1079	1655	2256	721
19396	Design custom breast implant	244	374	510	159

MUSCULOSKELETAL SYSTEM SURGERY

General

20000	Incision of abscess	142	193	245	108
20005	Incision of deep abscess	399	545	690	200
20100	Explore wound, neck	1265	1726	2184	608
20101	Explore wound, chest	397	541	685	192
20102	Explore wound, abdomen	493	673	852	235
20103	Explore wound, extremity	657	897	1135	317
20150	Excise epiphyseal bar	1675	2285	2891	1079
20200	Muscle biopsy	215	293	370	108
20205	Deep muscle biopsy	370	505	640	179
20206	Needle biopsy, muscle	169	231	292	82
20220	Bone biopsy, trocar/needle	191	261	330	87
20225	Bone biopsy, trocar/needle	440	600	760	148
20240	Bone biopsy, excisional	404	552	698	200
20245	Bone biopsy, excisional	561	765	968	303
20250	Open bone biopsy	1369	1868	2364	413
20251	Open bone biopsy	1420	1938	2452	471
20500	Injection of sinus tract	65	89	113	50
20501	Inject sinus tract for x-ray	101	138	175	34
20520	Remove foreign body	170	232	294	100
20525	Remove foreign body	459	627	793	226
20550	Inject tendon/ligament/cyst	62	83	104	41
20600	Drain/inject joint/bursa	65	83	101	46
20605	Drain/inject joint/bursa	65	84	102	46

MC = Medicare Fee

Code	Short Description	50th	75th	90th	MC
20610	Drain/inject joint/bursa	69	90	112	41
20615	Treatment of bone cyst	247	337	426	88
20650	Insert and remove bone pin	201	274	347	128
20660	Apply/remove fixation device	458	625	791	167
20661	Application of head brace	719	981	1241	343
20662	Application of pelvis brace	725	989	1251	517
20663	Application of thigh brace	637	869	1100	404
20665	Remove fixation device	89	122	154	71
20670	Remove support implant	199	272	344	98
20680	Remove support implant	502	685	867	279
20690	Apply bone fixation device	700	956	1209	306
20692	Apply bone fixation device	907	1238	1566	503
20693	Adjust bone fixation device	560	764	967	323
20694	Remove bone fixation device	391	533	674	266
20802	Replantation, arm, complete	7436	10149	12840	3284
20805	Replantation, forearm, complete	7501	10237	12951	4019
20808	Replantation, hand, complete	8124	11087	14027	4997
20816	Replantation digit, complete	3827	5223	6607	2463
20822	Replantation digit, complete	2888	3941	4986	2036
20824	Replantation thumb, complete	4006	5467	6917	2463
20827	Replantation thumb, complete	3430	4681	5922	2094
20838	Replantation, foot, complete	7329	10002	12654	3284
20900	Remove bone for graft	427	583	737	322
20902	Remove bone for graft	804	1098	1389	489
20910	Remove cartilage for graft	542	739	935	225
20912	Remove cartilage for graft	702	959	1213	442
20920	Remove fascia for graft	467	637	806	364
20922	Remove fascia for graft	631	861	1089	436
20924	Remove tendon for graft	596	814	1030	485
20926	Remove tissue for graft	420	573	725	311
20930	Spinal bone allograft	227	310	393	0
20931	Spinal bone allograft	287	392	496	150
20936	Spinal bone autograft	304	415	525	0
20937	Spinal bone autograft	433	591	748	232
20938	Spinal bone autograft	472	644	814	251
20950	Record fluid pressure, muscle	181	247	312	99
20955	Fibula bone graft, microvascular	6085	8305	10507	3120
20956	Iliac bone graft, microvascular	4221	5761	7289	2707
20957	Metatarsal bone graft, microvascular	4373	5968	7551	2804
20962	Other bone graft, microvascular	3778	5156	6523	2707
20969	Bone/skin graft, microvascular	5359	7314	9253	3493

SURGERY SERVICES

Code	Short Description	50th	75th	90th	MC
20970	Bone/skin graft, iliac crest	6448	8800	11133	3422
20972	Bone-skin graft, metatarsal	6441	8791	11121	3449
20973	Bone-skin graft, great toe	6735	9191	11628	3678
20974	Electrical bone stimulation	391	534	676	185
20975	Electrical bone stimulation	612	835	1057	257

Head

Code	Short Description	50th	75th	90th	MC
21010	Incision of jaw joint	1600	2175	2737	798
21015	Resection of facial tumor	927	1260	1585	491
21025	Excision of bone, lower jaw	915	1244	1565	522
21026	Excision of facial bone(s)	914	1242	1563	310
21029	Contour of face bone lesion	1245	1693	2130	681
21030	Remove face bone lesion	1058	1438	1810	376
21031	Remove exostosis, mandible	518	705	886	282
21032	Remove exostosis, maxilla	653	888	1117	291
21034	Remove face bone lesion	1805	2454	3087	890
21040	Remove jaw bone lesion	524	712	896	198
21041	Remove jaw bone lesion	968	1316	1655	483
21044	Remove jaw bone lesion	1764	2399	3018	853
21045	Extensive jaw surgery	3391	4611	5801	1199
21050	Remove jaw joint	2061	2802	3525	928
21060	Remove jaw joint cartilage	1876	2551	3209	876
21070	Remove coronoid process	1769	2405	3026	600
21076	Prepare face/oral prosthesis	2150	2923	3677	1213
21077	Prepare face/oral prosthesis	5240	7125	8964	3051
21079	Prepare face/oral prosthesis	1754	2385	3001	2020
21080	Prepare face/oral prosthesis	2161	2938	3697	2270
21081	Prepare face/oral prosthesis	2006	2728	3432	2068
21082	Prepare face/oral prosthesis	1662	2260	2844	1887
21083	Prepare face/oral prosthesis	1687	2293	2885	1745
21084	Prepare face/oral prosthesis	2030	2760	3472	2036
21085	Prepare face/oral prosthesis	797	1083	1363	814
21086	Prepare face/oral prosthesis	2197	2987	3758	2254
21087	Prepare face/oral prosthesis	2197	2987	3758	2254
21088	Prepare face/oral prosthesis	1080	1469	1848	0
21100	Maxillofacial fixation	375	510	642	200
21110	Interdental fixation	799	1086	1366	434
21116	Injection, jaw joint x-ray	134	182	229	63
21120	Reconstruction of chin	1066	1449	1824	343

MC = Medicare Fee

Code	Short Description	50th	75th	90th	MC
21121	Reconstruction of chin	1474	2004	2521	539
21122	Reconstruction of chin	1799	2445	3077	593
21123	Reconstruction of chin	2181	2965	3730	776
21125	Augmentation lower jaw bone	1280	1740	2189	591
21127	Augmentation lower jaw bone	1784	2425	3051	753
21137	Reduction of forehead	1753	2384	3000	678
21138	Reduction of forehead	2268	3083	3879	846
21139	Reduction of forehead	2493	3390	4265	1015
21141	Reconstruct midface, lefort	2656	3612	4544	1292
21142	Reconstruct midface, lefort	2739	3725	4686	1339
21143	Reconstruct midface, lefort	2863	3893	4898	1392
21145	Reconstruct midface, lefort	3326	4523	5690	1367
21146	Reconstruct midface, lefort	3720	5058	6363	1415
21147	Reconstruct midface, lefort	3985	5419	6818	1467
21150	Reconstruct midface, lefort	2964	4031	5071	1762
21151	Reconstruct midface, lefort	3321	4516	5682	1973
21154	Reconstruct midface, lefort	3730	5071	6381	2113
21155	Reconstruct midface, lefort	3987	5420	6820	2396
21159	Reconstruct midface, lefort	6545	8899	11197	2959
21160	Reconstruct midface, lefort	7174	9754	12273	3241
21172	Reconstruct orbit/forehead	4414	6001	7551	1937
21175	Reconstruct orbit/forehead	5344	7267	9143	2325
21179	Reconstruct entire forehead	3651	4964	6246	1549
21180	Reconstruct entire forehead	4243	5769	7258	1762
21181	Contour cranial bone lesion	1429	1942	2444	678
21182	Reconstruct cranial bone	4627	6291	7915	2254
21183	Reconstruct cranial bone	4990	6785	8536	2466
21184	Reconstruct cranial bone	5325	7240	9109	2677
21188	Reconstruction of midface	3650	4963	6245	1549
21193	Reconstruct lower jaw bone	3111	4229	5321	1173
21194	Reconstruct lower jaw bone	3707	5040	6342	1359
21195	Reconstruct lower jaw bone	3530	4799	6038	1176
21196	Reconstruct lower jaw bone	3697	5026	6324	1296
21198	Reconstruct lower jaw bone	2483	3375	4247	1180
21206	Reconstruct upper jaw bone	2617	3559	4477	966
21208	Augmentation of facial bones	1776	2414	3038	864
21209	Reduction of facial bones	1578	2146	2700	455
21210	Face bone graft	2134	2902	3651	913
21215	Lower jaw bone graft	2443	3321	4179	964
21230	Rib cartilage graft	1904	2589	3258	872
21235	Ear cartilage graft	1361	1851	2329	610

SURGERY SERVICES

Code	Short Description	50th	75th	90th	MC
21240	Reconstruction of jaw joint	2790	3793	4773	1265
21242	Reconstruction of jaw joint	2987	4061	5109	1184
21243	Reconstruction of jaw joint	3261	4434	5578	1372
21244	Reconstruction of lower jaw	2861	3890	4895	1076
21245	Reconstruction of jaw	2472	3361	4228	940
21246	Reconstruction of jaw	3024	4111	5173	842
21247	Reconstruct lower jaw bone	4269	5804	7303	1997
21248	Reconstruction of jaw	2434	3309	4164	1069
21249	Reconstruction of jaw	3472	4720	5939	1724
21255	Reconstruct lower jaw bone	2818	3832	4821	1475
21256	Reconstruction of orbit	4625	6288	7912	1428
21260	Revise eye sockets	3911	5318	6691	1457
21261	Revise eye sockets	5757	7828	9849	1901
21263	Revise eye sockets	6735	9157	11521	2507
21267	Revise eye sockets	4307	5856	7368	1349
21268	Revise eye sockets	5675	7716	9708	1616
21270	Augmentation cheek bone	2378	3233	4068	810
21275	Revision orbitofacial bones	3046	4141	5211	813
21280	Revision of eyelid	1612	2192	2757	531
21282	Revision of eyelid	1197	1628	2049	340
21295	Revision of jaw muscle/bone	573	780	981	98
21296	Revision of jaw muscle/bone	1164	1583	1992	306
21300	Treatment of skull fracture	197	266	334	69
21310	Treatment of nose fracture	145	197	247	46
21315	Treatment of nose fracture	239	324	407	136
21320	Treatment of nose fracture	513	695	872	178
21325	Repair nose fracture	641	867	1088	321
21330	Repair nose fracture	1139	1541	1934	488
21335	Repair nose fracture	1943	2630	3300	789
21336	Repair nasal septal fracture	847	1147	1439	390
21337	Repair nasal septal fracture	344	466	585	226
21338	Repair nasoethmoid fracture	1391	1882	2362	459
21339	Repair nasoethmoid fracture	1670	2260	2836	603
21340	Repair nose fracture	1825	2470	3099	786
21343	Repair sinus fracture	1685	2281	2862	874
21344	Repair sinus fracture	2653	3590	4504	1112
21345	Repair nose/jaw fracture	1236	1673	2100	643
21346	Repair nose/jaw fracture	1687	2283	2865	800
21347	Repair nose/jaw fracture	2065	2795	3507	926
21348	Repair nose/jaw fracture	2888	3908	4904	1141

MC = Medicare Fee

Code	Short Description	50th	75th	90th	MC
21355	Repair cheek bone fracture	597	808	1014	203
21356	Repair cheek bone fracture	828	1121	1406	385
21360	Repair cheek bone fracture	1303	1763	2213	562
21365	Repair cheek bone fracture	1951	2640	3312	1097
21366	Repair cheek bone fracture	2631	3561	4468	1215
21385	Repair eye socket fracture	1551	2099	2633	761
21386	Repair eye socket fracture	1853	2507	3146	744
21387	Repair eye socket fracture	1845	2497	3133	685
21390	Repair eye socket fracture	2027	2743	3442	899
21395	Repair eye socket fracture	2483	3360	4217	896
21400	Treat eye socket fracture	222	300	376	103
21401	Repair eye socket fracture	823	1113	1397	233
21406	Repair eye socket fracture	1372	1856	2329	490
21407	Repair eye socket fracture	1650	2232	2801	625
21408	Repair eye socket fracture	2024	2739	3437	823
21421	Treat mouth roof fracture	1171	1584	1988	457
21422	Repair mouth roof fracture	1662	2249	2822	742
21423	Repair mouth roof fracture	2195	2970	3727	815
21431	Treat craniofacial fracture	1418	1918	2407	523
21432	Repair craniofacial fracture	1902	2574	3230	614
21433	Repair craniofacial fracture	2977	4028	5054	1711
21435	Repair craniofacial fracture	2878	3894	4886	1225
21436	Repair craniofacial fracture	3683	4984	6253	1670
21440	Repair dental ridge fracture	828	1120	1405	232
21445	Repair dental ridge fracture	1364	1846	2316	462
21450	Treat lower jaw fracture	344	465	584	231
21451	Treat lower jaw fracture	1067	1444	1812	440
21452	Treat lower jaw fracture	336	454	570	133
21453	Treat lower jaw fracture	1151	1557	1954	489
21454	Treat lower jaw fracture	1666	2255	2829	620
21461	Repair lower jaw fracture	1640	2219	2785	733
21462	Repair lower jaw fracture	1934	2617	3283	878
21465	Repair lower jaw fracture	1933	2616	3282	804
21470	Repair lower jaw fracture	2262	3061	3841	1306
21480	Reset dislocated jaw	214	290	364	59
21485	Reset dislocated jaw	677	916	1150	238
21490	Repair dislocated jaw	1409	1906	2392	696
21493	Treat hyoid bone fracture	191	258	324	112
21494	Repair hyoid bone fracture	1273	1722	2161	554
21495	Repair hyoid bone fracture	1344	1819	2282	418
21497	Interdental wiring	978	1323	1660	314

SURGERY SERVICES

Code	Short Description	50th	75th	90th	MC
Neck (Soft Tissues) and Thorax					
21501	Drain neck/chest lesion	470	641	808	217
21502	Drain chest lesion	788	1074	1354	445
21510	Drainage of bone lesion	604	824	1038	366
21550	Biopsy of neck/chest	204	278	350	115
21555	Remove lesion neck/chest	419	571	720	229
21556	Remove lesion neck/chest	754	1029	1296	380
21557	Remove tumor, neck or chest	1879	2562	3229	727
21600	Partial removal of rib	804	1097	1382	456
21610	Partial removal of rib	1662	2267	2857	756
21615	Remove rib	1786	2435	3069	834
21616	Remove rib and nerves	2030	2768	3488	776
21620	Partial removal of sternum	1758	2398	3022	558
21627	Sternal debridement	1150	1568	1976	471
21630	Extensive sternum surgery	2714	3701	4664	1219
21632	Extensive sternum surgery	3696	5040	6352	1188
21700	Revision of neck muscle	863	1177	1484	410
21705	Revision of neck muscle/rib	1361	1856	2339	577
21720	Revision of neck muscle	803	1095	1380	383
21725	Revision of neck muscle	998	1361	1715	475
21740	Reconstruction of sternum	2550	3478	4383	1015
21750	Repair sternum separation	1819	2481	3126	737
21800	Treatment of rib fracture	139	189	238	57
21805	Treatment of rib fracture	598	815	1028	161
21810	Treatment of rib fracture(s)	1614	2201	2774	476
21820	Treat sternum fracture	291	396	500	108
21825	Repair sternum fracture	1155	1575	1984	585
Back and Flank					
21920	Biopsy soft tissue of back	170	232	292	112
21925	Biopsy soft tissue of back	468	639	805	252
21930	Remove lesion, back or flank	577	786	991	313
21935	Remove tumor of back	1837	2504	3156	966
Spine (Vertebral Column)					
22100	Remove part of neck vertebra	1192	1625	2048	698
22101	Remove part of thorax vertebra	1149	1567	1975	723

MC = Medicare Fee

Code	Short Description	50th	75th	90th	MC
22102	Remove part of lumbar vertebra	1040	1419	1788	550
22103	Remove extra spine segment	368	501	632	194
22110	Remove part of neck vertebra	1593	2172	2738	901
22112	Remove part of thorax vertebra	1592	2171	2736	908
22114	Remove part of lumbar vertebra	1449	1976	2490	780
22116	Remove extra spine segment	366	498	628	192
22210	Revision of neck spine	3860	5264	6633	1512
22212	Revision of thorax spine	3707	5055	6371	1505
22214	Revision of lumbar spine	3367	4591	5786	1410
22216	Revise, extra spine segment	926	1263	1592	471
22220	Revision of neck spine	3589	4893	6167	1546
22222	Revision of thorax spine	3473	4736	5969	1379
22224	Revision of lumbar spine	3462	4720	5949	1467
22226	Revise, extra spine segment	926	1263	1592	471
22305	Treat spine process fracture	344	469	592	183
22310	Treat spine fracture	606	826	1041	201
22315	Treat spine fracture	1046	1426	1797	575
22325	Repair spine fracture	2376	3240	4083	1041
22326	Repair neck spine fracture	2897	3951	4979	1457
22327	Repair thorax spine fracture	2795	3811	4803	1409
22328	Repair additional spine fracture	738	1006	1268	383
22505	Manipulation of spine	172	235	296	105
22548	Neck spine fusion	3758	5232	6671	1992
22554	Neck spine fusion	3052	4250	5418	1603
22556	Thorax spine fusion	3632	5056	6446	1871
22558	Lumbar spine fusion	3331	4638	5913	1762
22585	Additional spinal fusion	984	1370	1747	467
22590	Spine and skull spinal fusion	4008	5580	7115	1757
22595	Neck spinal fusion	3747	5217	6652	1762
22600	Neck spine fusion	3141	4374	5576	1483
22610	Thorax spine fusion	2827	3936	5018	1394
22612	Lumbar spine fusion	3241	4512	5752	1739
22614	Spine fusion, extra segment	969	1349	1720	511
22630	Lumbar spine fusion	3075	4281	5458	1637
22632	Spine fusion, extra segment	816	1136	1449	434
22800	Fusion of spine	3465	4824	6151	1669
22802	Fusion of spine	4765	6634	8458	2466
22804	Fusion of spine	5141	7157	9125	2663
22808	Fusion of spine	3591	5000	6375	1822
22810	Fusion of spine	4106	5717	7289	1972
22812	Fusion of spine	4841	6741	8594	2400

SURGERY SERVICES

Code	Short Description	50th	75th	90th	MC
22830	Exploration of spinal fusion	2717	3783	4824	1009
22840	Insert spine fixation device	1912	2662	3395	756
22842	Insert spine fixation device	4521	6294	8025	799
22843	Insert spine fixation device	5562	7744	9874	913
22844	Insert spine fixation device	6624	9223	11759	1116
22845	Insert spine fixation device	2561	3566	4547	721
22846	Insert spine fixation device	3242	4514	5755	843
22847	Insert spine fixation device	3504	4879	6220	937
22848	Insert pelvic fixation device	931	1296	1653	498
22849	Reinsert spinal fixation	1725	2402	3063	1222
22850	Remove spine fixation device	1315	1831	2335	774
22851	Apply spine prosthetic device	1041	1450	1849	557
22852	Remove spine fixation device	1644	2289	2918	781
22855	Remove spine fixation device	1883	2621	3342	887

Abdomen

Code	Short Description	50th	75th	90th	MC
22900	Remove abdominal wall lesion	685	954	1217	341

Shoulder

Code	Short Description	50th	75th	90th	MC
23000	Remove calcium deposits	681	940	1225	307
23020	Release shoulder joint	1312	1812	2361	652
23030	Drain shoulder lesion	439	606	790	222
23031	Drain shoulder bursa	383	529	690	124
23035	Drain shoulder bone lesion	1214	1676	2184	590
23040	Exploratory shoulder surgery	1416	1956	2549	755
23044	Exploratory shoulder surgery	909	1256	1636	572
23065	Biopsy shoulder tissues	220	304	396	115
23066	Biopsy shoulder tissues	381	526	685	203
23075	Remove shoulder lesion	350	483	630	169
23076	Remove shoulder lesion	693	957	1247	439
23077	Remove tumor of shoulder	2242	3096	4034	909
23100	Biopsy of shoulder joint	1162	1605	2091	557
23101	Shoulder joint surgery	1189	1641	2139	519
23105	Remove shoulder joint lining	1678	2318	3021	767
23106	Incision of collarbone joint	1237	1708	2226	436
23107	Explore/treat shoulder joint	1440	1988	2591	764
23120	Partial removal collar bone	849	1172	1527	469
23125	Remove collarbone	1700	2348	3060	734

MC = Medicare Fee

Code	Short Description	50th	75th	90th	MC
23130	Partial removal shoulder bone	1057	1460	1903	602
23140	Remove bone lesion	770	1063	1386	442
23145	Remove bone lesion	1201	1658	2161	708
23146	Remove bone lesion	940	1298	1691	531
23150	Remove humerus lesion	1279	1766	2302	606
23155	Remove humerus lesion	1610	2223	2897	776
23156	Remove humerus lesion	1395	1927	2511	665
23170	Remove collarbone lesion	792	1093	1425	464
23172	Remove shoulder blade lesion	828	1143	1490	476
23174	Remove humerus lesion	1479	2043	2662	727
23180	Remove collar bone lesion	877	1211	1578	497
23182	Remove shoulder blade lesion	896	1237	1612	595
23184	Remove humerus lesion	1265	1746	2276	746
23190	Partial removal of scapula	894	1234	1608	543
23195	Remove head of humerus	1576	2176	2836	762
23200	Remove collar bone	1515	2093	2727	842
23210	Remove shoulder blade	1809	2498	3255	855
23220	Partial removal of humerus	1960	2707	3528	1077
23221	Partial removal of humerus	2383	3291	4289	1416
23222	Partial removal of humerus	2381	3288	4285	1565
23330	Remove shoulder foreign body	232	320	417	93
23331	Remove shoulder foreign body	998	1379	1796	367
23332	Remove shoulder foreign body	1881	2598	3385	860
23350	Injection for shoulder x-ray	112	155	202	50
23395	Muscle transfer, shoulder/arm	1761	2297	2819	1132
23397	Muscle transfers	2108	2749	3374	1240
23400	Fixation of shoulder blade	1961	2557	3138	959
23405	Incision of tendon and muscle	1116	1455	1786	647
23406	Incise tendon(s) and muscle(s)	1506	1964	2410	838
23410	Repair tendon(s)	1725	2249	2761	967
23412	Repair tendon(s)	1965	2562	3145	1113
23415	Release of shoulder ligament	1135	1479	1816	603
23420	Repair shoulder	2306	3006	3690	1170
23430	Repair biceps tendon	1432	1867	2291	708
23440	Removal/transplant tendon	1439	1876	2302	720
23450	Repair shoulder capsule	2166	2824	3466	1088
23455	Repair shoulder capsule	2336	3046	3738	1259
23460	Repair shoulder capsule	2414	3147	3863	1219
23462	Repair shoulder capsule	2356	3072	3770	1270
23465	Repair shoulder capsule	2322	3028	3716	1241
23466	Repair shoulder capsule	2478	3231	3965	1299

SURGERY SERVICES

Code	Short Description	50th	75th	90th	MC
23470	Reconstruct shoulder joint	2633	3433	4214	1401
23472	Reconstruct shoulder joint	3917	5106	6268	1648
23480	Revision of collarbone	1278	1666	2045	708
23485	Revision of collar bone	1717	2238	2747	1018
23490	Reinforce clavicle	1234	1609	1974	866
23491	Reinforce shoulder bones	1585	2067	2537	1119
23500	Treat clavicle fracture	258	331	403	149
23505	Treat clavicle fracture	422	542	659	254
23515	Repair clavicle fracture	1109	1424	1734	593
23520	Treat clavicle dislocation	254	326	397	141
23525	Treat clavicle dislocation	350	450	548	220
23530	Repair clavicle dislocation	1055	1356	1650	570
23532	Repair clavicle dislocation	1280	1645	2002	630
23540	Treat clavicle dislocation	228	293	356	150
23545	Treat clavicle dislocation	333	427	520	208
23550	Repair clavicle dislocation	1350	1735	2111	658
23552	Repair clavicle dislocation	1458	1873	2279	641
23570	Treat shoulder blade fracture	268	344	418	159
23575	Treat shoulder blade fracture	413	531	646	276
23585	Repair scapula fracture	1374	1765	2148	684
23600	Treat humerus fracture	386	496	604	240
23605	Treat humerus fracture	675	867	1055	397
23615	Repair humerus fracture	1614	2073	2523	827
23616	Repair humerus fracture	3154	4051	4931	1806
23620	Treat humerus fracture	339	436	531	221
23625	Treat humerus fracture	467	601	731	318
23630	Repair humerus fracture	1205	1547	1883	677
23650	Treat shoulder dislocation	339	435	530	218
23655	Treat shoulder dislocation	506	651	792	298
23660	Repair shoulder dislocation	1384	1779	2165	695
23665	Treat dislocation/fracture	489	628	764	314
23670	Repair dislocation/fracture	1439	1849	2250	745
23675	Treat dislocation/fracture	643	826	1005	396
23680	Repair dislocation/fracture	1811	2326	2832	937
23700	Fixation of shoulder	419	538	655	192
23800	Fusion of shoulder joint	2410	3097	3769	1278
23802	Fusion of shoulder joint	2488	3196	3890	1255
23900	Amputation of arm and girdle	3021	3881	4723	1304
23920	Amputation at shoulder joint	2324	2986	3634	1182
23921	Amputation follow-up surgery	652	837	1019	394

MC = Medicare Fee

Code	Short Description	50th	75th	90th	MC

Humerus (Upper Arm) and Elbow

Code	Short Description	50th	75th	90th	MC
23930	Drainage of arm lesion	375	493	609	180
23931	Drainage of arm bursa	281	369	456	96
23935	Drain arm/elbow bone lesion	786	1034	1276	433
24000	Exploratory elbow surgery	1214	1597	1971	538
24006	Release elbow joint	1553	2043	2522	667
24065	Biopsy arm/elbow soft tissue	178	234	289	113
24066	Biopsy arm/elbow soft tissue	517	680	840	314
24075	Remove arm/elbow lesion	426	560	691	238
24076	Remove arm/elbow lesion	687	904	1116	404
24077	Remove tumor of arm/elbow	1691	2225	2746	898
24100	Biopsy elbow joint lining	795	1046	1291	377
24101	Explore/treat elbow joint	1260	1659	2047	583
24102	Remove elbow joint lining	1619	2131	2630	755
24105	Remove elbow bursa	681	897	1107	309
24110	Remove humerus lesion	1218	1603	1979	631
24115	Remove/graft bone lesion	1535	2020	2493	703
24116	Remove/graft bone lesion	1487	1957	2416	876
24120	Remove elbow lesion	1024	1347	1663	526
24125	Remove/graft bone lesion	1202	1582	1952	540
24126	Remove/graft bone lesion	1183	1557	1922	644
24130	Remove head of radius	1055	1388	1713	543
24134	Remove arm bone lesion	1447	1905	2351	744
24136	Remove radius bone lesion	1390	1830	2258	673
24138	Remove elbow bone lesion	1328	1747	2157	582
24140	Partial removal of arm bone	1445	1901	2346	740
24145	Partial removal of radius	1027	1352	1668	571
24147	Partial removal of elbow	982	1292	1595	578
24149	Radical resection of elbow	1739	2288	2824	1100
24150	Extensive humerus surgery	2103	2768	3416	1135
24151	Extensive humerus surgery	2358	3103	3829	1203
24152	Extensive radius surgery	1711	2251	2779	683
24153	Extensive radius surgery	2177	2865	3536	909
24155	Remove elbow joint	1677	2207	2724	928
24160	Remove elbow joint implant	1072	1411	1741	510
24164	Remove radius head implant	950	1250	1542	481
24200	Remove arm foreign body	201	264	326	74
24201	Remove arm foreign body	521	685	845	307
24220	Injection for elbow x-ray	117	154	190	60

SURGERY SERVICES

Code	Short Description	50th	75th	90th	MC
24301	Muscle/tendon transfer	1599	2104	2597	741
24305	Arm tendon lengthening	746	982	1212	407
24310	Revision of arm tendon	640	842	1040	355
24320	Repair arm tendon	1845	2428	2996	806
24330	Revision of arm muscles	1408	1852	2286	761
24331	Revision of arm muscles	1726	2271	2803	838
24340	Repair biceps tendon	1454	1913	2361	618
24341	Repair tendon/muscle arm	962	1266	1562	608
24342	Repair ruptured tendon	1699	2236	2760	878
24350	Repair tennis elbow	660	869	1072	391
24351	Repair tennis elbow	767	1010	1246	432
24352	Repair tennis elbow	952	1252	1546	502
24354	Repair tennis elbow	896	1179	1455	501
24356	Revision of tennis elbow	1046	1376	1699	587
24360	Reconstruct elbow joint	2437	3207	3958	1159
24361	Reconstruct elbow joint	2431	3198	3948	1127
24362	Reconstruct elbow joint	2502	3293	4064	1112
24363	Replace elbow joint	3477	4576	5648	1759
24365	Reconstruct head of radius	1224	1611	1988	655
24366	Reconstruct head of radius	1435	1888	2331	852
24400	Revision of humerus	1649	2170	2678	798
24410	Revision of humerus	2077	2733	3374	1196
24420	Revision of humerus	1957	2575	3178	1071
24430	Repair humerus	2151	2830	3493	1157
24435	Repair humerus with graft	2411	3172	3915	1214
24470	Revision of elbow joint	1215	1599	1973	690
24495	Decompression of forearm	1317	1733	2139	566
24498	Reinforce humerus	1531	2014	2486	916
24500	Treat humerus fracture	322	414	505	232
24505	Treat humerus fracture	693	893	1088	395
24515	Repair humerus fracture	1685	2171	2646	869
24516	Repair humerus fracture	1702	2193	2672	869
24530	Treat humerus fracture	390	503	613	253
24535	Treat humerus fracture	772	995	1212	475
24538	Treat humerus fracture	1253	1615	1968	711
24545	Repair humerus fracture	1706	2198	2678	836
24546	Repair humerus fracture	2326	2997	3652	1024
24560	Treat humerus fracture	351	453	551	199
24565	Treat humerus fracture	580	747	910	359
24566	Treat humerus fracture	981	1264	1540	557

MC = Medicare Fee

Code	Short Description	50th	75th	90th	MC
24575	Repair humerus fracture	1324	1705	2078	742
24576	Treat humerus fracture	295	381	464	202
24577	Treat humerus fracture	597	769	937	394
24579	Repair humerus fracture	1371	1767	2153	806
24582	Treat humerus fracture	1070	1379	1680	609
24586	Repair elbow fracture	2131	2746	3346	1239
24587	Repair elbow fracture	2479	3194	3892	1186
24600	Treat elbow dislocation	352	453	552	244
24605	Treat elbow dislocation	467	602	733	300
24615	Repair elbow dislocation	1354	1744	2126	770
24620	Treat elbow fracture	745	960	1170	427
24635	Repair elbow fracture	1679	2163	2636	992
24640	Treat elbow dislocation	201	259	316	73
24650	Treat radius fracture	321	413	504	181
24655	Treat radius fracture	495	638	777	298
24665	Repair radius fracture	1072	1381	1682	628
24666	Repair radius fracture	1322	1703	2075	819
24670	Treatment of ulna fracture	309	398	485	181
24675	Treatment of ulna fracture	567	730	890	336
24685	Repair ulna fracture	1280	1649	2009	712
24800	Fusion of elbow joint	1894	2440	2973	901
24802	Fusion/graft of elbow joint	2246	2894	3527	1061
24900	Amputation of upper arm	1275	1642	2001	701
24920	Amputation of upper arm	1165	1501	1829	653
24925	Amputation follow-up surgery	696	897	1093	536
24930	Amputation follow-up surgery	1209	1557	1897	735
24931	Amputate upper arm and implant	1590	2049	2496	973
24935	Revision of amputation	1990	2563	3124	1193
24940	Revision of upper arm	1835	2364	2880	0

Forearm and Wrist

Code	Short Description	50th	75th	90th	MC
25000	Incision of tendon sheath	630	822	1010	307
25020	Decompression of forearm	732	956	1175	418
25023	Decompression of forearm	991	1294	1590	705
25028	Drainage of forearm lesion	471	615	755	282
25031	Drainage of forearm bursa	323	422	519	177
25035	Treat forearm bone lesion	827	1080	1327	556
25040	Explore/treat wrist joint	836	1092	1341	518
25065	Biopsy forearm soft tissues	175	229	282	107

SURGERY SERVICES

Code	Short Description	50th	75th	90th	MC
25066	Biopsy forearm soft tissues	405	528	649	217
25075	Remove forearm lesion	407	531	652	240
25076	Remove forearm lesion	641	837	1029	361
25077	Remove tumor, forearm/wrist	1569	2049	2517	763
25085	Incision of wrist capsule	782	1022	1255	411
25100	Biopsy of wrist joint	667	871	1070	362
25101	Explore/treat wrist joint	817	1067	1310	436
25105	Remove wrist joint lining	1045	1365	1677	549
25107	Remove wrist joint cartilage	888	1160	1425	474
25110	Remove wrist tendon lesion	491	641	787	276
25111	Remove wrist tendon lesion	685	894	1098	276
25112	Re-remove wrist tendon lesion	691	903	1110	344
25115	Remove wrist/forearm lesion	1175	1535	1886	643
25116	Remove wrist/forearm lesion	1262	1649	2026	633
25118	Excise wrist tendon sheath	906	1183	1454	412
25119	Partial removal of ulna	1150	1501	1845	562
25120	Remove forearm lesion	1013	1324	1626	528
25125	Remove/graft forearm lesion	1225	1600	1966	588
25126	Remove/graft forearm lesion	1172	1530	1880	592
25130	Remove wrist lesion	797	1040	1278	391
25135	Remove and graft wrist lesion	1027	1341	1648	511
25136	Remove and graft wrist lesion	875	1143	1404	442
25145	Remove forearm bone lesion	1254	1637	2011	499
25150	Partial removal of ulna	947	1237	1520	565
25151	Partial removal of radius	982	1282	1575	535
25170	Extensive forearm surgery	1757	2295	2820	855
25210	Remove wrist bone	861	1125	1382	441
25215	Remove wrist bones	1284	1678	2061	692
25230	Partial removal of radius	754	985	1210	446
25240	Partial removal of ulna	801	1046	1285	437
25246	Injection for wrist x-ray	140	183	225	64
25248	Remove forearm foreign body	583	761	935	291
25250	Remove wrist prosthesis	1024	1338	1644	505
25251	Remove wrist prosthesis	1514	1977	2429	736
25260	Repair forearm tendon/muscle	920	1201	1476	496
25263	Repair forearm tendon/muscle	1002	1308	1607	555
25265	Repair forearm tendon/muscle	1267	1654	2032	741
25270	Repair forearm tendon/muscle	705	920	1130	375
25272	Repair forearm tendon/muscle	782	1022	1255	417
25274	Repair forearm tendon/muscle	1110	1450	1782	634

MC = Medicare Fee

Code	Short Description	50th	75th	90th	MC
25280	Revise wrist/forearm tendon	879	1148	1411	457
25290	Incise wrist/forearm tendon	563	736	904	307
25295	Release wrist/forearm tendon	718	937	1151	381
25300	Fusion of tendons at wrist	1247	1629	2002	668
25301	Fusion of tendons at wrist	1134	1481	1819	629
25310	Transplant forearm tendon	1229	1605	1972	629
25312	Transplant forearm tendon	1418	1852	2275	707
25315	Revise palsy hand tendon(s)	1399	1827	2244	740
25316	Revise palsy hand tendon(s)	1692	2209	2715	938
25320	Repair/revise wrist joint	1725	2253	2769	783
25332	Revise wrist joint	1589	2075	2549	882
25335	Realignment of hand	2477	3235	3974	986
25337	Reconstruct ulna/radioulnar	1488	1944	2388	768
25350	Revision of radius	1272	1661	2041	672
25355	Revision of radius	1514	1977	2429	793
25360	Revision of ulna	1220	1593	1957	599
25365	Revise radius and ulna	1772	2314	2843	923
25370	Revise radius or ulna	1669	2180	2678	1024
25375	Revise radius and ulna	2091	2732	3356	1045
25390	Shorten radius/ulna	1414	1846	2269	793
25391	Lengthen radius/ulna	1825	2383	2928	1019
25392	Shorten radius and ulna	1915	2501	3074	1083
25393	Lengthen radius and ulna	2226	2908	3573	1237
25400	Repair radius or ulna	1571	2051	2520	900
25405	Repair/graft radius or ulna	1931	2521	3098	1098
25415	Repair radius and ulna	2005	2618	3217	1021
25420	Repair/graft radius and ulna	2393	3125	3840	1272
25425	Repair/graft radius or ulna	1779	2324	2855	1036
25426	Repair/graft radius and ulna	2212	2889	3549	1128
25440	Repair/graft wrist bone	1598	2087	2565	806
25441	Reconstruct wrist joint	1736	2267	2785	1003
25442	Reconstruct wrist joint	1249	1632	2005	728
25443	Reconstruct wrist joint	1425	1861	2286	818
25444	Reconstruct wrist joint	1494	1951	2397	883
25445	Reconstruct wrist joint	1509	1971	2422	843
25446	Wrist replacement	2868	3746	4603	1539
25447	Repair wrist joint(s)	1767	2307	2835	830
25449	Remove wrist joint implant	1405	1835	2254	886
25450	Revision of wrist joint	927	1211	1488	636
25455	Revision of wrist joint	1208	1578	1939	759
25490	Reinforce radius	1118	1460	1794	757

SURGERY SERVICES

Code	Short Description	50th	75th	90th	MC
25491	Reinforce ulna	1137	1485	1825	792
25492	Reinforce radius and ulna	1350	1763	2166	975
25500	Treat fracture of radius	305	377	446	194
25505	Treat fracture of radius	568	703	831	353
25515	Repair fracture of radius	1213	1502	1776	687
25520	Repair fracture of radius	971	1202	1422	499
25525	Repair fracture of radius	1958	2423	2866	971
25526	Repair fracture of radius	2629	3254	3849	1032
25530	Treat fracture of ulna	381	471	558	187
25535	Treat fracture of ulna	582	720	852	353
25545	Repair fracture of ulna	1200	1485	1756	673
25560	Treat fracture radius and ulna	366	453	536	190
25565	Treat fracture radius and ulna	760	940	1112	418
25574	Treat fracture radius and ulna	1166	1443	1707	614
25575	Repair fracture radius/ulna	1739	2152	2546	865
25600	Treat fracture radius/ulna	393	486	575	227
25605	Treat fracture radius/ulna	632	783	926	388
25611	Repair fracture radius/ulna	1047	1296	1533	553
25620	Repair fracture radius/ulna	1251	1548	1831	645
25622	Treat wrist bone fracture	387	479	567	198
25624	Treat wrist bone fracture	576	713	844	334
25628	Repair wrist bone fracture	1028	1273	1506	633
25630	Treat wrist bone fracture	383	474	561	205
25635	Treat wrist bone fracture	560	693	820	314
25645	Repair wrist bone fracture	901	1115	1319	570
25650	Repair wrist bone fracture	589	729	863	231
25660	Treat wrist dislocation	420	519	614	255
25670	Repair wrist dislocation	1057	1308	1547	618
25675	Treat wrist dislocation	441	546	646	274
25676	Repair wrist dislocation	1045	1293	1530	629
25680	Treat wrist fracture	543	672	795	326
25685	Repair wrist fracture	1366	1691	2001	766
25690	Treat wrist dislocation	700	866	1024	424
25695	Repair wrist dislocation	1191	1474	1744	635
25800	Fusion of wrist joint	1618	2002	2369	868
25805	Fusion/graft of wrist joint	1871	2316	2740	1009
25810	Fusion/graft of wrist joint	1911	2365	2797	965
25820	Fusion of hand bones	1423	1761	2083	694
25825	Fusion hand bones with graft	1848	2288	2706	856
25830	Fusion radioulnar joint/ulna	1498	1854	2193	768

MC = Medicare Fee

Code	Short Description	50th	75th	90th	MC
25900	Amputation of forearm	1190	1473	1742	650
25905	Amputation of forearm	1094	1354	1602	654
25907	Amputation follow-up surgery	712	881	1042	549
25909	Amputation follow-up surgery	1142	1413	1672	585
25915	Amputation of forearm	1811	2242	2651	1378
25920	Amputate hand at wrist	1109	1372	1623	640
25922	Amputate hand at wrist	697	862	1020	531
25924	Amputation follow-up surgery	1120	1386	1640	653
25927	Amputation of hand	1211	1498	1772	618
25929	Amputation follow-up surgery	666	824	974	501
25931	Amputation follow-up surgery	1118	1383	1637	499

Hand and Fingers

Code	Short Description	50th	75th	90th	MC
26010	Drainage of finger abscess	101	138	167	64
26011	Drainage of finger abscess	320	435	528	153
26020	Drain hand tendon sheath	620	844	1024	329
26025	Drainage of palm bursa	663	902	1094	378
26030	Drainage of palm bursa(s)	1036	1409	1709	476
26034	Treat hand bone lesion	711	967	1174	412
26035	Decompress fingers/hand	1443	1962	2381	562
26037	Decompress fingers/hand	1280	1741	2113	555
26040	Release palm contracture	738	1004	1219	253
26045	Release palm contracture	746	1014	1231	429
26055	Incise finger tendon sheath	609	828	1005	253
26060	Incision of finger tendon	295	401	486	155
26070	Explore/treat hand joint	542	737	894	256
26075	Explore/treat finger joint	568	772	937	309
26080	Explore/treat finger joint	520	708	859	291
26100	Biopsy hand joint lining	575	782	949	274
26105	Biopsy finger joint lining	589	801	972	333
26110	Biopsy finger joint lining	502	683	829	268
26115	Remove hand lesion	420	572	694	234
26116	Remove hand lesion	694	944	1145	372
26117	Remove tumor, hand/finger	1441	1961	2379	554
26121	Release palm contracture	1400	1904	2311	727
26123	Release palm contracture	1605	2184	2650	760
26125	Release palm contracture	716	974	1182	299
26130	Remove wrist joint lining	915	1245	1510	433
26135	Revise finger joint, each	972	1322	1604	483

SURGERY SERVICES

Code	Short Description	50th	75th	90th	MC
26140	Revise finger joint, each	884	1202	1458	432
26145	Tendon excision, palm/finger	897	1220	1480	452
26160	Remove tendon sheath lesion	547	744	903	224
26170	Remove palm tendon, each	546	743	902	308
26180	Remove finger tendon	630	857	1039	381
26185	Remove finger bone	582	791	960	378
26200	Remove hand bone lesion	781	1062	1289	410
26205	Remove/graft bone lesion	978	1330	1614	576
26210	Remove finger lesion	642	873	1059	373
26215	Remove/graft finger lesion	875	1190	1444	522
26230	Partial removal of hand bone	706	961	1166	427
26235	Partial removal, finger bone	657	894	1085	418
26236	Partial removal, finger bone	603	820	995	371
26250	Extensive hand surgery	1110	1509	1831	562
26255	Extensive hand surgery	1545	2101	2550	867
26260	Extensive finger surgery	1122	1526	1852	528
26261	Extensive finger surgery	1365	1857	2254	690
26262	Partial removal of finger	1029	1400	1698	429
26320	Remove implant from hand	602	819	994	309
26350	Repair finger/hand tendon	993	1309	1617	492
26352	Repair/graft hand tendon	1334	1758	2173	588
26356	Repair finger/hand tendon	1299	1713	2117	611
26357	Repair finger/hand tendon	1336	1761	2176	625
26358	Repair/graft hand tendon	1557	2052	2536	682
26370	Repair finger/hand tendon	1045	1378	1702	573
26372	Repair/graft hand tendon	1305	1720	2126	619
26373	Repair finger/hand tendon	1112	1466	1812	614
26390	Revise hand/finger tendon	1158	1526	1886	704
26392	Repair/graft hand tendon	1400	1846	2281	771
26410	Repair hand tendon	597	787	972	320
26412	Repair/graft hand tendon	894	1178	1456	508
26415	Excision, hand/finger tendon	1071	1412	1745	616
26416	Graft hand or finger tendon	1288	1698	2099	752
26418	Repair finger tendon	611	805	994	322
26420	Repair/graft finger tendon	900	1186	1466	511
26426	Repair finger/hand tendon	950	1253	1548	522
26428	Repair/graft finger tendon	1100	1450	1792	525
26432	Repair finger tendon	620	818	1010	295
26433	Repair finger tendon	703	926	1145	354
26434	Repair/graft finger tendon	876	1155	1427	455

MC = Medicare Fee

Code	Short Description	50th	75th	90th	MC
26437	Realignment of tendons	771	1016	1255	401
26440	Release palm/finger tendon	715	943	1165	349
26442	Release palm and finger tendon	820	1080	1335	442
26445	Release hand/finger tendon	656	865	1068	311
26449	Release forearm/hand tendon	979	1291	1595	507
26450	Incision of palm tendon	480	633	782	241
26455	Incision of finger tendon	501	661	816	223
26460	Incise hand/finger tendon	410	541	669	208
26471	Fusion of finger tendons	835	1101	1361	406
26474	Fusion of finger tendons	693	914	1129	413
26476	Tendon lengthening	602	793	980	317
26477	Tendon shortening	654	862	1065	380
26478	Lengthening of hand tendon	801	1056	1305	417
26479	Shortening of hand tendon	819	1079	1334	461
26480	Transplant hand tendon	1086	1431	1768	557
26483	Transplant/graft hand tendon	1398	1843	2277	701
26485	Transplant palm tendon	1214	1601	1978	584
26489	Transplant/graft palm tendon	1298	1711	2114	498
26490	Revise thumb tendon	1263	1665	2057	672
26492	Tendon transfer with graft	1539	2029	2508	752
26494	Hand tendon/muscle transfer	1389	1831	2262	651
26496	Revise thumb tendon	1597	2105	2602	765
26497	Finger tendon transfer	1465	1931	2387	729
26498	Finger tendon transfer	2026	2671	3300	1075
26499	Revision of finger	1700	2241	2770	690
26500	Hand tendon reconstruction	755	995	1230	380
26502	Hand tendon reconstruction	970	1279	1580	508
26504	Hand tendon reconstruction	1121	1478	1827	586
26508	Release thumb contracture	899	1186	1465	410
26510	Thumb tendon transfer	1055	1391	1719	387
26516	Fusion of knuckle joint	894	1178	1456	451
26517	Fusion of knuckle joints	1177	1552	1917	653
26518	Fusion of knuckle joints	1336	1761	2176	637
26520	Release knuckle contracture	856	1128	1394	401
26525	Release finger contracture	798	1052	1300	364
26530	Revise knuckle joint	968	1276	1577	486
26531	Revise knuckle with implant	1265	1668	2061	602
26535	Revise finger joint	916	1208	1493	408
26536	Revise/implant finger joint	1204	1587	1961	572
26540	Repair hand joint	1166	1537	1899	544
26541	Repair hand joint with graft	1396	1840	2273	734

SURGERY SERVICES

Code	Short Description	50th	75th	90th	MC
26542	Repair hand joint with graft	1198	1579	1951	512
26545	Reconstruct finger joint	949	1251	1545	499
26546	Repair non-union hand	1116	1471	1818	706
26548	Reconstruct finger joint	1046	1379	1703	564
26550	Construct thumb replacement	2766	3646	4505	1724
26551	Great toe-hand transfer	5814	7665	9471	3678
26553	Single toe-hand transfer	5774	7612	9405	3653
26554	Double toe-hand transfer	6889	9082	11222	4358
26555	Positional change of finger	1827	2409	2977	1341
26556	Toe joint transfer	5872	7741	9565	3715
26560	Repair web finger	1042	1374	1698	414
26561	Repair web finger	1607	2119	2618	822
26562	Repair web finger	2054	2708	3346	830
26565	Correct metacarpal flaw	1007	1328	1641	515
26567	Correct finger deformity	869	1146	1416	448
26568	Lengthen metacarpal/finger	1288	1698	2098	715
26580	Repair hand deformity	2502	3298	4075	1470
26585	Repair finger deformity	1872	2468	3050	1127
26587	Reconstruct extra finger	767	1011	1250	0
26590	Repair finger deformity	1741	2295	2836	1448
26591	Repair muscles of hand	694	915	1131	219
26593	Release muscles of hand	732	965	1193	381
26596	Excision constricting tissue	1396	1841	2275	717
26597	Release of scar contracture	1496	1972	2437	737
26600	Treat metacarpal fracture	245	323	399	140
26605	Treat metacarpal fracture	384	506	625	209
26607	Treat metacarpal fracture	647	853	1054	361
26608	Treat metacarpal fracture	798	1051	1299	361
26615	Repair metacarpal fracture	699	922	1139	427
26641	Treat thumb dislocation	413	545	673	192
26645	Treat thumb fracture	402	530	655	263
26650	Repair thumb fracture	681	898	1110	397
26665	Repair thumb fracture	1204	1587	1961	575
26670	Treat hand dislocation	243	321	396	176
26675	Treat hand dislocation	472	622	768	369
26676	Pin hand dislocation	549	723	894	425
26685	Repair hand dislocation	839	1106	1366	519
26686	Repair hand dislocation	1096	1445	1785	582
26700	Treat knuckle dislocation	254	334	413	173
26705	Treat knuckle dislocation	352	464	573	234

MC = Medicare Fee

Code	Short Description	50th	75th	90th	MC
26706	Pin knuckle dislocation	606	798	987	407
26715	Repair knuckle dislocation	813	1072	1325	402
26720	Treat finger fracture, each	182	240	297	110
26725	Treat finger fracture, each	292	384	475	192
26727	Treat finger fracture, each	464	612	756	301
26735	Repair finger fracture, each	747	984	1216	393
26740	Treat finger fracture, each	272	359	443	122
26742	Treat finger fracture, each	419	552	682	233
26746	Repair finger fracture, each	758	1000	1235	436
26750	Treat finger fracture, each	144	189	234	98
26755	Treat finger fracture, each	228	301	372	162
26756	Pin finger fracture, each	323	426	526	249
26765	Repair finger fracture, each	512	675	834	279
26770	Treat finger dislocation	177	233	288	143
26775	Treat finger dislocation	260	343	423	185
26776	Pin finger dislocation	360	474	586	272
26785	Repair finger dislocation	457	603	745	295
26820	Thumb fusion with graft	1315	1734	2142	610
26841	Fusion of thumb	1034	1363	1684	549
26842	Thumb fusion with graft	1280	1688	2085	699
26843	Fusion of hand joint	1034	1363	1684	577
26844	Fusion/graft of hand joint	1253	1651	2040	659
26850	Fusion of knuckle	941	1241	1533	468
26852	Fusion of knuckle with graft	1123	1481	1830	575
26860	Fusion of finger joint	787	1038	1282	373
26861	Fusion of finger joint, added	323	426	526	174
26862	Fusion/graft of finger joint	961	1267	1566	511
26863	Fuse/graft added joint	485	640	791	308
26910	Amputate metacarpal bone	1006	1326	1638	519
26951	Amputation of finger/thumb	651	858	1061	303
26952	Amputation of finger/thumb	842	1110	1372	418

Pelvis and Hip Joint

Code	Short Description	50th	75th	90th	MC
26990	Drainage of pelvis lesion	640	845	1039	402
26991	Drainage of pelvis bursa	497	656	807	313
26992	Drainage of bone lesion	1058	1397	1718	766
27000	Incision of hip tendon	382	504	620	284
27001	Incision of hip tendon	561	740	910	356
27003	Incision of hip tendon	955	1261	1551	570

SURGERY SERVICES

Code	Short Description	50th	75th	90th	MC
27005	Incision of hip tendon	851	1124	1382	498
27006	Incision of hip tendons	959	1266	1557	560
27025	Incision of hip/thigh fascia	1286	1698	2088	674
27030	Drainage of hip joint	1786	2358	2900	998
27033	Exploration of hip joint	1837	2425	2982	1013
27035	Denervation of hip joint	2190	2891	3556	1167
27036	Excision of hip joint/muscle	1607	2122	2609	996
27040	Biopsy of soft tissues	180	237	292	112
27041	Biopsy of soft tissues	531	700	861	479
27047	Remove hip/pelvis lesion	507	669	823	359
27048	Remove hip/pelvis lesion	787	1039	1278	425
27049	Remove tumor, hip/pelvis	2176	2873	3533	962
27050	Biopsy of sacroiliac joint	735	970	1193	373
27052	Biopsy of hip joint	1462	1930	2373	555
27054	Remove hip joint lining	2082	2749	3380	776
27060	Remove ischial bursa	690	911	1120	366
27062	Remove femur lesion/bursa	651	859	1056	380
27065	Remove hip bone lesion	723	954	1173	453
27066	Remove hip bone lesion	1303	1720	2115	721
27067	Remove/graft hip bone lesion	1679	2217	2726	1030
27070	Partial removal of hip bone	1033	1364	1677	713
27071	Partial removal of hip bone	1507	1990	2447	792
27075	Extensive hip surgery	2400	3168	3896	1245
27076	Extensive hip surgery	3493	4612	5671	1537
27077	Extensive hip surgery	4600	6073	7468	1710
27078	Extensive hip surgery	1634	2157	2652	891
27079	Extensive hip surgery	1820	2403	2955	877
27080	Remove tail bone	793	1047	1287	443
27086	Remove hip foreign body	168	221	272	95
27087	Remove hip foreign body	651	859	1056	474
27090	Remove hip prosthesis	1603	2116	2602	821
27091	Remove hip prosthesis	3894	5141	6322	1710
27093	Injection for hip x-ray	173	228	280	87
27095	Injection for hip x-ray	266	351	432	82
27097	Revision of hip tendon	1021	1348	1658	671
27098	Transfer tendon to pelvis	1409	1860	2288	671
27100	Transfer of abdominal muscle	1740	2297	2824	770
27105	Transfer of spinal muscle	1773	2341	2879	720
27110	Transfer of iliopsoas muscle	2228	2942	3617	980
27111	Transfer of iliopsoas muscle	2136	2819	3467	974

MC = Medicare Fee

Code	Short Description	50th	75th	90th	MC
27120	Reconstruction of hip socket	3089	4078	5015	1479
27122	Reconstruction of hip socket	2767	3653	4492	1341
27125	Partial hip replacement	3113	4110	5054	1312
27130	Total hip replacement	4277	5570	6794	1869
27132	Total hip replacement	4736	6252	7688	2138
27134	Revise hip joint replacement	4374	5775	7101	2545
27137	Revise hip joint replacement	4171	5507	6772	1928
27138	Revise hip joint replacement	4315	5697	7006	1969
27140	Transplant of femur ridge	1590	2099	2582	952
27146	Incision of hip bone	2510	3314	4075	1123
27147	Revision of hip bone	3061	4041	4970	1548
27151	Incision of hip bones	3162	4174	5133	1652
27156	Revision of hip bones	3430	4528	5568	1764
27158	Revision of pelvis	3072	4055	4987	1379
27161	Incision of neck of femur	2397	3164	3891	1252
27165	Incision/fixation of femur	2926	3863	4751	1403
27170	Repair/graft femur head/neck	2954	3899	4795	1340
27175	Treat slipped epiphysis	1136	1500	1845	328
27176	Treat slipped epiphysis	2319	3061	3764	904
27177	Repair slipped epiphysis	2590	3419	4204	1108
27178	Repair slipped epiphysis	2453	3239	3983	896
27179	Revise head/neck of femur	2002	2643	3250	971
27181	Repair slipped epiphysis	2732	3607	4435	1145
27185	Revision of femur epiphysis	851	1123	1381	461
27187	Reinforce hip bones	3557	4696	5775	1244
27193	Treat pelvic ring fracture	623	807	986	289
27194	Treat pelvic ring fracture	969	1255	1533	508
27200	Treat tail bone fracture	244	316	386	134
27202	Repair tail bone fracture	682	884	1080	533
27215	Pelvic fracture(s) treatment	1756	2276	2779	940
27216	Treat pelvic ring fracture	2324	3010	3677	737
27217	Treat pelvic ring fracture	2697	3493	4267	1187
27218	Treat pelvic ring fracture	3481	4509	5508	1399
27220	Treat hip socket fracture	607	786	960	398
27222	Treat hip socket fracture	1168	1514	1849	714
27226	Treat hip wall fracture	2937	3806	4648	1273
27227	Treat hip fracture(s)	4016	5203	6354	1764
27228	Treat hip fracture(s)	5792	7503	9164	1909
27230	Treat fracture of thigh	505	654	799	338
27232	Treat fracture of thigh	1330	1723	2104	778
27235	Repair thigh fracture	2413	3126	3818	1098

SURGERY SERVICES

Code	Short Description	50th	75th	90th	MC
27236	Repair thigh fracture	2801	3668	4510	1335
27238	Treatment of thigh fracture	629	815	996	420
27240	Treatment of thigh fracture	1479	1915	2339	868
27244	Repair thigh fracture	2595	3299	3981	1314
27245	Repair thigh fracture	2800	3627	4430	1478
27246	Treatment of thigh fracture	514	666	813	347
27248	Repair thigh fracture	1276	1653	2019	962
27250	Treat hip dislocation	534	691	844	386
27252	Treat hip dislocation	758	982	1199	561
27253	Repair hip dislocation	2052	2658	3247	1075
27254	Repair hip dislocation	2687	3481	4251	1294
27256	Treatment of hip dislocation	791	1025	1252	229
27257	Treatment of hip dislocation	1090	1412	1725	400
27258	Repair hip dislocation	2238	2900	3542	1195
27259	Repair hip dislocation	2558	3313	4047	1590
27265	Treatment of hip dislocation	579	750	916	342
27266	Treatment of hip dislocation	783	1014	1239	473
27275	Manipulation of hip joint	352	456	557	164
27280	Fusion of sacroiliac joint	1763	2285	2790	928
27282	Fusion of pubic bones	1944	2518	3075	835
27284	Fusion of hip joint	2692	3487	4259	1279
27286	Fusion of hip joint	3254	4215	5149	1303
27290	Amputation of leg at hip	4674	6056	7396	2047
27295	Amputation of leg at hip	3257	4220	5154	1449

Femur (Thigh Region) and Knee Joint

Code	Short Description	50th	75th	90th	MC
27301	Drain thigh/knee lesion	495	641	773	341
27303	Drainage of bone lesion	894	1158	1397	568
27305	Incise thigh tendon and fascia	743	962	1161	387
27306	Incision of thigh tendon	397	514	620	255
27307	Incision of thigh tendons	523	677	817	342
27310	Exploration of knee joint	1510	1956	2359	765
27315	Partial removal, thigh nerve	1195	1548	1867	504
27320	Partial removal, thigh nerve	1165	1508	1820	464
27323	Biopsy thigh soft tissues	206	267	322	126
27324	Biopsy thigh soft tissues	442	572	690	296
27327	Remove thigh lesion	448	580	700	272
27328	Remove thigh lesion	743	962	1161	396
27329	Remove tumor, thigh/knee	1915	2481	2992	1055

MC = Medicare Fee

Code	Short Description	50th	75th	90th	MC
27330	Biopsy knee joint lining	1281	1659	2002	472
27331	Explore/treat knee joint	1373	1778	2145	557
27332	Remove knee cartilage	1785	2311	2788	777
27333	Remove knee cartilage	1910	2473	2984	728
27334	Remove knee joint lining	1937	2509	3027	788
27335	Remove knee joint lining	2020	2616	3156	911
27340	Remove kneecap bursa	820	1062	1282	330
27345	Remove knee cyst	1032	1336	1612	481
27350	Remove kneecap	1488	1928	2326	730
27355	Remove femur lesion	1328	1720	2075	626
27356	Remove femur lesion/graft	1576	2042	2463	714
27357	Remove femur lesion/graft	1755	2274	2743	781
27358	Remove femur lesion/fixation	1404	1818	2194	394
27360	Partial removal leg bone(s)	1486	1924	2321	755
27365	Extensive leg surgery	2447	3170	3824	1234
27370	Injection for knee x-ray	111	144	174	52
27372	Remove foreign body	650	842	1015	343
27380	Repair kneecap tendon	1335	1729	2086	627
27381	Repair/graft kneecap tendon	1672	2165	2612	899
27385	Repair thigh muscle	1542	1998	2410	690
27386	Repair/graft of thigh muscle	1961	2540	3063	957
27390	Incision of thigh tendon	748	969	1169	391
27391	Incision of thigh tendons	989	1281	1546	509
27392	Incision of thigh tendons	1438	1863	2247	687
27393	Lengthening of thigh tendon	933	1209	1458	494
27394	Lengthening of thigh tendons	1149	1488	1795	573
27395	Lengthening of thigh tendons	1701	2203	2657	909
27396	Transplant of thigh tendon	1696	2197	2651	610
27397	Transplants of thigh tendons	1970	2552	3078	819
27400	Revise thigh muscles/tendons	1705	2208	2664	692
27403	Repair knee cartilage	1862	2412	2909	712
27405	Repair knee ligament	1761	2281	2752	784
27407	Repair knee ligament	1928	2497	3012	776
27409	Repair knee ligaments	2432	3150	3800	1163
27418	Repair degenerated kneecap	2357	3053	3683	946
27420	Revision of unstable kneecap	1861	2410	2907	865
27422	Revision of unstable kneecap	1938	2510	3028	886
27424	Revision/removal of kneecap	1954	2531	3053	899
27425	Lateral retinacular release	1555	2014	2430	498
27427	Reconstruction, knee	2261	2929	3533	874
27428	Reconstruction, knee	2951	3823	4611	1170

SURGERY SERVICES

Code	Short Description	50th	75th	90th	MC
27429	Reconstruction, knee	3068	3975	4794	1088
27430	Revision of thigh muscles	1784	2311	2787	780
27435	Incision of knee joint	1613	2089	2520	663
27437	Revise kneecap	1745	2260	2726	760
27438	Revise kneecap with implant	2264	2932	3537	1012
27440	Revision of knee joint	2299	2978	3593	927
27441	Revision of knee joint	2283	2957	3567	805
27442	Revision of knee joint	2655	3439	4149	1127
27443	Revision of knee joint	2524	3269	3943	1053
27445	Revision of knee joint	3764	4876	5882	1647
27446	Revision of knee joint	3323	4304	5192	1512
27447	Total knee replacement	4336	5610	6763	1975
27448	Incision of thigh	2128	2757	3325	998
27450	Incision of thigh	2503	3242	3911	1196
27454	Realignment of thigh bone	2551	3304	3986	1380
27455	Realignment of knee	1799	2331	2812	1023
27457	Realignment of knee	2056	2663	3212	1106
27465	Shortening of thigh bone	2407	3118	3761	1066
27466	Lengthening of thigh bone	2997	3883	4683	1209
27468	Shorten/lengthen thighs	3989	5167	6232	1465
27470	Repair thigh	2603	3372	4068	1346
27472	Repair/graft of thigh	3152	4082	4924	1559
27475	Surgery to stop leg growth	1639	2123	2561	674
27477	Surgery to stop leg growth	2012	2606	3143	944
27479	Surgery to stop leg growth	2380	3082	3718	1011
27485	Surgery to stop leg growth	1409	1825	2201	689
27486	Revise knee joint replace	3594	4655	5615	1722
27487	Revise knee joint replace	4915	6366	7679	2283
27488	Remove knee prosthesis	2311	2993	3610	1311
27495	Reinforce thigh	2213	2867	3458	1373
27496	Decompression of thigh/knee	844	1093	1318	394
27497	Decompression of thigh/knee	1326	1717	2072	483
27498	Decompression of thigh/knee	1512	1958	2362	550
27499	Decompression of thigh/knee	1956	2534	3057	634
27500	Treatment of thigh fracture	883	1232	1572	454
27501	Treatment of thigh fracture	897	1251	1596	454
27502	Treatment of thigh fracture	1170	1632	2082	721
27503	Treatment of thigh fracture	1507	2101	2680	721
27506	Repair thigh fracture	2545	3548	4528	1359
27507	Treatment of thigh fracture	2259	3150	4019	1244

MC = Medicare Fee

Code	Short Description	50th	75th	90th	MC
27508	Treatment of thigh fracture	724	1009	1287	395
27509	Treatment of thigh fracture	1102	1536	1961	454
27510	Treatment of thigh fracture	1094	1526	1947	632
27511	Treatment of thigh fracture	2230	3109	3968	1230
27513	Treatment of thigh fracture	2722	3795	4843	1391
27514	Repair thigh fracture	2467	3439	4389	1349
27516	Repair thigh growth plate	802	1118	1426	411
27517	Repair thigh growth plate	1169	1630	2080	681
27519	Repair thigh growth plate	2392	3335	4256	1122
27520	Treat kneecap fracture	417	582	742	244
27524	Repair kneecap fracture	1543	2151	2744	843
27530	Treatment of knee fracture	488	681	869	281
27532	Treatment of knee fracture	796	1110	1417	526
27535	Treatment of knee fracture	1688	2354	3004	945
27536	Repair knee fracture	1996	2782	3551	1101
27538	Treat knee fracture(s)	705	983	1254	333
27540	Repair knee fracture	1803	2513	3207	985
27550	Treat knee dislocation	454	634	809	328
27552	Treat knee dislocation	604	842	1074	440
27556	Repair knee dislocation	1962	2735	3490	1097
27557	Repair knee dislocation	2275	3172	4048	1291
27558	Repair knee dislocation	2558	3566	4551	1327
27560	Treat kneecap dislocation	311	433	553	202
27562	Treat kneecap dislocation	583	813	1037	449
27566	Repair kneecap dislocation	1597	2227	2842	933
27570	Fixation of knee joint	418	583	743	145
27580	Fusion of knee	2479	3457	4411	1432
27590	Amputate leg at thigh	1724	2403	3067	831
27591	Amputate leg at thigh	1852	2583	3296	985
27592	Amputate leg at thigh	1684	2347	2996	727
27594	Amputation follow-up surgery	690	963	1228	414
27596	Amputation follow-up surgery	1527	2129	2717	722
27598	Amputate lower leg at knee	1664	2319	2960	843

Leg (Tibia and Fibula) and Ankle Joint

Code	Short Description	50th	75th	90th	MC
27600	Decompression of lower leg	675	858	1046	354
27601	Decompression of lower leg	825	1048	1278	353
27602	Decompression of lower leg	1071	1360	1659	446
27603	Drain lower leg lesion	526	668	815	280

SURGERY SERVICES

Code	Short Description	50th	75th	90th	MC
27604	Drain lower leg bursa	295	374	457	206
27605	Incision of achilles tendon	293	372	453	160
27606	Incision of achilles tendon	405	515	628	247
27607	Treat lower leg bone lesion	784	996	1214	551
27610	Explore/treat ankle joint	1136	1444	1761	624
27612	Exploration of ankle joint	1171	1488	1815	614
27613	Biopsy lower leg soft tissue	240	305	372	111
27614	Biopsy lower leg soft tissue	564	717	874	307
27615	Remove tumor, lower leg	1492	1895	2311	838
27618	Remove lower leg lesion	445	566	690	285
27619	Remove lower leg lesion	776	985	1202	496
27620	Explore, treat ankle joint	1041	1322	1613	500
27625	Remove ankle joint lining	1411	1793	2187	705
27626	Remove ankle joint lining	1544	1961	2392	815
27630	Remove tendon lesion	556	706	861	320
27635	Remove lower leg bone lesion	1248	1586	1934	655
27637	Remove/graft leg bone lesion	1518	1929	2352	748
27638	Remove/graft leg bone lesion	1531	1945	2373	809
27640	Partial removal of tibia	1512	1921	2343	850
27641	Partial removal of fibula	1303	1655	2019	654
27645	Extensive lower leg surgery	2128	2703	3296	1051
27646	Extensive lower leg surgery	1682	2137	2606	949
27647	Extensive ankle/heel surgery	1795	2281	2782	884
27648	Injection for ankle x-ray	123	156	190	49
27650	Repair achilles tendon	1411	1792	2185	766
27652	Repair/graft achilles tendon	1660	2108	2571	852
27654	Repair achilles tendon	1787	2270	2769	866
27656	Repair leg fascia defect	676	859	1047	314
27658	Repair leg tendon, each	744	945	1153	362
27659	Repair leg tendon, each	964	1224	1493	512
27664	Repair leg tendon, each	588	747	911	324
27665	Repair leg tendon, each	786	998	1217	426
27675	Repair lower leg tendons	821	1043	1272	555
27676	Repair lower leg tendons	955	1213	1480	652
27680	Release of lower leg tendon	665	845	1030	395
27681	Release of lower leg tendons	830	1054	1286	519
27685	Revision of lower leg tendon	825	1048	1279	402
27686	Revise lower leg tendons	1003	1275	1555	566
27687	Revision of calf tendon	898	1141	1392	474
27690	Revise lower leg tendon	1053	1337	1631	616

MC = Medicare Fee

Code	Short Description	50th	75th	90th	MC
27691	Revise lower leg tendon	1282	1628	1986	721
27692	Revise additional leg tendon	277	352	429	165
27695	Repair ankle ligament	1186	1506	1837	602
27696	Repair ankle ligaments	1503	1909	2328	627
27698	Repair ankle ligament	1760	2235	2727	874
27700	Revision of ankle joint	2029	2578	3144	843
27702	Reconstruct ankle joint	3177	4035	4922	1301
27703	Reconstruction, ankle joint	3096	3932	4796	1202
27704	Remove ankle implant	1224	1554	1896	550
27705	Incision of tibia	1578	2005	2445	874
27707	Incision of fibula	782	994	1212	366
27709	Incision of tibia and fibula	1823	2315	2824	910
27712	Realignment of lower leg	2063	2621	3197	1013
27715	Revision of lower leg	2600	3303	4029	1081
27720	Repair tibia	2074	2635	3214	1076
27722	Repair/graft of tibia	2078	2640	3220	907
27724	Repair/graft of tibia	2440	3099	3780	1274
27725	Repair lower leg	2651	3368	4108	1035
27727	Repair lower leg	2134	2711	3307	944
27730	Repair tibia epiphysis	1158	1470	1793	440
27732	Repair fibula epiphysis	773	982	1197	421
27734	Repair lower leg epiphyses	1475	1873	2285	656
27740	Repair leg epiphyses	1903	2417	2949	727
27742	Repair leg epiphyses	2252	2861	3490	808
27745	Reinforce tibia	1744	2216	2702	777
27750	Treatment of tibia fracture	525	667	814	271
27752	Treatment of tibia fracture	876	1113	1357	435
27756	Repair tibia fracture	1185	1505	1836	595
27758	Repair tibia fracture	1937	2461	3001	1037
27759	Repair tibia fracture	1981	2516	3069	1127
27760	Treatment of ankle fracture	379	482	588	226
27762	Treatment of ankle fracture	543	690	841	338
27766	Repair ankle fracture	1224	1554	1896	660
27780	Treatment of fibula fracture	300	381	465	184
27781	Treatment of fibula fracture	459	583	711	313
27784	Repair fibula fracture	986	1252	1527	507
27786	Treatment of ankle fracture	368	467	570	219
27788	Treatment of ankle fracture	529	672	820	314
27792	Repair ankle fracture	1145	1454	1773	615
27808	Treatment of ankle fracture	469	595	726	229
27810	Treatment of ankle fracture	777	987	1204	421

SURGERY SERVICES

Code	Short Description	50th	75th	90th	MC
27814	Repair ankle fracture	1557	1977	2412	846
27816	Treatment of ankle fracture	456	579	706	266
27818	Treatment of ankle fracture	894	1135	1384	501
27822	Repair ankle fracture	1734	2203	2686	832
27823	Repair ankle fracture	1945	2470	3013	1017
27824	Treat lower leg fracture	474	602	734	266
27825	Treat lower leg fracture	924	1174	1432	501
27826	Treat lower leg fracture	1402	1781	2172	745
27827	Treat lower leg fracture	2032	2581	3148	1043
27828	Treat lower leg fracture	2351	2987	3643	1176
27829	Treat lower leg joint	877	1113	1358	494
27830	Treat lower leg dislocation	395	502	612	283
27831	Treat lower leg dislocation	505	641	782	348
27832	Repair lower leg dislocation	965	1225	1494	494
27840	Treat ankle dislocation	321	407	497	246
27842	Treat ankle dislocation	453	575	702	320
27846	Repair ankle dislocation	1421	1805	2201	748
27848	Repair ankle dislocation	1462	1857	2265	789
27860	Fixation of ankle joint	225	286	349	152
27870	Fusion of ankle joint	2103	2671	3258	1126
27871	Fusion of tibiofibular joint	1050	1334	1627	690
27880	Amputation of lower leg	1628	2068	2523	809
27881	Amputation of lower leg	1838	2335	2848	929
27882	Amputation of lower leg	1357	1723	2102	653
27884	Amputation follow-up surgery	735	934	1139	441
27886	Amputation follow-up surgery	1503	1909	2328	662
27888	Amputation of foot at ankle	1495	1899	2317	783
27889	Amputation of foot at ankle	1405	1784	2176	740
27892	Decompression of leg	1175	1492	1820	392
27893	Decompression of leg	1174	1491	1819	391
27894	Decompression of leg	1400	1779	2170	540

Foot and Toes

28001	Drainage of bursa of foot	181	237	292	124
28002	Treatment of foot infection	352	462	568	247
28003	Treatment of foot infection	538	705	868	449
28005	Treat foot bone lesion	744	975	1200	479
28008	Incision of foot fascia	604	792	975	279
28010	Incision of toe tendon	279	366	451	264

MC = Medicare Fee

DOES YOUR DOCTOR CHARGE TOO MUCH?

Code	Short Description	50th	75th	90th	MC
28011	Incision of toe tendons	310	407	501	230
28020	Exploration of a foot joint	737	966	1190	382
28022	Exploration of a foot joint	517	677	834	291
28024	Exploration of a toe joint	422	553	681	262
28030	Remove foot nerve	1070	1402	1726	395
28035	Decompression of tibia nerve	1114	1461	1798	471
28043	Excision of foot lesion	378	495	609	207
28045	Excision of foot lesion	614	805	991	350
28046	Resection of tumor, foot	1389	1821	2243	605
28050	Biopsy of foot joint lining	704	922	1136	329
28052	Biopsy of foot joint lining	531	696	857	313
28054	Biopsy of toe joint lining	391	512	631	224
28060	Partial removal foot fascia	791	1037	1277	384
28062	Remove foot fascia	1223	1603	1974	558
28070	Remove foot joint lining	739	968	1192	381
28072	Remove foot joint lining	527	691	850	311
28080	Remove foot lesion	690	904	1113	305
28086	Excise foot tendon sheath	893	1170	1441	316
28088	Excise foot tendon sheath	692	907	1117	301
28090	Remove foot lesion	555	728	896	296
28092	Remove toe lesions	383	502	618	224
28100	Remove ankle/heel lesion	801	1049	1292	412
28102	Remove/graft foot lesion	988	1295	1594	590
28103	Remove/graft foot lesion	840	1102	1357	487
28104	Remove foot lesion	684	896	1104	380
28106	Remove/graft foot lesion	885	1159	1428	548
28107	Remove/graft foot lesion	726	952	1172	413
28108	Remove toe lesions	531	696	857	338
28110	Part removal of metatarsal	594	779	959	302
28111	Part removal of metatarsal	752	986	1215	407
28112	Part removal of metatarsal	644	845	1040	340
28113	Part removal of metatarsal	656	860	1059	360
28114	Remove metatarsal heads	1442	1890	2327	759
28116	Revision of foot	904	1185	1459	511
28118	Remove heel bone	885	1159	1428	470
28119	Remove heel spur	834	1093	1346	438
28120	Part removal of ankle/heel	836	1096	1350	415
28122	Partial removal of foot bone	737	966	1189	454
28124	Partial removal of toe	532	697	858	348
28126	Partial removal of toe	498	653	804	305
28130	Remove ankle bone	1205	1580	1945	599

SURGERY SERVICES

Code	Short Description	50th	75th	90th	MC
28140	Remove metatarsal	783	1027	1264	470
28150	Remove toe	530	694	855	294
28153	Partial removal of toe	545	715	880	306
28160	Partial removal of toe	533	699	860	319
28171	Extensive foot surgery	1278	1675	2063	701
28173	Extensive foot surgery	1147	1503	1851	573
28175	Extensive foot surgery	825	1082	1332	454
28190	Remove foot foreign body	146	194	242	95
28192	Remove foot foreign body	398	530	662	258
28193	Remove foot foreign body	579	771	964	314
28200	Repair foot tendon	745	991	1239	395
28202	Repair/graft of foot tendon	970	1292	1615	510
28208	Repair foot tendon	445	592	740	281
28210	Repair/graft of foot tendon	677	901	1126	477
28220	Release of foot tendon	577	768	959	337
28222	Release of foot tendons	805	1072	1340	489
28225	Release of foot tendon	397	529	661	236
28226	Release of foot tendons	500	665	832	315
28230	Incision of foot tendon(s)	375	500	625	259
28232	Incision of toe tendon	251	334	418	194
28234	Incision of foot tendon	247	329	411	188
28238	Revision of foot tendon	1000	1332	1664	604
28240	Release of big toe	457	608	760	251
28250	Revision of foot fascia	762	1014	1267	416
28260	Release of midfoot joint	1042	1388	1735	483
28261	Revision of foot tendon	1233	1641	2051	677
28262	Revision of foot and ankle	2126	2831	3538	1110
28264	Release of midfoot joint	1461	1946	2432	808
28270	Release of foot contracture	392	522	653	289
28272	Release of toe joint, each	316	420	525	229
28280	Fusion of toes	483	643	803	288
28285	Repair hammertoe	657	880	1103	361
28286	Repair hammertoe	612	815	1018	328
28288	Partial removal of foot bone	636	847	1058	330
28290	Correction of bunion	887	1182	1477	447
28292	Correction of bunion	1049	1397	1746	553
28293	Correction of bunion	1319	1756	2195	741
28294	Correction of bunion	1208	1609	2011	716
28296	Correction of bunion	1405	1871	2338	727
28297	Correction of bunion	1274	1696	2119	739

MC = Medicare Fee

Code	Short Description	50th	75th	90th	MC
28298	Correction of bunion	1011	1346	1683	679
28299	Correction of bunion	1430	1904	2379	777
28300	Incision of heel bone	1174	1564	1954	642
28302	Incision of ankle bone	1218	1622	2026	753
28304	Incision of midfoot bones	1060	1411	1764	618
28305	Incise/graft midfoot bones	1327	1767	2209	821
28306	Incision of metatarsal	872	1161	1451	421
28307	Incision of metatarsal	991	1319	1649	498
28308	Incision of metatarsal	749	997	1246	446
28309	Incision of metatarsals	1006	1339	1673	773
28310	Revision of big toe	602	801	1001	378
28312	Revision of toe	488	649	811	366
28313	Repair deformity of toe	540	719	898	296
28315	Remove sesamoid bone	613	817	1021	363
28320	Repair foot bones	1109	1477	1845	727
28322	Repair metatarsals	751	1000	1250	514
28340	Resect enlarged toe tissue	1108	1476	1844	544
28341	Resect enlarged toe	1327	1767	2209	648
28344	Repair extra toe(s)	663	883	1103	322
28345	Repair webbed toe(s)	898	1196	1495	456
28360	Reconstruct cleft foot	1689	2249	2811	1037
28400	Treatment of heel fracture	394	514	632	197
28405	Treatment of heel fracture	580	758	932	344
28406	Treatment of heel fracture	823	1075	1322	506
28415	Repair heel fracture	1489	1946	2392	990
28420	Repair/graft heel fracture	1833	2396	2946	1106
28430	Treatment of ankle fracture	345	451	555	188
28435	Treatment of ankle fracture	492	643	790	280
28436	Treatment of ankle fracture	625	816	1004	365
28445	Repair ankle fracture	1326	1734	2131	748
28450	Treat midfoot fracture, each	312	407	501	153
28455	Treat midfoot fracture, each	399	522	641	228
28456	Repair midfoot fracture	474	620	762	198
28465	Repair midfoot fracture, each	863	1129	1387	506
28470	Treat metatarsal fracture	275	360	442	149
28475	Treat metatarsal fracture	347	453	557	211
28476	Repair metatarsal fracture	506	661	812	275
28485	Repair metatarsal fracture	775	1013	1245	416
28490	Treat big toe fracture	158	206	253	79
28495	Treat big toe fracture	173	226	277	107
28496	Repair big toe fracture	291	380	468	179

SURGERY SERVICES

Code	Short Description	50th	75th	90th	MC
28505	Repair big toe fracture	510	666	819	273
28510	Treatment of toe fracture	129	168	207	78
28515	Treatment of toe fracture	165	216	265	101
28525	Repair toe fracture	411	538	661	212
28530	Treat sesamoid bone fracture	213	279	343	83
28531	Treat sesamoid bone fracture	349	456	560	167
28540	Treat foot dislocation	272	355	437	98
28545	Treat foot dislocation	388	507	623	142
28546	Treat foot dislocation	541	707	869	239
28555	Repair foot dislocation	947	1238	1522	478
28570	Treat foot dislocation	268	351	431	131
28575	Treat foot dislocation	453	592	727	240
28576	Treat foot dislocation	574	750	922	272
28585	Repair foot dislocation	1098	1435	1764	506
28600	Treat foot dislocation	216	282	347	97
28605	Treat foot dislocation	335	438	538	197
28606	Treat foot dislocation	519	678	833	334
28615	Repair foot dislocation	804	1051	1292	498
28630	Treat toe dislocation	208	272	335	109
28635	Treat toe dislocation	288	376	462	137
28636	Treat toe dislocation	445	582	715	222
28645	Repair toe dislocation	542	709	871	297
28660	Treat toe dislocation	138	180	221	73
28665	Treat toe dislocation	230	301	370	115
28666	Treat toe dislocation	423	553	680	212
28675	Repair toe dislocation	460	601	738	240
28705	Fusion of foot bones	2404	3142	3862	1250
28715	Fusion of foot bones	2071	2708	3328	1040
28725	Fusion of foot bones	1580	2066	2539	854
28730	Fusion of foot bones	1476	1930	2372	795
28735	Fusion of foot bones	1621	2119	2605	834
28737	Revision of foot bones	1405	1836	2257	744
28740	Fusion of foot bones	1015	1327	1632	518
28750	Fusion of big toe joint	934	1221	1501	511
28755	Fusion of big toe joint	698	912	1121	338
28760	Fusion of big toe joint	847	1107	1361	511
28800	Amputation of midfoot	1256	1642	2019	598
28805	Amputation through metatarsal	1240	1620	1992	592
28810	Amputation toe and metatarsal	796	1040	1279	399
28820	Amputation of toe	524	685	842	258

MC = Medicare Fee

Code	Short Description	50th	75th	90th	MC
28825	Partial amputation of toe	437	571	702	233

Application of Casts and Strapping

Code	Short Description	50th	75th	90th	MC
29000	Application of body cast	475	620	762	169
29010	Application of body cast	374	488	599	187
29015	Application of body cast	437	570	701	199
29020	Application of body cast	357	465	572	163
29025	Application of body cast	384	501	615	127
29035	Application of body cast	255	333	409	159
29040	Application of body cast	338	441	542	178
29044	Application of body cast	300	392	481	179
29046	Application of body cast	324	423	519	197
29049	Application of figure eight	125	163	200	53
29055	Application of shoulder cast	239	311	383	123
29058	Application of shoulder cast	149	194	238	80
29065	Application of long arm cast	121	157	193	71
29075	Application of forearm cast	94	121	147	58
29085	Apply hand/wrist cast	83	109	133	56
29105	Apply long arm splint	80	105	129	56
29125	Apply forearm splint	61	80	98	39
29126	Apply forearm splint	107	140	172	48
29130	Application of finger splint	46	60	73	27
29131	Application of finger splint	105	137	168	39
29200	Strapping of chest	48	63	78	30
29220	Strapping of low back	65	85	105	42
29240	Strapping of shoulder	61	80	98	39
29260	Strapping of elbow or wrist	42	54	67	31
29280	Strapping of hand or finger	38	49	60	29
29305	Application of hip cast	277	350	424	166
29325	Application of hip casts	317	400	485	178
29345	Application of long leg cast	166	209	253	101
29355	Application of long leg cast	172	217	263	109
29358	Apply long leg cast brace	208	263	319	143
29365	Application of long leg cast	140	176	214	85
29405	Apply short leg cast	124	156	189	70
29425	Apply short leg cast	150	189	229	83
29435	Apply short leg cast	184	232	281	100
29440	Addition of walker to cast	45	56	68	32
29445	Apply rigid leg cast	242	305	370	148

SURGERY SERVICES

Code	Short Description	50th	75th	90th	MC
29450	Application of leg cast	78	99	120	56
29505	Application long leg splint	90	114	138	52
29515	Application lower leg splint	74	94	114	49
29520	Strapping of hip	64	81	98	36
29530	Strapping of knee	54	69	83	38
29540	Strapping of ankle	39	48	58	33
29550	Strapping of toes	36	44	53	30
29580	Application of paste boot	63	78	93	55
29590	Application of foot splint	101	128	155	41
29700	Removal/revision of cast	63	80	97	37
29705	Removal/revision of cast	72	91	110	45
29710	Removal/revision of cast	98	124	150	72
29715	Removal/revision of cast	108	136	165	75
29720	Repair body cast	52	65	79	37
29730	Windowing of cast	52	65	79	40
29740	Wedging of cast	69	88	106	60
29750	Wedging of clubfoot cast	87	109	133	71

Arthroscopy

Code	Short Description	50th	75th	90th	MC
29800	Jaw arthroscopy/surgery	964	1263	1555	381
29804	Jaw arthroscopy/surgery	1675	2195	2702	779
29815	Shoulder arthroscopy	811	1063	1308	445
29819	Shoulder arthroscopy/surgery	1494	1958	2411	730
29820	Shoulder arthroscopy/surgery	1524	1997	2459	684
29821	Shoulder arthroscopy/surgery	1910	2502	3081	755
29822	Shoulder arthroscopy/surgery	1656	2170	2672	714
29823	Shoulder arthroscopy/surgery	1905	2496	3073	803
29825	Shoulder arthroscopy/surgery	1267	1661	2044	743
29826	Shoulder arthroscopy/surgery	2151	2819	3471	878
29830	Elbow arthroscopy	830	1087	1339	463
29834	Elbow arthroscopy/surgery	1278	1675	2062	509
29835	Elbow arthroscopy/surgery	1415	1854	2283	525
29836	Elbow arthroscopy/surgery	1763	2310	2845	612
29837	Elbow arthroscopy/surgery	1327	1739	2141	558
29838	Elbow arthroscopy/surgery	1544	2024	2492	614
29840	Wrist arthroscopy	869	1139	1403	359
29843	Wrist arthroscopy/surgery	1022	1339	1649	487
29844	Wrist arthroscopy/surgery	1053	1380	1699	502
29845	Wrist arthroscopy/surgery	1256	1646	2026	610

MC = Medicare Fee

Code	Short Description	50th	75th	90th	MC
29846	Wrist arthroscopy/surgery	1343	1760	2167	684
29847	Wrist arthroscopy/surgery	1384	1814	2233	578
29848	Wrist arthroscopy/surgery	1248	1636	2014	376
29850	Knee arthroscopy/surgery	1638	2146	2642	788
29851	Knee arthroscopy/surgery	2187	2865	3528	985
29855	Tibial arthroscopy/surgery	1804	2364	2911	912
29856	Tibial arthroscopy/surgery	2049	2685	3305	1055
29870	Knee arthroscopy/diagnostic	936	1226	1509	376
29871	Knee arthroscopy/drainage	1230	1611	1984	553
29874	Knee arthroscopy/surgery	1511	1980	2438	673
29875	Knee arthroscopy/surgery	1535	2012	2477	620
29876	Knee arthroscopy/surgery	1852	2427	2988	756
29877	Knee arthroscopy/surgery	1739	2279	2805	709
29879	Knee arthroscopy/surgery	1845	2417	2976	776
29880	Knee arthroscopy/surgery	2397	3141	3867	819
29881	Knee arthroscopy/surgery	1982	2597	3198	746
29882	Knee arthroscopy/surgery	2063	2704	3329	819
29883	Knee arthroscopy/surgery	2582	3383	4165	925
29884	Knee arthroscopy/surgery	1616	2117	2606	687
29885	Knee arthroscopy/surgery	1951	2556	3147	717
29886	Knee arthroscopy/surgery	1749	2292	2822	592
29887	Knee arthroscopy/surgery	2037	2669	3286	823
29888	Knee arthroscopy/surgery	3390	4442	5469	1325
29889	Knee arthroscopy/surgery	3015	3951	4864	1030
29894	Ankle arthroscopy/surgery	1370	1796	2211	686
29895	Ankle arthroscopy/surgery	1449	1899	2338	667
29897	Ankle arthroscopy/surgery	1457	1910	2351	695
29898	Ankle arthroscopy/surgery	1715	2247	2767	801

RESPIRATORY SYSTEM SURGERY

Nose

Code	Short Description	50th	75th	90th	MC
30000	Drainage of nose lesion	166	229	295	78
30020	Drainage of nose lesion	175	241	311	79
30100	Intranasal biopsy	122	168	217	67
30110	Remove nose polyp(s)	242	334	432	118
30115	Remove nose polyp(s)	610	842	1087	287
30117	Remove intranasal lesion	449	619	799	244
30118	Remove intranasal lesion	1208	1667	2152	712

SURGERY SERVICES

Code	Short Description	50th	75th	90th	MC
30120	Revision of nose	1118	1543	1993	504
30124	Remove nose lesion	311	429	555	174
30125	Remove nose lesion	1187	1639	2116	512
30130	Remove turbinate bones	403	556	718	194
30140	Remove turbinate bones	694	957	1236	262
30150	Partial removal of nose	1071	1478	1908	687
30160	Remove nose	1721	2375	3067	874
30200	Injection treatment of nose	62	86	111	46
30210	Nasal sinus therapy	94	130	168	51
30220	Insert nasal septal button	219	302	389	124
30300	Remove nasal foreign body	106	146	188	58
30310	Remove nasal foreign body	333	459	593	145
30320	Remove nasal foreign body	740	1021	1319	358
30400	Reconstruction of nose	1810	2497	3225	811
30410	Reconstruction of nose	2506	3458	4465	1143
30420	Reconstruction of nose	3103	4282	5529	1398
30430	Revision of nose	883	1218	1573	529
30435	Revision of nose	1630	2249	2904	883
30450	Revision of nose	2131	2940	3796	1176
30460	Revision of nose	1679	2317	2992	746
30462	Revision of nose	3041	4197	5419	1492
30520	Repair nasal septum	1509	2083	2690	539
30540	Repair nasal defect	1454	2006	2591	580
30545	Repair nasal defect	2074	2862	3695	891
30560	Release of nasal adhesions	130	179	231	70
30580	Repair upper jaw fistula	1150	1587	2049	523
30600	Repair mouth/nose fistula	982	1355	1749	390
30620	Intranasal reconstruction	1488	2053	2651	544
30630	Repair nasal septum defect	1278	1764	2277	541
30801	Cauterization inner nose	117	162	209	60
30802	Cauterization inner nose	234	323	417	117
30901	Control of nosebleed	114	150	189	71
30903	Control of nosebleed	168	232	299	96
30905	Control of nosebleed	290	401	517	154
30906	Repeat control of nosebleed	276	381	492	141
30915	Ligation nasal sinus artery	1284	1771	2287	476
30920	Ligation upper jaw artery	1686	2327	3004	775
30930	Therapy fracture of nose	157	217	280	78

MC = Medicare Fee

Code	Short Description	50th	75th	90th	MC

Accessory Sinuses

Code	Short Description	50th	75th	90th	MC
31000	Irrigation maxillary sinus	100	138	178	61
31002	Irrigation sphenoid sinus	162	223	288	91
31020	Exploration maxillary sinus	590	814	1051	226
31030	Exploration maxillary sinus	1384	1909	2465	539
31032	Explore sinus, remove polyps	1537	2121	2739	600
31040	Exploration behind upper jaw	2132	2942	3799	694
31050	Exploration sphenoid sinus	1178	1625	2099	461
31051	Sphenoid sinus surgery	1420	1959	2529	625
31070	Exploration of frontal sinus	1066	1471	1900	364
31075	Exploration of frontal sinus	1837	2535	3273	797
31080	Remove frontal sinus	2003	2765	3570	826
31081	Remove frontal sinus	1973	2722	3515	924
31084	Remove frontal sinus	2615	3609	4659	1149
31085	Remove frontal sinus	2672	3687	4761	1216
31086	Remove frontal sinus	2194	3028	3910	942
31087	Remove frontal sinus	2095	2891	3732	936
31090	Exploration of sinuses	2800	3863	4988	875
31200	Remove ethmoid sinus	816	1126	1454	385
31201	Remove ethmoid sinus	1343	1853	2393	615
31205	Remove ethmoid sinus	1659	2289	2956	725
31225	Remove upper jaw	2963	4088	5279	1551
31230	Remove upper jaw	3558	4909	6339	1743
31231	Nasal endoscopy, diagnostic	191	261	329	104
31233	Nasal/sinus endoscopy, diagnostic	345	492	635	209
31235	Nasal/sinus endoscopy, diagnostic	513	732	944	208
31237	Nasal/sinus endoscopy, surgical	412	588	758	265
31238	Nasal/sinus endoscopy, surgical	632	902	1164	312
31239	Nasal/sinus endoscopy, surgical	1590	2269	2928	813
31240	Nasal/sinus endoscopy, surgical	531	758	978	250
31254	Revision of ethmoid sinus	1108	1581	2039	447
31255	Remove ethmoid sinus	1674	2390	3083	673
31256	Exploration maxillary sinus	803	1146	1478	295
31267	Endoscopy, maxillary sinus	1231	1756	2266	452
31276	Sinus surgical endoscopy	1370	1956	2523	638
31287	Nasal/sinus endoscopy, surgical	882	1258	1623	379
31288	Nasal/sinus endoscopy, surgical	1037	1480	1909	444
31290	Nasal/sinus endoscopy, surgical	2397	3421	4413	1351
31291	Nasal/sinus endoscopy, surgical	2515	3589	4630	1425

SURGERY SERVICES

Code	Short Description	50th	75th	90th	MC
31292	Nasal/sinus endoscopy, surgical	1946	2778	3584	1127
31293	Nasal/sinus endoscopy, surgical	2156	3077	3970	1234
31294	Nasal/sinus endoscopy, surgical	2474	3530	4555	1436

Larynx

Code	Short Description	50th	75th	90th	MC
31300	Remove larynx lesion	2012	2657	3286	1026
31320	Diagnostic incision larynx	921	1217	1505	349
31360	Remove larynx	3168	4183	5173	1453
31365	Remove larynx	4530	5983	7398	2059
31367	Partial removal of larynx	3136	4142	5122	1495
31368	Partial removal of larynx	4491	5932	7335	2112
31370	Partial removal of larynx	3395	4484	5545	1476
31375	Partial removal of larynx	2856	3773	4665	1367
31380	Partial removal of larynx	2947	3892	4813	1479
31382	Partial removal of larynx	2905	3836	4744	1426
31390	Remove larynx and pharynx	4192	5536	6846	2214
31395	Reconstruct larynx and pharynx	4941	6525	8069	2606
31400	Revision of larynx	2075	2740	3388	697
31420	Remove epiglottis	1781	2352	2908	706
31500	Insert emergency airway	211	284	356	116
31502	Change of windpipe airway	123	163	201	51
31505	Diagnostic laryngoscopy	94	124	153	43
31510	Laryngoscopy with biopsy	201	265	328	98
31511	Remove foreign body, larynx	246	326	403	125
31512	Remove larynx lesion	272	359	444	159
31513	Injection into vocal cord	361	477	589	204
31515	Laryngoscopy for aspiration	213	281	348	120
31520	Diagnostic laryngoscopy	328	433	535	171
31525	Diagnostic laryngoscopy	389	513	635	198
31526	Diagnostic laryngoscopy	573	756	935	247
31527	Laryngoscopy for treatment	795	1049	1298	258
31528	Laryngoscopy and dilatation	526	695	860	210
31529	Laryngoscopy and dilatation	400	528	653	212
31530	Operative laryngoscopy	679	897	1109	292
31531	Operative laryngoscopy	874	1155	1428	355
31535	Operative laryngoscopy	739	977	1208	301
31536	Operative laryngoscopy	933	1232	1523	324
31540	Operative laryngoscopy	878	1159	1433	397
31541	Operative laryngoscopy	1132	1495	1848	388

MC = Medicare Fee

Code	Short Description	50th	75th	90th	MC
31560	Operative laryngoscopy	1450	1915	2368	430
31561	Operative laryngoscopy	1692	2235	2763	526
31570	Laryngoscopy with injection	817	1079	1334	373
31571	Laryngoscopy with injection	955	1262	1560	373
31575	Diagnostic laryngoscopy	232	301	369	112
31576	Laryngoscopy with biopsy	434	573	708	191
31577	Remove foreign body, larynx	696	919	1136	237
31578	Remove larynx lesion	808	1067	1320	275
31579	Diagnostic laryngoscopy	458	604	747	191
31580	Revision of larynx	2652	3502	4330	1057
31582	Revision of larynx	3018	3986	4928	1552
31584	Repair larynx fracture	2817	3720	4600	1271
31585	Repair larynx fracture	483	638	788	336
31586	Repair larynx fracture	839	1108	1370	569
31587	Revision of larynx	2220	2932	3625	703
31588	Revision of larynx	2009	2654	3282	930
31590	Re-innervate larynx	1811	2391	2957	500
31595	Larynx nerve surgery	1785	2357	2915	595

Trachea and Bronchi

Code	Short Description	50th	75th	90th	MC
31600	Incision of windpipe	754	954	1159	328
31601	Incision of windpipe	823	1042	1265	400
31603	Incision of windpipe	858	1086	1318	356
31605	Incision of windpipe	793	1004	1219	327
31610	Incision of windpipe	1080	1367	1660	606
31611	Surgery/speech prosthesis	844	1068	1297	496
31612	Puncture/clear windpipe	126	160	194	87
31613	Repair windpipe opening	581	736	894	261
31614	Repair windpipe opening	1266	1603	1946	535
31615	Visualization of windpipe	365	462	561	167
31622	Diagnostic bronchoscopy	545	679	817	219
31625	Bronchoscopy with biopsy	620	773	929	246
31628	Bronchoscopy with biopsy	710	886	1065	296
31629	Bronchoscopy with biopsy	628	794	965	262
31630	Bronchoscopy with repair	726	919	1115	316
31631	Bronchoscopy with dilation	718	909	1104	285
31635	Remove foreign body, airway	784	992	1205	345
31640	Bronchoscopy and remove lesion	862	1092	1326	419
31641	Bronchoscopy, treat blockage	1112	1407	1709	403

SURGERY SERVICES

Code	Short Description	50th	75th	90th	MC
31645	Bronchoscopy, clear airways	579	732	889	231
31646	Bronchoscopy, re-clear airways	504	638	775	197
31656	Bronchoscopy, inject for x-ray	485	614	745	172
31700	Insertion of airway catheter	289	366	445	94
31708	Instill airway contrast dye	139	176	213	73
31710	Insertion of airway catheter	165	209	254	75
31715	Injection for bronchus x-ray	115	145	176	52
31717	Bronchial brush biopsy	175	221	269	93
31720	Clearance of airways	83	105	127	61
31725	Clearance of airways	322	407	495	114
31730	Introduction windpipe wire/tube	417	528	641	180
31750	Repair windpipe	2281	2888	3507	849
31755	Repair windpipe	2832	3585	4354	1156
31760	Repair windpipe	2926	3704	4498	1336
31766	Reconstruction of windpipe	3533	4472	5431	1882
31770	Repair/graft of bronchus	3171	4014	4874	1497
31775	Reconstruct bronchus	3186	4033	4897	1581
31780	Reconstruct windpipe	3115	3944	4789	1401
31781	Reconstruct windpipe	3466	4388	5328	1605
31785	Remove windpipe lesion	2818	3567	4331	1020
31786	Remove windpipe lesion	3589	4543	5517	1483
31800	Repair windpipe injury	1705	2159	2621	486
31805	Repair windpipe injury	2368	2998	3640	933
31820	Closure of windpipe lesion	548	693	842	319
31825	Repair windpipe defect	793	1004	1219	466
31830	Revise windpipe scar	549	695	844	327

Lungs and Pleura

Code	Short Description	50th	75th	90th	MC
32000	Drainage of chest	195	255	316	81
32002	Treatment of collapsed lung	353	467	582	121
32005	Treat lung lining chemically	246	326	406	133
32020	Insertion of chest tube	472	612	754	275
32035	Exploration of chest	1174	1553	1937	574
32036	Exploration of chest	1350	1785	2227	630
32095	Biopsy through chest wall	1352	1788	2230	665
32100	Exploration/biopsy of chest	1829	2419	3018	925
32110	Explore/repair chest	2060	2725	3399	995
32120	Re-exploration of chest	1845	2441	3045	819
32124	Explore chest, free adhesions	2012	2662	3320	949

MC = Medicare Fee

Code	Short Description	50th	75th	90th	MC
32140	Remove lung lesion(s)	2125	2811	3506	1062
32141	Remove/treat lung lesions	2111	2792	3482	1109
32150	Remove lung lesion(s)	1895	2506	3126	972
32151	Remove lung foreign body	1902	2516	3138	897
32160	Open chest heart massage	1740	2302	2871	704
32200	Drainage of lung lesion	1727	2284	2850	812
32215	Treat chest lining	1774	2347	2927	743
32220	Release of lung	2651	3507	4375	1433
32225	Partial release of lung	1988	2630	3281	1033
32310	Remove chest lining	2669	3531	4404	1015
32320	Free/remove chest lining	3032	4011	5003	1600
32400	Needle biopsy chest lining	222	294	367	109
32402	Open biopsy chest lining	1239	1639	2044	611
32405	Biopsy, lung or mediastinum	384	507	633	138
32420	Puncture/clear lung	250	331	413	123
32440	Remove lung, total	3168	4191	5228	1215
32442	Remove lung, resect trachea	4206	5564	6940	1805
32445	Remove lung	3953	5228	6522	1875
32480	Partial removal of lung	2999	3967	4949	1467
32482	Partial removal of lung	3255	4306	5371	1531
32484	Partial removal of lung	3382	4474	5581	1568
32486	Partial removal of lung	3624	4794	5980	1664
32488	Partial removal of lung	4048	5355	6679	1785
32491	Partial removal of lung	2885	3816	4761	0
32500	Partial removal of lung	2277	3012	3758	1149
32501	Repair bronchus	811	1073	1338	381
32520	Remove lung and revise chest	3650	4828	6023	1737
32522	Remove lung and revise chest	4158	5499	6860	1893
32525	Remove lung and revise chest	4457	5895	7354	2065
32540	Remove lung lesion	2409	3187	3975	1062
32601	Thoracoscopy, diagnostic	842	1113	1389	371
32602	Thoracoscopy, diagnostic	1019	1348	1682	409
32603	Thoracoscopy, diagnostic	1347	1782	2222	459
32604	Thoracoscopy, diagnostic	1499	1983	2474	515
32605	Thoracoscopy, diagnostic	1022	1352	1687	426
32606	Thoracoscopy, diagnostic	1317	1742	2173	500
32650	Thoracoscopy, surgical	1637	2166	2702	743
32651	Thoracoscopy, surgical	2260	2990	3729	1033
32652	Thoracoscopy, surgical	3004	3973	4956	1433
32653	Thoracoscopy, surgical	1660	2196	2739	972
32654	Thoracoscopy, surgical	2027	2681	3345	995

SURGERY SERVICES

Code	Short Description	50th	75th	90th	MC
32655	Thoracoscopy, surgical	2186	2891	3607	1120
32656	Thoracoscopy, surgical	2035	2692	3358	1098
32657	Thoracoscopy, surgical	2262	2993	3733	1149
32658	Thoracoscopy, surgical	2164	2862	3570	1063
32659	Thoracoscopy, surgical	2078	2748	3428	1088
32660	Thoracoscopy, surgical	3051	4036	5035	1586
32661	Thoracoscopy, surgical	2005	2652	3308	916
32662	Thoracoscopy, surgical	2376	3143	3920	1300
32663	Thoracoscopy, surgical	3241	4288	5348	1489
32664	Thoracoscopy, surgical	2268	3000	3742	1028
32665	Thoracoscopy, surgical	2545	3367	4200	1248
32800	Repair lung hernia	1772	2343	2923	858
32810	Close chest after drainage	1954	2585	3224	750
32815	Close bronchial fistula	3470	4590	5725	1533
32820	Reconstruct injured chest	3596	4756	5933	1654
32850	Remove lung for transplant	2089	2764	3447	0
32851	Lung transplant, single	5803	7675	9574	2571
32852	Lung transplant, with bypass	6660	8809	10989	2788
32853	Lung transplant, double	7327	9692	12090	3214
32854	Lung transplant, with bypass	7896	10443	13027	3432
32900	Remove rib(s)	2001	2647	3302	1095
32905	Revise and repair chest wall	2292	3031	3781	1348
32906	Revise and repair chest wall	2961	3917	4886	1697
32940	Revision of lung	3072	4063	5069	1219
32960	Therapeutic pneumothorax	174	230	287	93

CARDIOVASCULAR SYSTEM SURGERY

Heart and Pericardium

Code	Short Description	50th	75th	90th	MC
33010	Drainage of heart sac	320	426	535	126
33011	Repeat drainage of heart sac	249	331	416	111
33015	Incision of heart sac	603	803	1007	412
33020	Incision of heart sac	2102	2799	3513	1063
33025	Incision of heart sac	2135	2843	3569	1088
33030	Partial removal of heart sac	3032	4037	5067	1646
33031	Partial removal of heart sac	3542	4716	5919	1383
33050	Remove heart sac lesion	2159	2874	3608	916
33120	Remove heart lesion	5380	7163	8991	2243
33130	Remove heart lesion	3251	4329	5434	1377

MC = Medicare Fee

DOES YOUR DOCTOR CHARGE TOO MUCH?

Code	Short Description	50th	75th	90th	MC
33200	Insertion of heart pacemaker	2332	3105	3898	997
33201	Insertion of heart pacemaker	1892	2519	3162	862
33206	Insertion of heart pacemaker	1642	2187	2745	598
33207	Insertion of heart pacemaker	1676	2232	2801	697
33208	Insertion of heart pacemaker	2032	2648	3280	600
33210	Insertion of heart electrode	548	730	916	223
33211	Insertion of heart electrode	615	819	1028	226
33212	Insertion of pulse generator	908	1209	1518	452
33213	Insertion of pulse generator	1018	1356	1702	403
33214	Upgrade of pacemaker system	1248	1662	2086	449
33216	Revision implanted electrode	1010	1345	1688	346
33217	Insert/revise electrode	953	1269	1592	357
33218	Repair pacemaker electrodes	855	1139	1430	402
33220	Repair pacemaker electrode	870	1158	1454	335
33222	Pacemaker skin pocket	910	1211	1520	447
33223	Pacemaker skin pocket	1136	1513	1899	505
33233	Remove pacemaker system	442	588	738	183
33234	Remove pacemaker system	1300	1731	2173	407
33235	Remove pacemaker electrode	1338	1782	2237	389
33236	Remove electrode/thoracotomy	1813	2414	3030	628
33237	Remove electrode/thoracotomy	2258	3007	3774	916
33238	Remove electrode/thoracotomy	2496	3323	4171	1035
33240	Insert/replace pulse generator	1255	1672	2098	527
33241	Remove pulse generator only	658	876	1100	218
33242	Repair pulse generator/leads	1536	2045	2567	590
33243	Remove generator/thoracotomy	3422	4556	5719	1239
33244	Remove generator	2079	2769	3475	746
33245	Implant heart defibrillator	2787	3711	4658	1228
33246	Implant heart defibrillator	3702	4929	6187	1706
33247	Insert/replace leads	1970	2624	3293	806
33249	Insert/replace leads/generator	3290	4381	5499	1285
33250	Ablate heart dysrhythm focus	3078	4098	5144	1243
33251	Ablate heart dysrhythm focus	3849	5125	6433	1651
33253	Reconstruct atria	4810	6405	8039	2195
33261	Ablate heart dysrhythm focus	3546	4722	5927	1531
33300	Repair heart wound	2953	3931	4935	1303
33305	Repair heart wound	3711	4942	6203	1560
33310	Exploratory heart surgery	2757	3671	4607	1184
33315	Exploratory heart surgery	4143	5516	6924	1455
33320	Repair major blood vessel(s)	3440	4581	5750	1260
33321	Repair major vessel	4077	5429	6814	1743

SURGERY SERVICES

Code	Short Description	50th	75th	90th	MC
33322	Repair major blood vessel(s)	4587	6108	7667	1730
33330	Insert major vessel graft	4047	5389	6764	1317
33332	Insert major vessel graft	4139	5511	6917	1560
33335	Insert major vessel graft	5400	7190	9024	1754
33400	Repair aortic valve	4652	6629	8654	2059
33401	Repair aortic valve	4544	6475	8452	2033
33403	Repair aortic valve	4788	6823	8907	2070
33404	Prepare heart-aorta conduit	5304	7558	9866	2509
33405	Replace aortic valve	4755	6776	8845	2536
33406	Replace aortic valve	6114	8713	11373	3061
33411	Replace aortic valve	6036	8602	11229	3029
33412	Replace aortic valve	6015	8572	11190	3100
33413	Replace aortic valve	6571	9364	12223	3263
33414	Repair aortic valve	5804	8271	10797	2988
33415	Revision, subvalvular tissue	4947	7050	9202	2407
33416	Revise ventricle muscle	5041	7184	9378	2416
33417	Repair aortic valve	5228	7450	9725	2702
33420	Revision of mitral valve	3680	5245	6846	1689
33422	Revision of mitral valve	5136	7319	9554	2398
33425	Repair mitral valve	5116	7291	9518	2463
33426	Repair mitral valve	5323	7585	9901	2652
33427	Repair mitral valve	5600	7980	10417	2884
33430	Replace mitral valve	4800	6840	8929	2783
33460	Revision of tricuspid valve	4640	6613	8632	2073
33463	Valvuloplasty, tricuspid	5285	7532	9832	2489
33464	Valvuloplasty, tricuspid	5527	7876	10281	2554
33465	Replace tricuspid valve	5201	7412	9676	2580
33468	Revision of tricuspid valve	5244	7473	9755	2739
33470	Revision of pulmonary valve	3776	5382	7025	1645
33471	Valvotomy, pulmonary valve	4050	5772	7534	1983
33472	Revision of pulmonary valve	4179	5956	7775	2077
33474	Revision of pulmonary valve	4530	6456	8427	2077
33475	Replacement, pulmonary valve	5490	7824	10213	2705
33476	Revision of heart chamber	4912	7000	9138	2274
33478	Revision of heart chamber	5106	7277	9499	2456
33500	Repair heart vessel fistula	4472	6240	7657	2321
33501	Repair heart vessel fistula	2847	3973	4875	1288
33502	Coronary artery correction	3242	4524	5551	1426
33503	Coronary artery graft	4126	5757	7064	2180
33504	Coronary artery graft	4981	6951	8529	2293

MC = Medicare Fee

DOES YOUR DOCTOR CHARGE TOO MUCH?

Code	Short Description	50th	75th	90th	MC
33505	Repair artery w/tunnel	5491	7662	9402	2603
33506	Repair artery, translocation	5433	7581	9302	2603
33510	CABG, vein, single	4236	5912	7254	2298
33511	CABG, vein, two	5148	7184	8814	2523
33512	CABG, vein, three	5488	7657	9396	2748
33513	CABG, vein, four	5644	7876	9664	2972
33514	CABG, vein, five	6156	8590	10540	3196
33516	CABG, vein, six+	6391	8918	10943	3420
33517	CABG, artery-vein, single	678	947	1162	224
33518	CABG, artery-vein, two	980	1367	1678	449
33519	CABG, artery-vein, three	1303	1818	2231	673
33521	CABG, artery-vein, four	1711	2388	2930	898
33522	CABG, artery-vein, five	2214	3089	3791	1122
33523	CABG, artery-vein, six+	2873	4009	4919	1347
33530	Coronary artery, bypass/re-op	1218	1700	2085	617
33533	CABG, arterial, single	4804	6577	7997	2368
33534	CABG, arterial, two	4810	6712	8236	2663
33535	CABG, arterial, three	5912	8250	10123	2958
33536	CABG, arterial, four+	7042	9827	12058	3253
33542	Remove heart lesion	5346	7460	9153	2483
33545	Repair heart damage	6567	9163	11244	2963
33572	Open coronary endarterectomy	826	1153	1415	325
33600	Closure of valve	5785	8072	9905	2741
33602	Closure of valve	5496	7669	9410	2494
33606	Anastomosis/artery-aorta	6043	8432	10346	2988
33608	Repair anomaly w/conduit	6188	8635	10596	3016
33610	Repair by enlargement	6086	8492	10420	2988
33611	Repair double ventricle	6382	8906	10928	3061
33612	Repair double ventricle	6488	9053	11109	3092
33615	Repair complex cardiac anomalies	6272	8752	10739	3034
33617	Repair complex cardiac anomalies	6531	9113	11182	3098
33619	Repair single ventricle	7186	10027	12304	3473
33641	Repair heart septum defect	4229	5902	7242	1993
33645	Revision of heart veins	4597	6415	7871	2186
33647	Repair heart septum defects	5401	7536	9247	2718
33660	Repair heart defects	5382	7510	9215	2420
33665	Repair heart defects	5736	8003	9820	2530
33670	Repair heart chambers	6335	8840	10847	3061
33681	Repair heart septum defect	5252	7329	8993	2678
33684	Repair heart septum defect	5693	7943	9747	2751
33688	Repair heart septum defect	5428	7575	9295	2787

SURGERY SERVICES

Code	Short Description	50th	75th	90th	MC
33690	Reinforce pulmonary artery	3229	4506	5529	1769
33692	Repair heart defects	5929	8273	10151	2988
33694	Repair heart defects	6133	8558	10501	3025
33697	Repair heart defects	6524	9104	11171	3098
33702	Repair heart defects	5228	7295	8951	2420
33710	Repair heart defects	5628	7853	9636	2752
33720	Repair heart defect	5252	7328	8992	2420
33722	Repair heart defect	5498	7672	9414	2494
33730	Repair heart-vein defect(s)	5697	7949	9754	3011
33732	Repair heart-vein defect	5302	7399	9079	2520
33735	Revision of heart chamber	3697	5159	6330	2002
33736	Revision of heart chamber	4239	5916	7259	2095
33737	Revision of heart chamber	3868	5397	6623	2022
33750	Major vessel shunt	3798	5300	6504	1838
33755	Major vessel shunt	3829	5342	6555	1851
33762	Major vessel shunt	3812	5319	6526	1851
33764	Major vessel shunt and graft	3598	5021	6161	1851
33766	Major vessel shunt	3831	5345	6559	1887
33767	Atrial septectomy/septostomy	4382	6114	7502	2132
33770	Repair great vessels defect	6341	8848	10856	3089
33771	Repair great vessels defect	6535	9119	11189	3135
33774	Repair great vessels defect	5595	7808	9580	2603
33775	Repair great vessels defect	5771	8053	9882	2648
33776	Repair great vessels defect	6135	8561	10504	2897
33777	Repair great vessels defect	5895	8226	10094	2695
33778	Repair great vessels defect	6680	9321	11438	3298
33779	Repair great vessels defect	6756	9427	11567	3307
33780	Repair great vessels defect	6993	9758	11973	3335
33781	Repair great vessels defect	6852	9561	11732	3316
33786	Repair arterial trunk	6522	9100	11166	3135
33788	Revision of pulmonary artery	4293	5990	7350	2377
33800	Aortic suspension	2645	3691	4529	1252
33802	Repair vessel defect	3218	4490	5510	1704
33803	Repair vessel defect	3617	5048	6194	1777
33813	Repair septal defect	3693	5153	6323	1814
33814	Repair septal defect	5046	7041	8640	2384
33820	Revise major vessel	2897	4043	4961	1668
33822	Revise major vessel	2980	4158	5102	1704
33824	Revise major vessel	3434	4792	5880	1777
33840	Remove aorta constriction	4102	5724	7023	2242

MC = Medicare Fee

Code	Short Description	50th	75th	90th	MC
33845	Remove aorta constriction	4501	6280	7706	2297
33851	Remove aorta constriction	4604	6425	7883	2261
33852	Repair septal defect	4847	6763	8298	2352
33853	Repair septal defect	5922	8264	10140	3025
33860	Ascending aorta graft	5695	7947	9752	2848
33861	Ascending aorta graft	6524	9103	11170	2922
33863	Ascending aorta graft	6820	9517	11678	2995
33870	Transverse aortic arch graft	7604	10610	13019	3561
33875	Thoracic aorta graft	5282	7370	9044	2682
33877	Thoracoabdominal graft	6664	9299	11410	3663
33910	Remove lung artery emboli	4203	5864	7196	1535
33915	Remove lung artery emboli	3142	4385	5381	1291
33916	Surgery of great vessel	4507	6289	7717	1768
33917	Repair pulmonary artery	5170	7214	8852	2560
33918	Repair pulmonary atresia	5198	7253	8900	2377
33919	Repair pulmonary atresia	6242	8710	10688	3057
33920	Repair pulmonary atresia	6146	8576	10524	3043
33922	Transect pulmonary artery	4604	6425	7883	2033
33924	Remove pulmonary shunt	912	1273	1562	402
33930	Remove donor heart/lung	3269	4561	5597	0
33935	Transplantation, heart/lung	16905	23589	28945	5868
33940	Remove donor heart	2684	3745	4595	0
33945	Transplantation of heart	12809	17873	21931	4593
33960	External circulation assist	3141	4383	5378	1053
33961	External circulation assist	2025	2826	3468	736
33970	Aortic circulation assist	1273	1776	2179	603
33971	Aortic circulation assist	953	1330	1632	564
33973	Insert balloon device	1642	2291	2812	716
33974	Remove intra-aortic balloon	1965	2742	3365	742
33975	Implant ventricular device	3135	4375	5369	1428
33976	Implant ventricular device	4364	6089	7472	1946
33977	Remove ventricular device	2744	3829	4698	1249
33978	Remove ventricular device	3136	4376	5370	1428

Arteries and Veins

Code	Short Description	50th	75th	90th	MC
34001	Remove artery clot	1648	2151	2655	908
34051	Remove artery clot	2303	3007	3711	938
34101	Remove artery clot	1442	1882	2323	740
34111	Remove arm artery clot	1364	1780	2197	646

SURGERY SERVICES

Code	Short Description	50th	75th	90th	MC
34151	Remove artery clot	2266	2958	3651	1160
34201	Remove artery clot	1686	2202	2717	739
34203	Remove leg artery clot	1727	2254	2782	839
34401	Remove vein clot	1867	2437	3008	825
34421	Remove vein clot	1361	1777	2193	701
34451	Remove vein clot	2118	2765	3413	1019
34471	Remove vein clot	1258	1643	2028	509
34490	Remove vein clot	1275	1664	2054	605
34501	Repair valve, femoral vein	1752	2287	2823	701
34502	Reconstruct, vena cava	4518	5898	7280	1876
34510	Transposition of vein valve	2090	2729	3368	848
34520	Cross-over vein graft	2725	3558	4391	890
34530	Leg vein fusion	2412	3149	3886	1178
35001	Repair defect of artery	2849	3720	4591	1463
35002	Repair artery rupture, neck	3121	4075	5029	1346
35005	Repair defect of artery	2759	3602	4445	1135
35011	Repair defect of artery	2443	3189	3936	1052
35013	Repair artery rupture, arm	2894	3779	4663	1326
35021	Repair defect of artery	2888	3770	4653	1530
35022	Repair artery rupture, chest	3181	4153	5126	1514
35045	Repair defect of arm artery	2389	3119	3850	983
35081	Repair defect of artery	3719	4856	5993	2035
35082	Repair artery rupture, aorta	4416	5766	7116	2411
35091	Repair defect of artery	4339	5665	6991	2348
35092	Repair artery rupture, aorta	5411	7065	8719	2644
35102	Repair defect of artery	3981	5198	6415	2166
35103	Repair artery rupture, groin	4562	5955	7350	2461
35111	Repair defect of artery	2812	3672	4532	1440
35112	Repair artery rupture, spleen	3258	4254	5250	1172
35121	Repair defect of artery	3832	5003	6174	1860
35122	Repair artery rupture, belly	4193	5474	6756	2101
35131	Repair defect of artery	2886	3768	4650	1418
35132	Repair artery rupture, groin	3700	4831	5962	1678
35141	Repair defect of artery	2522	3293	4064	1219
35142	Repair artery rupture, thigh	2941	3839	4738	1341
35151	Repair defect of artery	2791	3644	4498	1342
35152	Repair artery rupture, knee	2802	3658	4515	1040
35161	Repair defect of artery	2578	3366	4154	1435
35162	Repair artery rupture	2788	3640	4492	1605
35180	Repair blood vessel lesion	2366	3089	3813	819

MC = Medicare Fee

Code	Short Description	50th	75th	90th	MC
35182	Repair blood vessel lesion	2935	3832	4729	1108
35184	Repair blood vessel lesion	2274	2969	3664	884
35188	Repair blood vessel lesion	2548	3327	4106	889
35189	Repair blood vessel lesion	3374	4405	5437	1198
35190	Repair blood vessel lesion	2329	3041	3753	954
35201	Repair blood vessel lesion	2232	2914	3597	826
35206	Repair blood vessel lesion	2092	2731	3371	818
35207	Repair blood vessel lesion	2279	2975	3672	862
35211	Repair blood vessel lesion	3578	4671	5765	1411
35216	Repair blood vessel lesion	2815	3675	4536	1166
35221	Repair blood vessel lesion	3018	3940	4862	1112
35226	Repair blood vessel lesion	2105	2748	3391	808
35231	Repair blood vessel lesion	2947	3848	4749	1088
35236	Repair blood vessel lesion	2798	3653	4509	950
35241	Repair blood vessel lesion	4119	5377	6637	1453
35246	Repair blood vessel lesion	3255	4250	5245	1464
35251	Repair blood vessel lesion	3357	4382	5409	1075
35256	Repair blood vessel lesion	2615	3414	4214	987
35261	Repair blood vessel lesion	2404	3139	3874	1038
35266	Repair blood vessel lesion	2468	3222	3976	914
35271	Repair blood vessel lesion	3755	4902	6050	1375
35276	Repair blood vessel lesion	2834	3700	4567	1180
35281	Repair blood vessel lesion	2939	3837	4735	1413
35286	Repair blood vessel lesion	2327	3038	3749	980
35301	Rechanneling of artery	2810	3631	4452	1376
35311	Rechanneling of artery	3610	4714	5818	1942
35321	Rechanneling of artery	2480	3237	3995	1057
35331	Rechanneling of artery	3233	4221	5210	1487
35341	Rechanneling of artery	3402	4441	5481	1745
35351	Rechanneling of artery	2867	3744	4620	1453
35355	Rechanneling of artery	2984	3896	4809	1322
35361	Rechanneling of artery	3574	4666	5759	1784
35363	Rechanneling of artery	3928	5129	6330	1983
35371	Rechanneling of artery	2258	2947	3638	1009
35372	Rechanneling of artery	2198	2870	3542	1013
35381	Rechanneling of artery	2552	3332	4112	1216
35390	Re-operation, carotid	631	824	1017	204
35450	Repair arterial blockage	1722	2215	2720	796
35452	Repair arterial blockage	1177	1514	1859	463
35454	Repair arterial blockage	1505	1936	2377	606
35456	Repair arterial blockage	1634	2103	2582	731

SURGERY SERVICES

Code	Short Description	50th	75th	90th	MC
35458	Repair arterial blockage	1639	2108	2589	846
35459	Repair arterial blockage	1577	2029	2492	819
35460	Repair venous blockage	1200	1544	1896	387
35470	Repair arterial blockage	1409	1813	2226	677
35471	Repair arterial blockage	1595	2052	2520	796
35472	Repair arterial blockage	1090	1402	1722	365
35473	Repair arterial blockage	1239	1595	1958	501
35474	Repair arterial blockage	1415	1820	2235	604
35475	Repair arterial blockage	1383	1779	2185	699
35476	Repair venous blockage	879	1131	1388	319
35480	Atherectomy, open	2041	2626	3225	1023
35481	Atherectomy, open	1272	1636	2009	489
35482	Atherectomy, open	1293	1664	2043	661
35483	Atherectomy, open	1609	2070	2542	798
35484	Atherectomy, open	1854	2386	2930	882
35485	Atherectomy, open	1510	1943	2386	585
35490	Atherectomy, percutaneous	1909	2455	3015	845
35491	Atherectomy, percutaneous	1198	1542	1893	404
35492	Atherectomy, percutaneous	1181	1519	1866	546
35493	Atherectomy, percutaneous	1535	1976	2426	659
35494	Atherectomy, percutaneous	1744	2243	2755	729
35495	Atherectomy, percutaneous	1432	1843	2263	483
35501	Artery bypass graft	2822	3631	4459	1620
35506	Artery bypass graft	3074	3955	4856	1619
35507	Artery bypass graft	3041	3913	4805	1567
35508	Artery bypass graft	2930	3770	4630	1529
35509	Artery bypass graft	3057	3933	4830	1562
35511	Artery bypass graft	2620	3370	4139	1083
35515	Artery bypass graft	2760	3551	4360	1190
35516	Artery bypass graft	2851	3668	4505	1415
35518	Artery bypass graft	2936	3778	4639	1382
35521	Artery bypass graft	2859	3678	4517	1411
35526	Artery bypass graft	3321	4273	5247	1330
35531	Artery bypass graft	3676	4730	5808	1897
35533	Artery bypass graft	3601	4633	5689	1763
35536	Artery bypass graft	3534	4547	5584	1859
35541	Artery bypass graft	3579	4605	5655	1858
35546	Artery bypass graft	3658	4706	5779	1958
35548	Artery bypass graft	3440	4426	5435	1706
35549	Artery bypass graft	3935	5062	6217	1874

MC = Medicare Fee

Code	Short Description	50th	75th	90th	MC
35551	Artery bypass graft	3823	4919	6041	1892
35556	Artery bypass graft	3166	4073	5002	1664
35558	Artery bypass graft	2815	3621	4447	1286
35560	Artery bypass graft	3697	4757	5842	1820
35563	Artery bypass graft	2650	3409	4187	930
35565	Artery bypass graft	3148	4050	4974	1388
35566	Artery bypass graft	3424	4405	5410	1951
35571	Artery bypass graft	3354	4315	5299	1595
35582	Vein bypass graft	3833	4931	6056	2138
35583	Vein bypass graft	3275	4214	5174	1776
35585	Vein bypass graft	3660	4709	5783	2124
35587	Vein bypass graft	3371	4337	5326	1709
35601	Artery bypass graft	3102	4126	5203	1516
35606	Artery bypass graft	2905	3864	4873	1516
35612	Artery bypass graft	2857	3800	4792	1362
35616	Artery bypass graft	2861	3805	4799	1368
35621	Artery bypass graft	2942	3913	4935	1346
35623	Bypass graft, not vein	2582	3434	4330	986
35626	Artery bypass graft	3591	4777	6024	1843
35631	Artery bypass graft	3394	4514	5692	1748
35636	Artery bypass graft	3281	4363	5503	1448
35641	Artery bypass graft	3619	4813	6069	1861
35642	Artery bypass graft	3260	4336	5468	1140
35645	Artery bypass graft	3271	4350	5485	1149
35646	Artery bypass graft	3755	4994	6298	2069
35650	Artery bypass graft	2831	3766	4748	1320
35651	Artery bypass graft	4063	5405	6815	2068
35654	Artery bypass graft	3559	4733	5969	1748
35656	Artery bypass graft	2983	3968	5003	1566
35661	Artery bypass graft	2677	3561	4490	1198
35663	Artery bypass graft	2919	3882	4896	1309
35665	Artery bypass graft	2867	3814	4809	1403
35666	Artery bypass graft	3265	4343	5476	1647
35671	Artery bypass graft	2796	3719	4690	1309
35681	Artery bypass graft	1935	2573	3245	873
35691	Arterial transposition	3172	4219	5321	1587
35693	Arterial transposition	2629	3496	4409	989
35694	Arterial transposition	2946	3919	4942	1140
35695	Arterial transposition	2946	3919	4942	1140
35700	Re-operation, bypass graft	653	869	1096	197
35701	Exploration, carotid artery	1058	1407	1774	460

SURGERY SERVICES

Code	Short Description	50th	75th	90th	MC
35721	Exploration, femoral artery	1001	1332	1680	444
35741	Exploration popliteal artery	921	1225	1545	452
35761	Exploration of artery/vein	1067	1420	1790	455
35800	Explore neck vessels	1138	1514	1909	483
35820	Explore chest vessels	1809	2406	3035	820
35840	Explore abdominal vessels	1599	2126	2682	679
35860	Explore limb vessels	1171	1557	1964	456
35870	Repair vessel graft defect	3736	4970	6267	1301
35875	Remove clot in graft	1679	2233	2816	745
35876	Remove clot in graft	1967	2617	3300	889
35901	Excision, graft, neck	1595	2122	2676	626
35903	Excision, graft, extremity	1624	2160	2724	678
35905	Excision, graft, thorax	3121	4151	5234	988
35907	Excision, graft, abdomen	3217	4278	5395	1018
36000	Place needle in vein	70	100	133	15
36005	Injection, venography	168	237	312	47
36010	Place catheter in vein	354	495	648	157
36011	Place catheter in vein	396	558	734	169
36012	Place catheter in vein	516	728	957	210
36013	Place catheter in artery	393	555	729	160
36014	Place catheter in artery	491	693	911	180
36015	Place catheter in artery	521	735	967	210
36100	Establish access to artery	374	528	694	192
36120	Establish access to artery	395	558	733	151
36140	Establish access to artery	318	449	590	118
36145	Artery to vein shunt	473	668	878	166
36160	Establish access to aorta	424	598	787	204
36200	Place catheter in aorta	484	643	816	196
36215	Place catheter in artery	570	804	1057	247
36216	Place catheter in artery	705	940	1194	284
36217	Place catheter in artery	786	1108	1457	339
36218	Place catheter in artery	214	302	397	54
36245	Place catheter in artery	631	891	1171	261
36246	Place catheter in artery	691	975	1282	284
36247	Place catheter in artery	765	1080	1420	339
36248	Place catheter in artery	227	320	420	54
36260	Insertion of infusion pump	1137	1604	2109	682
36261	Revision of infusion pump	753	1063	1397	298
36262	Remove infusion pump	564	796	1047	234
36400	Drawing blood	34	48	63	9

MC = Medicare Fee

Code	Short Description	50th	75th	90th	MC
36405	Drawing blood	61	86	113	22
36406	Drawing blood	40	57	75	14
36410	Drawing blood	40	57	75	14
36415	Drawing blood	12	17	22	0
36420	Establish access to vein	118	167	219	50
36425	Establish access to vein	53	74	98	27
36430	Blood transfusion service	83	122	164	35
36440	Blood transfusion service	154	218	286	80
36450	Exchange transfusion service	534	754	991	139
36455	Exchange transfusion service	626	883	1161	160
36460	Transfusion service, fetal	979	1381	1816	401
36468	Injection(s); spider veins	96	135	178	0
36469	Injection(s); spider veins	115	162	213	0
36470	Injection therapy of vein	78	109	144	51
36471	Injection therapy of veins	118	167	219	74
36481	Insertion of catheter, vein	896	1264	1661	505
36488	Insertion of catheter, vein	200	283	372	79
36489	Insertion of catheter, vein	224	315	413	82
36490	Insertion of catheter, vein	279	393	517	105
36491	Insertion of catheter, vein	350	494	649	113
36493	Repositioning of catheter, vein	200	283	372	64
36500	Insertion of catheter, vein	285	402	528	112
36510	Insertion of catheter, vein	111	156	205	46
36520	Plasma and/or cell exchange	369	520	684	123
36522	Photopheresis	405	572	752	179
36530	Insertion of infusion pump	790	1114	1465	421
36531	Revision of infusion pump	863	1218	1601	370
36532	Remove infusion pump	547	772	1015	209
36533	Insertion of access port	830	1162	1520	398
36534	Revision of access port	690	973	1280	253
36535	Remove access port	419	591	777	173
36600	Withdrawal of arterial blood	52	73	96	20
36620	Insertion catheter, artery	155	218	285	63
36625	Insertion catheter, artery	192	271	357	101
36640	Insertion catheter, artery	345	487	641	157
36660	Insertion catheter, artery	156	221	290	61
36680	Insert needle, bone cavity	221	312	410	83
36800	Insertion of cannula	406	538	681	160
36810	Insertion of cannula	909	1210	1535	378
36815	Insertion of cannula	696	926	1175	264
36821	Artery-vein fusion	1407	1873	2375	671

SURGERY SERVICES

Code	Short Description	50th	75th	90th	MC
36822	Insertion of cannula(s)	1190	1583	2008	450
36825	Artery-vein graft	1729	2301	2919	901
36830	Artery-vein graft	1879	2430	3025	927
36832	Revise artery-vein fistula	1651	2198	2788	623
36834	Repair A-V aneurysm	1634	2174	2758	738
36835	Artery to vein shunt	1410	1877	2381	418
36860	Cannula declotting	293	390	495	164
36861	Cannula declotting	578	770	976	268
37140	Revision of circulation	3627	4827	6123	1636
37145	Revision of circulation	3617	4813	6106	1642
37160	Revision of circulation	3655	4864	6170	1639
37180	Revision of circulation	3602	4794	6081	1564
37181	Splice spleen/kidney veins	4391	5844	7413	1762
37200	Transcatheter biopsy	699	930	1180	200
37201	Transcatheter therapy infuse	1045	1391	1764	363
37202	Transcatheter therapy infuse	804	1070	1357	339
37203	Transcatheter retrieval	818	1089	1382	301
37204	Transcatheter occlusion	2438	3244	4115	1083
37205	Transcatheter stent	1350	1797	2279	540
37206	Transcatheter stent	756	1006	1276	269
37207	Transcatheter stent	1695	2255	2861	540
37208	Transcatheter stent	861	1146	1454	269
37209	Exchange arterial catheter	387	515	653	122
37250	Intravascular us	172	229	291	90
37251	Intravascular us	131	175	222	69
37565	Ligation of neck vein	958	1274	1616	332
37600	Ligation of neck artery	894	1190	1510	383
37605	Ligation of neck artery	1003	1335	1693	444
37606	Ligation of neck artery	1143	1521	1929	446
37607	Ligation of fistula	911	1213	1539	374
37609	Temporal artery procedure	410	546	693	192
37615	Ligation of neck artery	976	1299	1648	441
37616	Ligation of chest artery	2027	2697	3421	758
37617	Ligation of abdomen artery	1711	2277	2888	924
37618	Ligation of extremity artery	1101	1465	1858	394
37620	Revision of major vein	1788	2379	3018	769
37650	Revision of major vein	813	1082	1372	351
37660	Revision of major vein	1302	1733	2199	642
37700	Revise leg vein	680	905	1148	311
37720	Remove leg vein	1060	1411	1790	448

MC = Medicare Fee

Code	Short Description	50th	75th	90th	MC
37730	Remove leg veins	1270	1690	2144	591
37735	Remove leg veins/lesion	1967	2618	3321	782
37760	Revision of leg veins	1888	2512	3186	740
37780	Revision of leg vein	359	478	607	224
37785	Revise secondary varicosity	294	391	496	181
37788	Re-vascularization, penis	2130	2834	3595	1482
37790	Penile venous occlusion	1851	2463	3125	557

SPLEEN AND LYMPHATIC SYSTEMS SURGERY

Spleen

Code	Short Description	50th	75th	90th	MC
38100	Remove spleen, total	1669	2298	2942	875
38101	Remove spleen, partial	1942	2674	3424	821
38102	Remove spleen, total	956	1317	1686	307
38115	Repair ruptured spleen	1960	2699	3456	847
38200	Injection for spleen x-ray	309	425	544	175

Bone Marrow or Stem Cell Transplantation Services

Code	Short Description	50th	75th	90th	MC
38230	Bone marrow collection	854	1177	1507	232
38231	Stem cell collection	245	338	432	96
38240	Bone marrow/stem transplant	624	859	1100	145
38241	Bone marrow/stem transplant	613	845	1082	143

Lymph Nodes and Lymphatic Channels

Code	Short Description	50th	75th	90th	MC
38300	Drainage lymph node lesion	155	214	273	83
38305	Drainage lymph node lesion	397	547	700	254
38308	Incision of lymph channels	663	913	1170	327
38380	Thoracic duct procedure	837	1152	1475	458
38381	Thoracic duct procedure	1804	2484	3181	826
38382	Thoracic duct procedure	1598	2201	2818	592
38500	Biopsy/removal, lymph node(s)	344	474	607	184
38505	Needle biopsy, lymph node(s)	207	285	365	96
38510	Biopsy/removal, lymph node(s)	554	763	977	269
38520	Biopsy/removal, lymph node(s)	639	880	1127	328
38525	Biopsy/removal, lymph node(s)	626	862	1103	292
38530	Biopsy/removal, lymph node(s)	841	1159	1484	375
38542	Explore deep node(s), neck	794	1093	1400	402

SURGERY SERVICES

Code	Short Description	50th	75th	90th	MC
38550	Removal neck/armpit lesion	794	1093	1400	399
38555	Removal neck/armpit lesion	1541	2122	2717	844
38562	Removal, pelvic lymph nodes	1475	2032	2602	693
38564	Removal, abdomen lymph nodes	1654	2277	2916	740
38700	Remove lymph nodes, neck	1514	2085	2669	732
38720	Remove lymph nodes, neck	2602	3584	4589	1189
38724	Remove lymph nodes, neck	2625	3615	4629	1167
38740	Remove armpit lymph nodes	927	1276	1634	470
38745	Remove armpits lymph nodes	1562	2151	2755	715
38746	Remove thoracic lymph nodes	699	963	1233	280
38747	Remove abdominal lymph nodes	778	1071	1372	313
38760	Remove groin lymph nodes	1193	1642	2103	634
38765	Remove groin lymph nodes	2408	3316	4246	1181
38770	Remove pelvis lymph nodes	2218	3054	3911	1156
38780	Remove abdomen lymph nodes	3220	4435	5679	1356
38790	Injection for lymphatic x-ray	318	438	561	102
38794	Access thoracic lymph duct	525	722	925	284

MEDIASTINUM AND DIAPHRAGM SURGERY

Mediastinum

Code	Short Description	50th	75th	90th	MC
39000	Exploration of chest	870	1174	1486	481
39010	Exploration of chest	1591	2149	2720	960
39200	Removal chest lesion	2177	2940	3720	1028
39220	Removal chest lesion	2531	3417	4325	1335
39400	Visualization of chest	889	1201	1520	441

Diaphragm

Code	Short Description	50th	75th	90th	MC
39501	Repair diaphragm laceration	2141	2891	3659	977
39502	Repair paraesophageal hernia	2135	2883	3649	1159
39503	Repair diaphragm hernia	3603	4865	6157	2400
39520	Repair diaphragm hernia	2267	3062	3875	1184
39530	Repair diaphragm hernia	2371	3201	4051	1221
39531	Repair diaphragm hernia	2200	2971	3760	1055
39540	Repair diaphragm hernia	2250	3039	3846	1048
39541	Repair diaphragm hernia	2266	3060	3872	1087
39545	Revision of diaphragm	1727	2332	2951	832

MC = Medicare Fee

Code	Short Description	50th	75th	90th	MC

DIGESTIVE SYSTEM SURGERY

Lips

Code	Short Description	50th	75th	90th	MC
40490	Biopsy of lip	120	160	201	79
40500	Partial excision of lip	969	1294	1627	406
40510	Partial excision of lip	904	1207	1518	445
40520	Partial excision of lip	793	1059	1331	383
40525	Reconstruct lip with flap	1332	1779	2236	712
40527	Reconstruct lip with flap	2213	2955	3715	852
40530	Partial removal of lip	891	1190	1496	432
40650	Repair lip	540	722	907	341
40652	Repair lip	670	895	1126	400
40654	Repair lip	914	1220	1534	503
40700	Repair cleft lip/nasal	1930	2577	3240	851
40701	Repair cleft lip/nasal	2896	3868	4863	1425
40702	Repair cleft lip/nasal	1822	2433	3059	892
40720	Repair cleft lip/nasal	1991	2659	3343	951
40761	Repair cleft lip/nasal	2680	3579	4499	1041

Vestibule of Mouth

Code	Short Description	50th	75th	90th	MC
40800	Drainage of mouth lesion	121	162	204	75
40801	Drainage of mouth lesion	304	406	511	169
40804	Removal foreign body, mouth	125	167	210	71
40805	Removal foreign body, mouth	357	477	600	214
40806	Incision of lip fold	101	135	170	28
40808	Biopsy of mouth lesion	123	164	206	69
40810	Excision of mouth lesion	158	210	264	100
40812	Excise/repair mouth lesion	223	297	374	152
40814	Excise/repair mouth lesion	388	519	652	268
40816	Excision of mouth lesion	489	653	821	278
40818	Excise oral mucosa for graft	330	441	554	185
40819	Excise lip or cheek fold	255	340	428	141
40820	Treatment of mouth lesion	112	149	187	70
40830	Repair mouth laceration	159	212	267	95
40831	Repair mouth laceration	332	444	558	179
40840	Reconstruction of mouth	1062	1418	1782	599
40842	Reconstruction of mouth	1063	1419	1785	599
40843	Reconstruction of mouth	1437	1920	2413	839

SURGERY SERVICES

Code	Short Description	50th	75th	90th	MC
40844	Reconstruction of mouth	1816	2425	3048	1109
40845	Reconstruction of mouth	2535	3385	4255	1736

Tongue and Floor of Mouth

Code	Short Description	50th	75th	90th	MC
41000	Drainage of mouth lesion	129	172	216	81
41005	Drainage of mouth lesion	125	166	209	74
41006	Drainage of mouth lesion	237	316	398	160
41007	Drainage of mouth lesion	327	437	550	240
41008	Drainage of mouth lesion	265	354	445	167
41009	Drainage of mouth lesion	390	521	655	275
41010	Incision of tongue fold	149	199	251	55
41015	Drainage of mouth lesion	292	390	490	179
41016	Drainage of mouth lesion	429	573	721	306
41017	Drainage of mouth lesion	338	452	568	203
41018	Drainage of mouth lesion	503	671	844	355
41100	Biopsy of tongue	142	189	238	95
41105	Biopsy of tongue	181	241	304	99
41108	Biopsy of floor of mouth	141	188	237	76
41110	Excision of tongue lesion	202	270	339	114
41112	Excision of tongue lesion	331	443	557	206
41113	Excision of tongue lesion	379	506	636	271
41114	Excision of tongue lesion	916	1224	1538	588
41115	Excision of tongue fold	199	265	333	143
41116	Excision of mouth lesion	446	595	749	202
41120	Partial removal of tongue	1274	1701	2139	666
41130	Partial removal of tongue	1560	2083	2619	804
41135	Tongue and neck surgery	2932	3916	4924	1652
41140	Remove tongue	2843	3797	4774	1755
41145	Tongue removal; neck surgery	3847	5138	6460	2090
41150	Tongue, mouth, jaw surgery	3032	4050	5091	1666
41153	Tongue, mouth, neck surgery	3820	5102	6414	1944
41155	Tongue, jaw, and neck surgery	4431	5917	7439	2342
41250	Repair tongue laceration	189	252	317	118
41251	Repair tongue laceration	261	348	438	177
41252	Repair tongue laceration	415	554	697	217
41500	Fixation of tongue	592	790	993	277
41510	Tongue to lip surgery	870	1162	1460	247
41520	Reconstruction, tongue fold	368	492	619	228

MC = Medicare Fee

Code	Short Description	50th	75th	90th	MC

Dentoalveolar Structures

Code	Short Description	50th	75th	90th	MC
41800	Drainage of gum lesion	129	172	216	73
41805	Removal foreign body, gum	141	188	237	82
41806	Removal foreign body, jawbone	266	356	447	172
41820	Excision, gum, each quadrant	463	618	777	0
41821	Excision of gum flap	110	146	184	0
41822	Excision of gum lesion	298	398	500	219
41823	Excision of gum lesion	437	584	734	304
41825	Excision of gum lesion	189	252	317	114
41826	Excision of gum lesion	243	325	408	177
41827	Excision of gum lesion	499	666	837	293
41828	Excision of gum lesion	407	544	684	294
41830	Remove gum tissue	408	545	685	319
41850	Treatment of gum lesion	102	136	171	0
41870	Gum graft	540	722	907	0
41872	Repair gum	486	648	815	236
41874	Repair tooth socket	443	592	744	285

Palate and Uvula

Code	Short Description	50th	75th	90th	MC
42000	Drainage mouth roof lesion	129	169	210	72
42100	Biopsy roof of mouth	141	185	230	83
42104	Excision lesion, mouth roof	233	306	380	133
42106	Excision lesion, mouth roof	298	390	485	177
42107	Excision lesion, mouth roof	1235	1620	2015	379
42120	Remove palate/lesion	1573	2064	2566	526
42140	Excision of uvula	203	266	331	119
42145	Repair, palate, pharynx/uvula	1602	2101	2612	693
42160	Treatment mouth roof lesion	215	282	350	135
42180	Repair palate	289	380	472	194
42182	Repair palate	499	654	813	300
42200	Reconstruct cleft palate	1844	2419	3008	752
42205	Reconstruct cleft palate	2207	2894	3599	812
42210	Reconstruct cleft palate	2528	3316	4123	1068
42215	Reconstruct cleft palate	1816	2383	2962	666
42220	Reconstruct cleft palate	1671	2192	2725	504
42225	Reconstruct cleft palate	1864	2445	3039	668
42226	Lengthening of palate	2025	2656	3302	712
42227	Lengthening of palate	1970	2584	3213	653

SURGERY SERVICES

Code	Short Description	50th	75th	90th	MC
42235	Repair palate	1072	1406	1748	529
42260	Repair nose to lip fistula	774	1015	1262	526
42280	Preparation, palate mold	204	267	332	144
42281	Insertion, palate prosthesis	189	247	308	133

Salivary Gland and Ducts

Code	Short Description	50th	75th	90th	MC
42300	Drainage of salivary gland	228	299	371	115
42305	Drainage of salivary gland	485	636	791	310
42310	Drainage of salivary gland	180	236	293	104
42320	Drainage of salivary gland	326	428	532	170
42325	Create salivary cyst drain	274	359	446	195
42326	Create salivary cyst drain	458	601	747	328
42330	Remove salivary stone	205	269	334	131
42335	Remove salivary stone	409	536	667	233
42340	Remove salivary stone	764	1002	1246	360
42400	Biopsy of salivary gland	137	180	224	66
42405	Biopsy of salivary gland	339	444	553	193
42408	Excision of salivary cyst	551	722	898	314
42409	Drainage of salivary cyst	407	534	663	229
42410	Excise parotid gland/lesion	1072	1406	1748	615
42415	Excise parotid gland/lesion	2256	2959	3679	1194
42420	Excise parotid gland/lesion	2766	3628	4510	1383
42425	Excise parotid gland/lesion	2034	2668	3317	977
42426	Excise parotid gland/lesion	3901	5117	6362	1866
42440	Excision submaxillary gland	1404	1842	2290	616
42450	Excision sublingual gland	942	1236	1537	319
42500	Repair salivary duct	840	1102	1370	362
42505	Repair salivary duct	1260	1653	2055	558
42507	Parotid duct diversion	1300	1706	2121	442
42508	Parotid duct diversion	1541	2022	2514	675
42509	Parotid duct diversion	2139	2806	3489	766
42510	Parotid duct diversion	1708	2240	2785	637
42550	Injection for salivary x-ray	108	141	176	55
42600	Closure of salivary fistula	1022	1341	1667	350
42650	Dilation of salivary duct	84	110	136	47
42660	Dilation of salivary duct	110	145	180	65
42665	Ligation of salivary duct	278	364	453	185

MC = Medicare Fee

Code	Short Description	50th	75th	90th	MC

Pharynx, Adenoids and Tonsils

Code	Short Description	50th	75th	90th	MC
42700	Drainage of tonsil abscess	181	248	316	98
42720	Drainage of throat abscess	338	463	591	257
42725	Drainage of throat abscess	823	1128	1439	561
42800	Biopsy of throat	147	201	257	84
42802	Biopsy of throat	207	284	362	103
42804	Biopsy of upper nose/throat	169	232	296	95
42806	Biopsy of upper nose/throat	211	289	369	121
42808	Excise pharynx lesion	413	565	721	200
42809	Remove pharynx foreign body	189	258	330	103
42810	Excision of neck cyst	530	726	927	268
42815	Excision of neck cyst	1348	1845	2355	646
42820	Remove tonsils and adenoids	626	857	1094	277
42821	Remove tonsils and adenoids	701	960	1225	334
42825	Remove tonsils	581	795	1015	242
42826	Remove tonsils	685	939	1198	296
42830	Remove adenoids	399	546	697	181
42831	Remove adenoids	428	586	748	205
42835	Remove adenoids	348	476	608	164
42836	Remove adenoids	431	590	753	243
42842	Extensive surgery of throat	1911	2617	3340	609
42844	Extensive surgery of throat	2513	3442	4392	975
42845	Extensive surgery of throat	3117	4269	5447	1675
42860	Excision of tonsil tags	375	514	656	166
42870	Excision of lingual tonsil	638	874	1115	299
42890	Partial removal of pharynx	1674	2293	2926	849
42892	Revision of pharyngeal walls	2170	2971	3791	1023
42894	Revision of pharyngeal walls	2986	4089	5218	1510
42900	Repair throat wound	742	1016	1297	381
42950	Reconstruction of throat	1589	2176	2776	738
42953	Repair throat, esophagus	1581	2165	2763	606
42955	Surgical opening of throat	681	933	1191	398
42960	Control throat bleeding	230	314	401	135
42961	Control throat bleeding	386	529	675	274
42962	Control throat bleeding	761	1042	1330	522
42970	Control nose/throat bleeding	347	475	607	187
42971	Control nose/throat bleeding	538	737	941	342
42972	Control nose/throat bleeding	681	933	1191	462

SURGERY SERVICES

Code	Short Description	50th	75th	90th	MC

Esophagus

Code	Short Description	50th	75th	90th	MC
43020	Incision of esophagus	1547	1950	2375	589
43030	Throat muscle surgery	1589	2004	2440	693
43045	Incision of esophagus	2593	3269	3981	1314
43100	Excision of esophagus lesion	1687	2127	2590	611
43101	Excision of esophagus lesion	2529	3188	3883	1033
43107	Remove esophagus	4997	6299	7671	2124
43108	Remove esophagus	5774	7278	8864	2456
43112	Remove esophagus	5164	6510	7928	2174
43113	Remove esophagus	5919	7462	9087	2494
43116	Partial removal of esophagus	5385	6788	8267	2345
43117	Partial removal of esophagus	5275	6650	8098	2300
43118	Partial removal of esophagus	5582	7037	8570	2419
43121	Partial removal of esophagus	4973	6268	7634	2087
43122	Partial removal of esophagus	4973	6268	7634	2087
43123	Partial removal of esophagus	5582	7037	8570	2419
43124	Remove esophagus	4681	5900	7186	2032
43130	Remove esophagus pouch	1849	2331	2839	897
43135	Remove esophagus pouch	2481	3128	3810	1136
43200	Esophagus endoscopy	442	557	679	154
43202	Esophagus endoscopy, biopsy	489	617	751	151
43204	Esophagus endoscopy and inject	707	891	1086	293
43205	Esophagus endoscopy/ligation	647	816	993	215
43215	Esophagus endoscopy	613	773	941	209
43216	Esophagus endoscopy/lesion	524	660	804	208
43217	Esophagus endoscopy	601	758	923	224
43219	Esophagus endoscopy	615	775	944	220
43220	Esophagus endoscopy, dilation	523	659	803	165
43226	Esophagus endoscopy, dilation	525	661	805	183
43227	Esophagus endoscopy, repair	713	899	1095	279
43228	Esophagus endoscopy, ablation	677	854	1040	292
43234	Upper GI endoscopy, exam	455	574	699	160
43235	Upper GI endoscopy, diagnosis	510	631	759	188
43239	Upper GI endoscopy, biopsy	575	716	865	211
43241	Upper GI endoscopy with tube	677	853	1039	205
43243	Upper GI endoscopy and inject	778	980	1194	346
43244	Upper GI endoscopy/ligation	765	965	1175	274
43245	Operative upper GI endoscopy	667	841	1024	266
43246	Place gastrostomy tube	865	1087	1321	339

MC = Medicare Fee

Code	Short Description	50th	75th	90th	MC
43247	Operative upper GI endoscopy	681	858	1045	265
43248	Upper GI endoscopy/guide wire	578	729	888	246
43249	Esophagus endoscopy, dilation	540	680	829	226
43250	Upper GI endoscopy/tumor	702	885	1077	270
43251	Operative upper GI endoscopy	720	907	1105	285
43255	Operative upper GI endoscopy	794	1001	1220	340
43258	Operative upper GI endoscopy	821	1035	1260	337
43259	Endoscopic ultrasound exam	853	1075	1309	300
43260	Endoscopy, bile duct/pancreas	912	1150	1400	401
43261	Endoscopy, bile duct/pancreas	921	1161	1414	410
43262	Endoscopy, bile duct/pancreas	1238	1561	1901	554
43263	Endoscopy, bile duct/pancreas	1045	1317	1604	402
43264	Endoscopy, bile duct/pancreas	1319	1663	2025	599
43265	Endoscopy, bile duct/pancreas	1402	1767	2152	524
43267	Endoscopy, bile duct/pancreas	1186	1495	1821	496
43268	Endoscopy, bile duct/pancreas	1234	1555	1894	543
43269	Endoscopy, bile duct/pancreas	1073	1352	1647	453
43271	Endoscopy, bile duct/pancreas	1232	1553	1891	505
43272	Endoscopy, bile duct/pancreas	1167	1471	1791	433
43300	Repair esophagus	2176	2988	3882	855
43305	Repair esophagus and fistula	2591	3557	4621	1241
43310	Repair esophagus	3249	4461	5795	1737
43312	Repair esophagus and fistula	3469	4763	6187	1680
43320	Fuse esophagus and stomach	2592	3558	4622	1107
43324	Revise esophagus and stomach	2141	2939	3819	1160
43325	Revise esophagus and stomach	2522	3463	4499	1119
43326	Revise esophagus and stomach	2371	3255	4228	919
43330	Repair esophagus	2350	3226	4191	1099
43331	Repair esophagus	2449	3363	4369	1248
43340	Fuse esophagus and intestine	2670	3666	4763	1145
43341	Fuse esophagus and intestine	2651	3640	4728	1043
43350	Surgical opening, esophagus	1748	2400	3117	792
43351	Surgical opening, esophagus	1810	2485	3228	926
43352	Surgical opening, esophagus	1731	2377	3088	833
43360	Gastrointestinal repair	4424	6074	7891	2025
43361	Gastrointestinal repair	5061	6949	9027	2345
43400	Ligate esophagus veins	2361	3241	4210	1094
43401	Esophagus surgery for veins	2411	3311	4301	1083
43405	Ligate/staple esophagus	2519	3458	4493	1252
43410	Repair esophagus wound	1725	2368	3077	789
43415	Repair esophagus wound	2422	3325	4320	1221

SURGERY SERVICES

Code	Short Description	50th	75th	90th	MC
43420	Repair esophagus opening	1527	2097	2724	656
43425	Repair esophagus opening	2479	3404	4422	1062
43450	Dilate esophagus	187	257	333	68
43453	Dilate esophagus	314	431	560	102
43456	Dilate esophagus	450	618	803	171
43458	Dilation of esophagus	439	603	784	156
43460	Pressure treatment esophagus	423	580	754	180

Stomach

Code	Short Description	50th	75th	90th	MC
43500	Surgical opening of stomach	1429	1858	2305	586
43501	Surgical repair of stomach	1924	2503	3104	947
43502	Surgical repair of stomach	2209	2872	3563	1021
43510	Surgical opening of stomach	1530	1990	2469	600
43520	Incision of pyloric muscle	1223	1591	1973	482
43600	Biopsy of stomach	174	226	280	78
43605	Biopsy of stomach	1471	1913	2373	604
43610	Excision of stomach lesion	1708	2221	2756	784
43611	Excision of stomach lesion	2249	2925	3628	872
43620	Remove stomach	3336	4338	5382	1551
43621	Remove stomach	3477	4522	5609	1567
43622	Remove stomach	3667	4769	5915	1618
43631	Remove stomach, partial	2328	3028	3756	1298
43632	Removal stomach, partial	2538	3301	4094	1298
43633	Removal stomach, partial	2915	3791	4703	1314
43634	Removal stomach, partial	3530	4591	5695	1787
43635	Partial removal of stomach	872	1133	1406	132
43638	Partial removal of stomach	3043	3957	4909	1391
43639	Removal stomach, partial	3317	4314	5351	1409
43640	Vagotomy and pylorus repair	1967	2558	3173	1012
43641	Vagotomy and pylorus repair	2328	3027	3755	1012
43750	Place gastrostomy tube	748	972	1206	299
43760	Change gastrostomy tube	143	192	243	61
43761	Reposition gastrostomy tube	258	335	416	107
43800	Reconstruction of pylorus	1592	2071	2569	694
43810	Fusion of stomach and bowel	1735	2256	2799	754
43820	Fusion of stomach and bowel	1657	2155	2673	803
43825	Fusion of stomach and bowel	2216	2882	3575	1047
43830	Place gastrostomy tube	1227	1596	1980	547
43831	Place gastrostomy tube	1064	1383	1716	492

MC = Medicare Fee

Code	Short Description	50th	75th	90th	MC
43832	Place gastrostomy tube	1515	1971	2445	782
43840	Repair stomach lesion	1584	2060	2556	782
43842	Gastroplasty for obesity	2456	3195	3963	1199
43843	Gastroplasty for obesity	2438	3170	3932	1199
43846	Gastric bypass for obesity	2998	3899	4836	1411
43847	Gastric bypass for obesity	2850	3706	4597	1488
43848	Revision gastroplasty	3108	4042	5015	1571
43850	Revise stomach-bowel fusion	2504	3256	4039	1250
43855	Revise stomach-bowel fusion	2811	3655	4534	1240
43860	Revise stomach-bowel fusion	2467	3209	3980	1254
43865	Revise stomach-bowel fusion	2817	3664	4545	1390
43870	Repair stomach opening	1194	1553	1926	529
43880	Repair stomach-bowel fistula	2134	2776	3443	1091

Intestines (Except Rectum)

Code	Short Description	50th	75th	90th	MC
44005	Freeing of bowel adhesion	1671	2139	2601	881
44010	Incision of small bowel	1713	2192	2665	688
44015	Insert needle catheter, bowel	758	970	1179	249
44020	Exploration of small bowel	1722	2203	2679	789
44021	Decompress small bowel	1514	1937	2356	754
44025	Incision of large bowel	1786	2285	2778	799
44050	Reduce bowel obstruction	1670	2137	2598	763
44055	Correct malrotation of bowel	1847	2364	2874	827
44100	Biopsy of bowel	298	381	463	113
44110	Excision of bowel lesion(s)	1623	2077	2526	717
44111	Excision of bowel lesion(s)	2126	2721	3308	899
44120	Remove small intestine	2059	2635	3204	964
44121	Remove small intestine	694	888	1079	284
44125	Remove small intestine	2169	2776	3375	1028
44130	Bowel to bowel fusion	1904	2436	2962	848
44139	Mobilization of colon	377	483	587	143
44140	Partial removal of colon	2318	3085	3843	1201
44141	Partial removal of colon	2429	3109	3779	1242
44143	Partial removal of colon	2439	3121	3795	1262
44144	Partial removal of colon	2541	3251	3953	1235
44145	Partial removal of colon	2726	3489	4241	1456
44146	Partial removal of colon	3139	4017	4885	1577
44147	Partial removal of colon	3096	3961	4816	1373
44150	Remove colon	3053	3907	4750	1453

SURGERY SERVICES

Code	Short Description	50th	75th	90th	MC
44151	Remove colon/ileostomy	3262	4174	5075	1183
44152	Remove colon/ileostomy	3931	5030	6115	1633
44153	Remove colon/ileostomy	4858	6217	7559	1869
44155	Remove colon	3719	4759	5786	1655
44156	Remove colon/ileostomy	3863	4943	6010	1339
44160	Remove colon	2473	3165	3848	1149
44300	Open bowel to skin	1201	1537	1869	592
44310	Ileostomy/jejunostomy	1704	2180	2650	769
44312	Revision of ileostomy	595	761	925	345
44314	Revision of ileostomy	1807	2313	2812	690
44316	Devise bowel pouch	2548	3261	3965	964
44320	Colostomy	1477	1890	2298	798
44322	Colostomy with biopsies	1660	2125	2583	836
44340	Revision of colostomy	526	673	818	268
44345	Revision of colostomy	1335	1708	2077	618
44346	Revision of colostomy	1524	1951	2372	747
44360	Small bowel endoscopy	622	826	1034	228
44361	Small bowel endoscopy, biopsy	624	828	1036	252
44363	Small bowel endoscopy	624	828	1038	236
44364	Small bowel endoscopy	715	949	1189	315
44365	Small bowel endoscopy	688	913	1143	300
44366	Small bowel endoscopy	839	1114	1395	368
44369	Small bowel endoscopy	863	1146	1435	396
44372	Small bowel endoscopy	832	1104	1383	374
44373	Small bowel endoscopy	825	1095	1371	309
44376	Small bowel endoscopy	969	1286	1610	322
44377	Small bowel endoscopy	1020	1353	1695	339
44378	Small bowel endoscopy	1207	1601	2006	430
44380	Small bowel endoscopy	379	503	630	120
44382	Small bowel endoscopy	436	578	724	145
44385	Endoscopy, bowel pouch	438	581	728	178
44386	Endoscopy, bowel pouch, biopsy	416	552	691	123
44388	Colon endoscopy	582	772	967	274
44389	Colonoscopy with biopsy	643	854	1069	248
44390	Colonoscopy for foreign body	651	864	1082	217
44391	Colonoscopy for bleeding	800	1061	1329	330
44392	Colonoscopy and polypectomy	768	1019	1277	317
44393	Colonoscopy, lesion removal	841	1116	1397	357
44394	Colonoscopy w/snare	785	1042	1305	336
44500	Intro, gastrointestinal tube	86	115	144	28

MC = Medicare Fee

Code	Short Description	50th	75th	90th	MC
44602	Suture, small intestine	1467	1947	2438	745
44603	Suture, small intestine	2128	2824	3536	939
44604	Suture, large intestine	1993	2645	3312	877
44605	Repair bowel lesion	2019	2679	3355	989
44615	Intestinal stricturoplasty	2010	2667	3340	825
44620	Repair bowel opening	1317	1748	2189	659
44625	Repair bowel opening	1919	2547	3190	930
44640	Repair bowel-skin fistula	1678	2227	2789	824
44650	Repair bowel fistula	1810	2403	3009	877
44660	Repair bowel-bladder fistula	1810	2402	3008	885
44661	Repair bowel-bladder fistula	2716	3605	4515	1254
44680	Surgical revision, intestine	2193	2911	3646	952

Meckel's Diverticulum and the Mesentery

Code	Short Description	50th	75th	90th	MC
44800	Excision of bowel pouch	1419	1883	2359	639
44820	Excision of mesentery lesion	1296	1720	2154	637
44850	Repair mesentery	1336	1773	2221	602

Appendix

Code	Short Description	50th	75th	90th	MC
44900	Drainage of appendix abscess	1142	1515	1897	507
44950	Appendectomy	1053	1398	1751	552
44955	Appendectomy	409	543	680	162
44960	Appendectomy	1301	1726	2162	659

Rectum

Code	Short Description	50th	75th	90th	MC
45000	Drainage of pelvic abscess	475	616	761	236
45005	Drainage of rectal abscess	305	395	489	135
45020	Drainage of rectal abscess	577	749	925	293
45100	Biopsy of rectum	457	594	733	218
45108	Remove anorectal lesion	874	1134	1402	291
45110	Remove rectum	3108	4035	4986	1623
45111	Partial removal of rectum	2362	3066	3788	1146
45112	Remove rectum	3598	4671	5772	1698
45113	Partial proctectomy	3903	5067	6261	1723
45114	Partial removal of rectum	3386	4395	5431	1559
45116	Partial removal of rectum	2687	3488	4310	1254
45120	Remove rectum	3689	4789	5918	1672

SURGERY SERVICES

Code	Short Description	50th	75th	90th	MC
45121	Remove rectum and colon	3317	4306	5321	1462
45123	Partial proctectomy	2380	3089	3817	1083
45130	Excision of rectal prolapse	1916	2487	3074	928
45135	Excision of rectal prolapse	3061	3974	4911	1374
45150	Excision of rectal stricture	965	1253	1548	362
45160	Excision of rectal lesion	2047	2658	3284	833
45170	Excision of rectal lesion	832	1080	1335	582
45190	Destruction, rectal tumor	1298	1685	2082	549
45300	Proctosigmoidoscopy	88	112	136	52
45303	Proctosigmoidoscopy	119	155	192	61
45305	Proctosigmoidoscopy; biopsy	174	226	279	78
45307	Proctosigmoidoscopy	291	378	468	124
45308	Proctosigmoidoscopy	265	344	425	111
45309	Proctosigmoidoscopy	315	409	505	130
45315	Proctosigmoidoscopy	342	444	548	152
45317	Proctosigmoidoscopy	366	475	587	162
45320	Proctosigmoidoscopy	383	497	614	199
45321	Proctosigmoidoscopy	357	464	573	151
45330	Sigmoidoscopy, diagnostic	173	224	276	75
45331	Sigmoidoscopy and biopsy	247	318	390	99
45332	Sigmoidoscopy	299	388	480	126
45333	Sigmoidoscopy and polypectomy	363	472	583	145
45334	Sigmoidoscopy for bleeding	440	571	706	192
45337	Sigmoidoscopy, decompression	452	587	726	189
45338	Sigmoidoscopy	392	508	628	164
45339	Sigmoidoscopy	496	644	796	218
45355	Surgical colonoscopy	428	555	686	152
45378	Diagnostic colonoscopy	684	866	1052	268
45379	Colonoscopy	903	1172	1448	342
45380	Colonoscopy and biopsy	762	975	1195	300
45382	Colonoscopy, control bleeding	874	1135	1403	390
45383	Colonoscopy, lesion removal	916	1189	1469	399
45384	Colonoscopy	909	1157	1410	391
45385	Colonoscopy, lesion removal	1013	1283	1560	410
45500	Repair rectum	1227	1593	1969	541
45505	Repair rectum	1263	1639	2025	516
45520	Treatment of rectal prolapse	101	131	162	41
45540	Correct rectal prolapse	2163	2807	3469	941
45541	Correct rectal prolapse	2054	2667	3295	868
45550	Repair rectum;remove sigmoid	2627	3410	4214	1206

MC = Medicare Fee

Code	Short Description	50th	75th	90th	MC
45560	Repair rectocele	1040	1350	1669	517
45562	Exploration/repair of rectum	1886	2448	3025	814
45563	Exploration/repair of rectum	2936	3812	4710	1284
45800	Repair rectum/bladder fistula	2259	2933	3624	941
45805	Repair fistula; colostomy	2610	3388	4187	1169
45820	Repair recto-urethral fistula	2241	2910	3595	918
45825	Repair fistula; colostomy	2514	3264	4033	1053
45900	Reduction of rectal prolapse	220	285	352	91
45905	Dilation of anal sphincter	194	252	311	91
45910	Dilation of rectal narrowing	228	296	366	111
45915	Remove rectal obstruction	240	311	384	94

Anus

Code	Short Description	50th	75th	90th	MC
46030	Remove rectal marker	103	136	168	64
46040	Incision of rectal abscess	393	519	645	249
46045	Incision of rectal abscess	399	528	656	238
46050	Incision of anal abscess	136	180	224	72
46060	Incision of rectal abscess	987	1305	1620	454
46070	Incision of anal septum	279	368	457	168
46080	Incision of anal sphincter	366	484	601	193
46083	Incise external hemorrhoid	114	151	187	66
46200	Remove anal fissure	592	782	971	275
46210	Remove anal crypt	227	301	373	132
46211	Remove anal crypts	597	789	980	246
46220	Remove anal tab	143	189	235	87
46221	Ligation of hemorrhoid(s)	166	219	272	85
46230	Remove anal tabs	185	245	305	134
46250	Hemorrhoidectomy	610	807	1002	299
46255	Hemorrhoidectomy	844	1116	1386	414
46257	Remove hemorrhoids and fissure	1066	1410	1751	479
46258	Remove hemorrhoids and fistula	1232	1629	2023	526
46260	Hemorrhoidectomy	1105	1461	1814	551
46261	Remove hemorrhoids and fissure	1155	1527	1896	612
46262	Remove hemorrhoids and fistula	1247	1649	2048	633
46270	Remove anal fistula	573	758	942	224
46275	Remove anal fistula	923	1221	1516	435
46280	Remove anal fistula	1091	1442	1791	511
46285	Remove anal fistula	382	505	627	257
46288	Repair anal fistula	1054	1393	1730	437

SURGERY SERVICES

Code	Short Description	50th	75th	90th	MC
46320	Remove hemorrhoid clot	149	197	245	93
46500	Injection into hemorrhoids	74	98	122	73
46600	Diagnostic anoscopy	55	72	89	26
46604	Anoscopy and dilation	133	176	218	67
46606	Anoscopy and biopsy	117	154	192	48
46608	Anoscopy;remove foreign body	205	271	337	87
46610	Anoscopy; remove lesion	194	256	318	91
46611	Anoscopy	258	341	423	109
46612	Anoscopy; remove lesions	292	386	480	153
46614	Anoscopy; control bleeding	262	347	431	149
46615	Anoscopy	421	557	691	174
46700	Repair anal stricture	1061	1403	1742	543
46705	Repair anal stricture	1004	1327	1648	419
46715	Repair ano-vaginal fistula	1205	1593	1978	430
46716	Repair ano-vaginal fistula	1553	2053	2550	740
46730	Construction of absent anus	2817	3725	4626	1314
46735	Construction of absent anus	3416	4517	5609	1594
46740	Construction of absent anus	2984	3946	4900	1412
46742	Repair, imperforated anus	4262	5637	6999	1933
46744	Repair, cloacal anomaly	4836	6395	7941	2170
46746	Repair, cloacal anomaly	5301	7010	8705	2374
46748	Repair, cloacal anomaly	5897	7798	9683	2645
46750	Repair anal sphincter	1236	1634	2029	572
46751	Repair anal sphincter	1234	1631	2026	498
46753	Reconstruction of anus	1313	1736	2155	469
46754	Remove suture from anus	293	388	482	130
46760	Repair anal sphincter	1595	2109	2618	735
46761	Repair anal sphincter	2018	2669	3314	717
46762	Implant artificial sphincter	2177	2879	3575	632
46900	Destruction, anal lesion(s)	111	147	183	86
46910	Destruction, anal lesion(s)	133	176	218	97
46916	Cryosurgery, anal lesion(s)	138	182	226	98
46917	Laser surgery,anal lesion(s)	288	381	473	160
46922	Excision of anal lesion(s)	214	283	351	130
46924	Destruction, anal lesion(s)	538	712	884	225
46934	Destruction of hemorrhoids	254	336	418	165
46935	Destruction of hemorrhoids	226	299	371	137
46936	Destruction of hemorrhoids	339	448	556	215
46937	Cryotherapy of rectal lesion	312	412	512	215
46938	Cryotherapy of rectal lesion	488	646	802	290

MC = Medicare Fee

Code	Short Description	50th	75th	90th	MC
46940	Treatment of anal fissure	196	259	321	111
46942	Treatment of anal fissure	210	277	344	98
46945	Ligation of hemorrhoids	196	260	322	102
46946	Ligation of hemorrhoids	320	423	525	149

Liver

Code	Short Description	50th	75th	90th	MC
47000	Needle biopsy of liver	302	418	536	111
47001	Needle biopsy, liver	241	334	428	134
47010	Drainage of liver lesion	1467	2028	2601	651
47015	Inject/aspirate liver cyst	1483	2050	2630	653
47100	Wedge biopsy of liver	990	1368	1755	416
47120	Partial removal of liver	3067	4239	5437	1344
47122	Extensive removal of liver	4450	6150	7888	2089
47125	Partial removal of liver	4209	5817	7461	1939
47130	Partial removal of liver	4481	6193	7944	2131
47133	Remove donor liver	5169	7144	9163	0
47134	Partial removal, donor liver	6199	8568	10990	2505
47135	Transplantation of liver	13076	18072	23181	5494
47136	Transplantation of liver	12618	17439	22369	4097
47300	Surgery for liver lesion	1744	2411	3092	708
47350	Repair liver wound	1760	2432	3120	791
47360	Repair liver wound	2408	3328	4269	1113
47361	Repair liver wound	4151	5737	7359	1791
47362	Repair liver wound	1492	2062	2645	640

Biliary Tract

Code	Short Description	50th	75th	90th	MC
47400	Incision of liver duct	2532	3263	4042	1115
47420	Incision of bile duct	2109	2718	3367	1045
47425	Incision of bile duct	2622	3380	4187	1136
47460	Incise bile duct sphincter	2485	3203	3968	1035
47480	Incision of gallbladder	1519	1958	2425	679
47490	Incision of gallbladder	716	923	1144	321
47500	Injection for liver x-rays	349	450	557	117
47505	Injection for liver x-rays	213	274	340	61
47510	Insert catheter, bile duct	692	892	1105	335
47511	Insert bile duct drain	948	1222	1513	413
47525	Change bile duct catheter	368	474	587	227
47530	Revise, reinsert bile tube	598	771	955	225

SURGERY SERVICES

Code	Short Description	50th	75th	90th	MC
47550	Bile duct endoscopy	496	640	793	192
47552	Biliary endoscopy, through skin	693	893	1106	291
47553	Biliary endoscopy, through skin	801	1033	1279	347
47554	Biliary endoscopy, through skin	1129	1455	1802	529
47555	Biliary endoscopy, through skin	893	1151	1425	334
47556	Biliary endoscopy, through skin	1068	1377	1705	365
47600	Remove gallbladder	1674	2157	2672	774
47605	Remove gallbladder	1813	2338	2895	838
47610	Remove gallbladder	2150	2771	3433	1029
47612	Remove gallbladder	2698	3478	4308	1262
47620	Remove gallbladder	2617	3374	4179	1150
47630	Remove bile duct stone	871	1122	1390	398
47700	Exploration of bile ducts	2090	2693	3336	894
47701	Bile duct revision	2825	3641	4510	1412
47711	Excision of bile duct tumor	2902	3741	4634	1277
47712	Excision of bile duct tumor	3665	4724	5852	1486
47715	Excision of bile duct cyst	2286	2946	3649	951
47716	Fusion of bile duct cyst	1942	2503	3101	802
47720	Fuse gallbladder and bowel	1889	2434	3015	901
47721	Fuse upper gi structures	2425	3126	3872	1110
47740	Fuse gallbladder and bowel	2176	2805	3475	1029
47741	Fuse gallbladder and bowel	2951	3804	4712	1321
47760	Fuse bile ducts and bowel	2524	3254	4030	1328
47765	Fuse liver ducts and bowel	2706	3488	4320	1435
47780	Fuse bile ducts and bowel	2895	3731	4622	1413
47785	Fuse bile ducts and bowel	3815	4918	6092	1564
47800	Reconstruction of bile ducts	2760	3557	4406	1306
47801	Placement, bile duct support	1485	1914	2370	681
47802	Fuse liver duct and intestine	2377	3064	3795	1094
47900	Suture bile duct injury	2735	3525	4366	1228

Pancreas

Code	Short Description	50th	75th	90th	MC
48000	Drainage of abdomen	1838	2369	2934	838
48001	Placement of drain, pancreas	2352	3031	3755	994
48005	Resect/debride pancreas	2297	2960	3667	1124
48020	Remove pancreatic stone	2211	2849	3529	830
48100	Biopsy of pancreas	1617	2084	2581	588
48102	Needle biopsy, pancreas	500	644	798	228
48120	Remove pancreas lesion	2106	2714	3362	963

MC = Medicare Fee

Code	Short Description	50th	75th	90th	MC
48140	Partial removal of pancreas	2701	3481	4312	1347
48145	Partial removal of pancreas	3068	3954	4898	1490
48146	Pancreatectomy	3626	4674	5790	1570
48148	Remove pancreatic duct	2308	2975	3685	947
48150	Partial removal of pancreas	4740	6109	7567	2630
48152	Pancreatectomy	4739	6108	7566	2489
48153	Pancreatectomy	5020	6471	8016	2630
48154	Pancreatectomy	4737	6106	7563	2489
48155	Remove pancreas	3601	4641	5749	1740
48160	Pancreas removal, transplant	4215	5433	6730	0
48180	Fuse pancreas and bowel	3121	4023	4983	1408
48400	Injection, intraoperative	275	355	440	104
48500	Surgery of pancreas cyst	1877	2419	2996	870
48510	Drain pancreatic pseudocyst	2090	2693	3336	789
48520	Fuse pancreas cyst and bowel	2240	2888	3577	1050
48540	Fuse pancreas cyst and bowel	2546	3282	4066	1219
48545	Pancreatorrhaphy	2215	2856	3537	937
48547	Duodenal exclusion	3148	4058	5026	1355
48554	Transplant allograft pancreas	4563	5882	7285	0
48556	Removal, allograft pancreas	1856	2392	2963	888

Abdomen, Peritoneum, and Omentum

Code	Short Description	50th	75th	90th	MC
49000	Exploration of abdomen	1376	1813	2291	749
49002	Reopening of abdomen	1273	1678	2120	650
49010	Exploration behind abdomen	1429	1883	2379	759
49020	Drain abdominal abscess	1101	1452	1834	770
49021	Drain abdominal abscess	929	1224	1547	475
49040	Drain abdominal abscess	1476	1945	2457	648
49060	Drain abdominal abscess	1247	1644	2077	665
49080	Puncture, peritoneal cavity	192	254	323	74
49081	Remove abdominal fluid	166	219	277	67
49085	Remove abdomen foreign body	1073	1414	1786	466
49180	Biopsy, abdominal mass	365	481	608	122
49200	Remove abdominal lesion	1605	2116	2674	758
49201	Remove abdominal lesion	2506	3303	4173	1109
49215	Excise sacral spine tumor	2363	3115	3936	1204
49220	Multiple surgery, abdomen	2651	3494	4415	1121
49250	Excision of umbilicus	1074	1416	1789	503
49255	Remove omentum	1156	1524	1926	643

SURGERY SERVICES

Code	Short Description	50th	75th	90th	MC
49400	Air injection into abdomen	203	267	337	123
49420	Insert abdominal drain	336	443	559	156
49421	Insert abdominal drain	765	1008	1273	386
49422	Remove perm cannula/catheter	812	1071	1353	422
49425	Insert abdomen-venous drain	1643	2166	2737	804
49426	Revise abdomen-venous shunt	1705	2247	2839	586
49427	Injection, abdominal shunt	203	267	337	45
49428	Ligation of shunt	407	537	678	127
49429	Remove shunt	1002	1321	1669	406
49495	Repair inguinal hernia	1263	1664	2103	460
49496	Repair inguinal hernia	1585	2090	2640	565
49500	Repair inguinal hernia	1006	1326	1676	409
49501	Repair inguinal hernia	1339	1766	2231	523
49505	Repair inguinal hernia	1108	1427	1776	455
49507	Repair inguinal hernia	1185	1562	1974	529
49520	Re-repair inguinal hernia	1297	1709	2160	555
49521	Repair inguinal hernia	1532	2020	2552	605
49525	Repair inguinal hernia	1183	1559	1970	537
49540	Repair lumbar hernia	1316	1735	2192	556
49550	Repair femoral hernia	1084	1430	1806	490
49553	Repair femoral hernia	1303	1718	2170	507
49555	Repair femoral hernia	1316	1734	2191	574
49557	Repair femoral hernia	1637	2158	2726	628
49560	Repair abdominal hernia	1371	1808	2284	636
49561	Repair incisional hernia	1640	2162	2732	708
49565	Re-repair abdominal hernia	1436	1893	2391	674
49566	Repair incisional hernia	1767	2330	2944	745
49568	Hernia repair w/mesh	469	618	780	313
49570	Repair epigastric hernia	788	1039	1313	384
49572	Repair epigastric hernia	992	1308	1653	479
49580	Repair umbilical hernia	834	1099	1389	330
49582	Repair umbilical hernia	1164	1534	1939	420
49585	Repair umbilical hernia	953	1256	1586	404
49587	Repair umbilical hernia	1208	1592	2012	441
49590	Repair abdominal hernia	1193	1572	1986	527
49600	Repair umbilical lesion	1369	1804	2279	603
49605	Repair umbilical lesion	2871	3784	4781	1247
49606	Repair umbilical lesion	2389	3149	3979	1053
49610	Repair umbilical lesion	1513	1995	2520	646
49611	Repair umbilical lesion	1553	2047	2586	702

MC = Medicare Fee

Code	Short Description	50th	75th	90th	MC
49900	Repair abdominal wall	830	1094	1382	534
49905	Omental flap	1325	1746	2206	419

URINARY SYSTEM SURGERY

Kidney

Code	Short Description	50th	75th	90th	MC
50010	Exploration of kidney	1635	2123	2615	816
50020	Drainage of kidney abscess	1428	1854	2284	779
50040	Drainage of kidney	1722	2235	2754	692
50045	Exploration of kidney	1906	2475	3049	982
50060	Remove kidney stone	2180	2830	3486	1227
50065	Incision of kidney	2595	3369	4150	1363
50070	Incision of kidney	2551	3311	4079	1302
50075	Remove kidney stone	2886	3746	4616	1661
50080	Remove kidney stone	2178	2827	3483	1072
50081	Remove kidney stone	2792	3624	4465	1445
50100	Revise kidney blood vessels	1823	2366	2915	1046
50120	Exploration of kidney	2007	2606	3210	1061
50125	Explore and drain kidney	2023	2626	3235	1078
50130	Remove kidney stone	2152	2793	3441	1181
50135	Exploration of kidney	2651	3442	4240	1446
50200	Biopsy of kidney	433	563	693	177
50205	Biopsy of kidney	1075	1396	1720	654
50220	Remove kidney	2289	2972	3661	1204
50225	Remove kidney	2610	3388	4174	1457
50230	Remove kidney	3080	3998	4926	1601
50234	Remove kidney and ureter	2785	3615	4453	1542
50236	Remove kidney and ureter	2928	3801	4683	1674
50240	Partial removal of kidney	2693	3496	4307	1485
50280	Remove kidney lesion	1841	2390	2944	1042
50290	Remove kidney lesion	1744	2263	2789	926
50300	Remove donor kidney	2861	3714	4576	0
50320	Remove donor kidney	3093	4015	4947	1571
50340	Remove kidney	2256	2929	3608	1006
50360	Transplantation of kidney	4749	6165	7595	2191
50365	Transplantation of kidney	5224	6782	8356	2639
50370	Remove transplanted kidney	2205	2863	3527	950
50380	Re-implantation of kidney	3116	4045	4983	1104
50390	Drainage of kidney lesion	326	423	521	123

SURGERY SERVICES

Code	Short Description	50th	75th	90th	MC
50392	Insert kidney drain	548	712	877	192
50393	Insert ureteral tube	579	752	927	240
50394	Injection for kidney x-ray	137	178	220	44
50395	Create passage to kidney	662	859	1058	227
50396	Measure kidney pressure	109	142	175	83
50398	Change kidney tube	168	219	269	79
50400	Revision of kidney/ureter	2448	3178	3916	1294
50405	Revision of kidney/ureter	2877	3735	4601	1623
50500	Repair kidney wound	2302	2988	3681	1264
50520	Close kidney-skin fistula	2235	2901	3574	1083
50525	Repair renal-abdomen fistula	2559	3322	4093	1371
50526	Repair renal-abdomen fistula	2469	3205	3949	1230
50540	Revision of horseshoe kidney	2775	3602	4438	1332
50551	Kidney endoscopy	591	768	946	309
50553	Kidney endoscopy	581	754	929	300
50555	Kidney endoscopy and biopsy	720	935	1152	456
50557	Kidney endoscopy and treatment	707	918	1131	462
50559	Renal endoscopy; radio tracer	648	842	1037	315
50561	Kidney endoscopy and treatment	845	1097	1351	515
50570	Kidney endoscopy	827	1073	1322	423
50572	Kidney endoscopy	1133	1471	1813	716
50574	Kidney endoscopy and biopsy	1190	1544	1903	730
50575	Kidney endoscopy	1653	2145	2643	972
50576	Kidney endoscopy and treatment	1238	1607	1979	800
50578	Renal endoscopy; radio tracer	1142	1482	1826	630
50580	Kidney endoscopy and treatment	1154	1498	1845	606
50590	Fragmenting of kidney stone	2484	3225	3973	784

Ureter

Code	Short Description	50th	75th	90th	MC
50600	Exploration of ureter	1854	2404	2981	993
50605	Insert ureteral support	1606	2082	2582	816
50610	Remove ureter stone	1994	2585	3206	1088
50620	Remove ureter stone	1899	2461	3052	1050
50630	Remove ureter stone	2037	2641	3275	1096
50650	Remove ureter	2077	2693	3340	1159
50660	Remove ureter	2556	3314	4110	1267
50684	Injection for ureter x-ray	89	115	142	51
50686	Measure ureter pressure	93	120	149	74
50688	Change of ureter tube	95	123	152	60

MC = Medicare Fee

Code	Short Description	50th	75th	90th	MC
50690	Injection for ureter x-ray	82	106	131	58
50700	Revision of ureter	1996	2587	3208	1097
50715	Release of ureter	1938	2513	3116	1182
50722	Release of ureter	1667	2161	2680	1071
50725	Release/revise ureter	2424	3142	3896	1208
50727	Revise ureter	1226	1589	1971	525
50728	Revise ureter	1527	1980	2455	773
50740	Fusion of ureter and kidney	2272	2945	3652	1254
50750	Fusion of ureter and kidney	2467	3198	3966	1308
50760	Fusion of ureters	2349	3044	3776	1255
50770	Splicing of ureters	2487	3224	3998	1368
50780	Re-implant ureter in bladder	2271	2944	3651	1267
50782	Re-implant ureter in bladder	2535	3286	4076	1309
50783	Re-implant ureter in bladder	2639	3421	4242	1344
50785	Re-implant ureter in bladder	2506	3248	4029	1425
50800	Implant ureter in bowel	2200	2852	3537	1155
50810	Fusion of ureter and bowel	2848	3692	4579	1268
50815	Urine shunt to bowel	2858	3705	4595	1603
50820	Construct bowel bladder	2957	3832	4753	1636
50825	Construct bowel bladder	3973	5150	6386	2371
50830	Revise urine flow	4243	5499	6820	2050
50840	Replace ureter by bowel	2751	3566	4423	1282
50845	Appendico-vesicostomy	2710	3513	4356	1357
50860	Transplant ureter to skin	1850	2398	2974	1020
50900	Repair ureter	1899	2462	3054	928
50920	Closure ureter/skin fistula	1896	2458	3048	927
50930	Closure ureter/bowel fistula	2310	2994	3713	1223
50940	Release of ureter	1466	1900	2357	950
50951	Endoscopy of ureter	373	484	600	295
50953	Endoscopy of ureter	403	523	649	309
50955	Ureter endoscopy and biopsy	457	592	734	368
50957	Ureter endoscopy and treatment	465	603	747	368
50959	Ureter endoscopy and tracer	407	527	654	316
50961	Ureter endoscopy and treatment	469	608	754	345
50970	Ureter endoscopy	572	741	919	501
50972	Ureter endoscopy and catheter	427	554	687	328
50974	Ureter endoscopy and biopsy	735	953	1182	658
50976	Ureter endoscopy and treatment	709	919	1139	627
50978	Ureter endoscopy and tracer	472	611	758	377
50980	Ureter endoscopy and treatment	493	639	792	398

SURGERY SERVICES

Code	Short Description	50th	75th	90th	MC
Bladder					
51000	Drainage of bladder	76	100	125	51
51005	Drainage of bladder	74	97	122	59
51010	Drainage of bladder	229	299	375	140
51020	Incise and treat bladder	1201	1566	1966	537
51030	Incise and treat bladder	1143	1491	1871	430
51040	Incise and drain bladder	1034	1349	1692	398
51045	Incise bladder, drain ureter	913	1192	1495	451
51050	Remove bladder stone	1169	1525	1913	547
51060	Remove ureter stone	1838	2398	3009	773
51065	Remove ureter stone	1617	2110	2647	621
51080	Drainage of bladder abscess	813	1061	1331	439
51500	Remove bladder cyst	1358	1772	2223	689
51520	Remove bladder lesion	1442	1881	2361	711
51525	Remove bladder lesion	1929	2517	3159	960
51530	Remove bladder lesion	1542	2012	2524	846
51535	Repair ureter lesion	1507	1967	2468	794
51550	Partial removal of bladder	1727	2253	2827	1025
51555	Partial removal of bladder	2155	2812	3528	1292
51565	Revise bladder and ureter(s)	2553	3330	4179	1469
51570	Remove bladder	2784	3632	4557	1540
51575	Remove bladder and nodes	3843	5014	6292	2078
51580	Remove bladder; revise tract	3780	4932	6189	1960
51585	Remove bladder and nodes	4426	5775	7247	2338
51590	Remove bladder; revise tract	4393	5732	7192	2244
51595	Remove bladder; revise tract	4982	6500	8156	2808
51596	Remove bladder; create pouch	5433	7088	8895	2933
51597	Remove pelvic structures	5105	6660	8357	2756
51600	Injection for bladder x-ray	72	94	118	46
51605	Preparation for bladder x-ray	72	94	118	38
51610	Injection for bladder x-ray	87	114	143	51
51700	Irrigation of bladder	49	63	78	43
51705	Change of bladder tube	74	96	121	54
51710	Change of bladder tube	166	217	272	81
51715	Endoscopic injection/implant	561	732	919	260
51720	Treatment of bladder lesion	97	121	147	94
51725	Simple cystometrogram	155	210	272	103
51726	Complex cystometrogram	193	262	340	122
51736	Urine flow measurement	64	87	113	41

MC = Medicare Fee

Code	Short Description	50th	75th	90th	MC
51741	Electro-uroflowmetry; first	104	135	170	68
51772	Urethra pressure profile	183	248	322	103
51784	Anal/urinary muscle study	181	244	317	105
51785	Anal/urinary muscle study	172	232	302	105
51792	Urinary reflex study	249	337	437	129
51795	Urine voiding pressure study	172	232	302	123
51797	Intra-abdominal pressure test	179	242	315	104
51800	Revision of bladder/urethra	2112	2704	3325	1165
51820	Revision of urinary tract	2602	3330	4096	983
51840	Attach bladder/urethra	1489	1906	2345	797
51841	Attach bladder/urethra	1867	2389	2939	966
51845	Repair bladder neck	1633	2090	2570	824
51860	Repair bladder wound	1445	1849	2275	769
51865	Repair bladder wound	1879	2405	2958	1026
51880	Repair bladder opening	795	1018	1252	495
51900	Repair bladder/vagina lesion	2428	3108	3823	973
51920	Close bladder-uterus fistula	1727	2210	2718	735
51925	Hysterectomy/bladder repair	2352	3011	3703	1038
51940	Correction of bladder defect	3657	4681	5757	1806
51960	Revision of bladder and bowel	3155	4038	4966	1764
51980	Construct bladder opening	1669	2137	2628	728
52000	Cystoscopy	247	312	377	136
52005	Cystoscopy and ureter catheter	389	500	611	188
52007	Cystoscopy and biopsy	437	561	685	240
52010	Cystoscopy and duct catheter	326	419	511	199
52204	Cystoscopy	401	515	629	196
52214	Cystoscopy and treatment	514	660	806	266
52224	Cystoscopy and treatment	458	589	718	249
52234	Cystoscopy and treatment	705	905	1104	385
52235	Cystoscopy and treatment	1189	1528	1863	523
52240	Cystoscopy and treatment	1723	2213	2699	844
52250	Cystoscopy and radio tracer	476	612	746	298
52260	Cystoscopy and treatment	401	515	628	243
52265	Cystoscopy and treatment	305	392	478	171
52270	Cystoscopy and revise urethra	504	647	789	283
52275	Cystoscopy and revise urethra	557	715	872	331
52276	Cystoscopy and treatment	797	1024	1249	394
52277	Cystoscopy and treatment	868	1115	1360	448
52281	Cystoscopy and treatment	382	484	584	209
52283	Cystoscopy and treatment	351	451	550	208
52285	Cystoscopy and treatment	430	552	673	268

SURGERY SERVICES

Code	Short Description	50th	75th	90th	MC
52290	Cystoscopy and treatment	454	583	711	278
52300	Cystoscopy and treatment	639	820	1001	356
52301	Cystoscopy and treatment	567	729	889	364
52305	Cystoscopy and treatment	673	865	1055	357
52310	Cystoscopy and treatment	469	602	734	240
52315	Cystoscopy and treatment	701	901	1099	379
52317	Remove bladder stone	1002	1286	1569	530
52318	Remove bladder stone	1311	1684	2054	699
52320	Cystoscopy and treatment	833	1070	1305	395
52325	Cystoscopy, stone removal	1033	1327	1619	546
52327	Cystoscopy, inject material	628	806	983	361
52330	Cystoscopy and treatment	630	809	987	346
52332	Cystoscopy and treatment	573	736	898	251
52334	Create passage to kidney	669	859	1048	332
52335	Endoscopy of urinary tract	971	1247	1522	431
52336	Cystoscopy, stone removal	1550	1991	2428	660
52337	Cystoscopy, stone removal	1872	2404	2932	762
52338	Cystoscopy and treatment	1315	1689	2060	542
52339	Cystoscopy and treatment	1326	1704	2078	597
52340	Cystoscopy and treatment	1001	1285	1568	569
52450	Incision of prostate	1070	1374	1676	489
52500	Revision of bladder neck	1161	1491	1818	628
52510	Dilation prostatic urethra	1172	1506	1836	570
52601	Prostatectomy (TURP)	1950	2492	3030	966
52606	Control post-op bleeding	550	706	862	432
52612	Prostatectomy, first stage	1856	2384	2907	675
52614	Prostatectomy, second stage	848	1089	1329	545
52620	Remove residual prostate	930	1194	1457	466
52630	Remove prostate regrowth	1686	2165	2641	636
52640	Relieve bladder contracture	971	1247	1522	516
52647	Laser surgery of prostate	1574	2022	2466	903
52648	Laser surgery of prostate	1700	2184	2664	935
52700	Drainage of prostate abscess	788	1012	1235	386

Urethra

Code	Short Description	50th	75th	90th	MC
53000	Incision of urethra	267	331	398	155
53010	Incision of urethra	562	696	837	273
53020	Incision of urethra	192	237	285	104
53025	Incision of urethra	103	127	153	78

MC = Medicare Fee

Code	Short Description	50th	75th	90th	MC
53040	Drainage of urethra abscess	411	509	612	309
53060	Drainage of urethra abscess	169	209	251	121
53080	Drainage of urinary leakage	530	657	789	402
53085	Drainage of urinary leakage	1301	1612	1938	668
53200	Biopsy of urethra	239	297	357	147
53210	Remove urethra	1382	1713	2058	739
53215	Remove urethra	1826	2262	2719	997
53220	Treatment of urethra lesion	957	1186	1425	463
53230	Remove urethra lesion	1268	1571	1888	697
53235	Remove urethra lesion	1166	1445	1737	484
53240	Surgery for urethra pouch	558	692	832	422
53250	Remove urethra gland	639	791	951	396
53260	Treatment of urethra lesion	213	264	317	162
53265	Treatment of urethra lesion	302	374	450	201
53270	Remove urethra gland	233	288	347	152
53275	Repair urethra defect	401	496	597	271
53400	Revise urethra, 1st stage	1208	1497	1799	780
53405	Revise urethra, 2nd stage	1575	1952	2345	989
53410	Reconstruction of urethra	1681	2083	2503	971
53415	Reconstruction of urethra	2270	2813	3381	1228
53420	Reconstruct urethra, stage 1	1911	2368	2846	987
53425	Reconstruct urethra, stage 2	1919	2378	2858	985
53430	Reconstruction of urethra	1525	1890	2271	908
53440	Correct bladder function	1946	2412	2899	1027
53442	Remove perineal prosthesis	727	901	1083	555
53443	Reconstruction of urethra	2137	2649	3183	1168
53445	Correct urine flow control	2891	3582	4305	1266
53447	Remove artificial sphincter	1244	1542	1853	876
53449	Correct artificial sphincter	1102	1366	1641	722
53450	Revision of urethra	497	616	740	338
53460	Revision of urethra	550	682	820	362
53502	Repair urethra injury	981	1215	1460	497
53505	Repair urethra injury	979	1213	1457	504
53510	Repair urethra injury	1308	1621	1948	672
53515	Repair urethra injury	1846	2288	2749	883
53520	Repair urethra defect	784	972	1168	573
53600	Dilate urethra stricture	70	87	104	60
53601	Dilate urethra stricture	61	76	91	50
53605	Dilate urethra stricture	154	191	229	69
53620	Dilate urethra stricture	113	140	168	82
53621	Dilate urethra stricture	77	95	115	68

SURGERY SERVICES

Code	Short Description	50th	75th	90th	MC
53660	Dilation of urethra	53	65	77	39
53661	Dilation of urethra	47	57	68	39
53665	Dilation of urethra	106	131	158	45
53670	Insert urinary catheter	40	51	63	29
53675	Insert urinary catheter	90	111	134	77

MALE GENITAL SYSTEM SURGERY

Penis

Code	Short Description	50th	75th	90th	MC
54000	Slitting of prepuce	110	147	190	85
54001	Slitting of prepuce	182	243	315	118
54015	Drain penis lesion	275	368	476	231
54050	Destruction, penis lesion(s)	77	103	134	61
54055	Destruction, penis lesion(s)	114	153	197	72
54056	Cryosurgery, penis lesion(s)	111	149	193	68
54057	Laser surgery, penis lesion(s)	233	312	403	116
54060	Excision of penis lesion(s)	212	283	366	123
54065	Destruction, penis lesion(s)	359	480	621	200
54100	Biopsy of penis	146	196	253	101
54105	Biopsy of penis	226	303	391	175
54110	Treatment of penis lesion	962	1287	1664	635
54111	Treat penis lesion, graft	1695	2266	2931	905
54112	Treat penis lesion, graft	1960	2621	3390	1059
54115	Treatment of penis lesion	614	821	1063	403
54120	Partial removal of penis	1090	1457	1885	637
54125	Remove penis	1936	2588	3348	1002
54130	Remove penis and nodes	2698	3606	4665	1365
54135	Remove penis and nodes	3339	4464	5774	1738
54150	Circumcision	121	162	209	91
54152	Circumcision	236	316	409	168
54160	Circumcision	199	267	345	168
54161	Circumcision	432	577	747	219
54200	Treatment of penis lesion	71	94	122	52
54205	Treatment of penis lesion	708	947	1225	500
54220	Treatment of penis lesion	242	324	419	163
54230	Prepare penis study	171	229	296	111
54231	Dynamic cavernosometry	342	457	591	141
54235	Penile injection	125	167	216	64
54240	Penis study	142	190	246	95

MC = Medicare Fee

Code	Short Description	50th	75th	90th	MC
54250	Penis study	161	215	279	119
54300	Revision of penis	1000	1337	1729	695
54304	Revision of penis	1473	1969	2547	847
54308	Reconstruction of urethra	1426	1906	2465	704
54312	Reconstruction of urethra	1692	2262	2926	915
54316	Reconstruction of urethra	1955	2614	3381	1110
54318	Reconstruction of urethra	1181	1578	2041	747
54322	Reconstruction of urethra	1360	1818	2351	806
54324	Reconstruction of urethra	1678	2244	2902	1075
54326	Reconstruction of urethra	1769	2365	3059	1029
54328	Revise penis, urethra	2068	2764	3575	1046
54332	Revise penis, urethra	2226	2976	3849	1166
54336	Revise penis, urethra	2703	3614	4674	1539
54340	Secondary urethral surgery	1107	1480	1915	594
54344	Secondary urethral surgery	1905	2547	3294	1297
54348	Secondary urethral surgery	2052	2743	3548	1138
54352	Reconstruct urethra, penis	3184	4256	5505	1619
54360	Penis plastic surgery	1046	1399	1809	745
54380	Repair penis	1224	1636	2116	889
54385	Repair penis	1518	2030	2626	1019
54390	Repair penis and bladder	1872	2502	3236	1408
54400	Insert semi-rigid prosthesis	1718	2297	2972	824
54401	Insert self-contained prosthesis	1874	2505	3240	941
54402	Remove penis prosthesis	946	1264	1635	595
54405	Insert multi-comp prosthesis	3067	4100	5303	1223
54407	Remove multi-comp prosthesis	1667	2228	2882	978
54409	Revise penis prosthesis	1257	1681	2174	836
54420	Revision of penis	1317	1761	2277	756
54430	Revision of penis	1259	1683	2177	673
54435	Revision of penis	563	753	974	397
54450	Preputial stretching	124	165	214	73

Testis

Code	Short Description	50th	75th	90th	MC
54500	Biopsy of testis	85	112	139	69
54505	Biopsy of testis	350	463	573	213
54510	Remove testis lesion	620	819	1013	336
54520	Remove testis	796	1052	1302	424
54530	Remove testis	1123	1484	1836	633
54535	Extensive testis surgery	1368	1808	2237	821

SURGERY SERVICES

Code	Short Description	50th	75th	90th	MC
54550	Exploration for testis	891	1177	1456	516
54560	Exploration for testis	1247	1647	2038	722
54600	Reduce testis torsion	928	1226	1517	456
54620	Suspension of testis	486	642	795	326
54640	Suspension of testis	1150	1520	1880	604
54650	Suspension of testis	1612	2131	2636	768
54660	Revision of testis	490	647	800	333
54670	Repair testis injury	817	1080	1337	421
54680	Relocation of testis	1204	1591	1968	801

Epididymis

Code	Short Description	50th	75th	90th	MC
54700	Drainage of scrotum	244	322	399	168
54800	Biopsy of epididymis	192	254	314	176
54820	Exploration of epididymis	570	753	931	296
54830	Remove epididymis lesion	631	833	1031	350
54840	Remove epididymis lesion	801	1059	1310	406
54860	Remove epididymis	832	1100	1361	458
54861	Remove epididymis	1194	1577	1951	649
54900	Fusion of spermatic ducts	1718	2271	2810	876
54901	Fusion of spermatic ducts	2489	3289	4070	1202

Tunica Vaginalis

Code	Short Description	50th	75th	90th	MC
55000	Drainage of hydrocele	79	104	129	72
55040	Remove hydrocele	813	1075	1330	416
55041	Remove hydroceles	1202	1588	1965	616
55060	Repair hydrocele	676	894	1106	385

Scrotum

Code	Short Description	50th	75th	90th	MC
55100	Drainage of scrotum abscess	134	177	219	105
55110	Explore scrotum	610	807	998	356
55120	Remove scrotum lesion	354	467	578	261
55150	Remove scrotum	693	915	1132	495
55175	Revision of scrotum	796	1052	1301	389
55180	Revision of scrotum	1264	1671	2067	692
55200	Incision of sperm duct	403	533	659	244
55250	Remove sperm duct(s)	445	588	727	240
55300	Preparation, sperm duct x-ray	413	546	676	254

MC = Medicare Fee

Code	Short Description	50th	75th	90th	MC
55400	Repair sperm duct	1537	2031	2513	604
55450	Ligation of sperm duct	308	407	504	267

Spermatic Cord

55500	Remove hydrocele	688	910	1126	396
55520	Remove sperm cord lesion	642	849	1050	364
55530	Revise spermatic cord veins	835	1104	1365	442
55535	Revise spermatic cord veins	917	1212	1500	433
55540	Revise hernia and sperm veins	963	1273	1575	496

Seminal Vesicles

55600	Incise sperm duct pouch	760	1004	1242	427
55605	Incise sperm duct pouch	1118	1477	1827	539
55650	Remove sperm duct pouch	1811	2393	2961	750
55680	Remove sperm pouch lesion	1356	1792	2217	378

Prostate

55700	Biopsy of prostate	275	359	442	127
55705	Biopsy of prostate	741	980	1212	318
55720	Drainage of prostate abscess	849	1121	1388	442
55725	Drainage of prostate abscess	1272	1681	2080	542
55801	Remove prostate	2151	2509	2884	1192
55810	Extensive prostate surgery	2919	3404	3913	1602
55812	Extensive prostate surgery	3138	3659	4207	1767
55815	Extensive prostate surgery	3930	4582	5268	2201
55821	Remove prostate	2080	2426	2789	1100
55831	Remove prostate	2189	2552	2934	1192
55840	Extensive prostate surgery	2877	3355	3857	1543
55842	Extensive prostate surgery	3208	3741	4302	1714
55845	Extensive prostate surgery	3711	4328	4975	2132
55859	Place needles/catheter, prostate	1400	1633	1878	716
55860	Surgical exposure, prostate	1441	1681	1932	821
55862	Extensive prostate surgery	2033	2370	2725	1170
55865	Extensive prostate surgery	3199	3731	4289	1915
55870	Electroejaculation	195	228	262	148

SURGERY SERVICES

Code	Short Description	50th	75th	90th	MC
LAPAROSCOPY AND HYSTEROSCOPY					
56300	Pelvis laparoscopy, diagnostic	909	1194	1465	357
56301	Laparoscopy; tubal cautery	987	1296	1590	384
56302	Laparoscopy; tubal block	1048	1377	1690	424
56303	Laparoscopy; excise lesions	1113	1461	1794	488
56304	Laparoscopy; lysis	1209	1587	1948	443
56305	Pelvic laparoscopy; biopsy	1047	1375	1687	382
56306	Laparoscopy; aspiration	999	1312	1610	391
56307	Laparoscopy; remove adnexa	1580	2074	2546	760
56308	Laparoscopy; hysterectomy	2551	3350	4112	990
56309	Laparoscopy; remove myoma	1411	1853	2274	755
56311	Laparoscopic lymph node biopsy	1387	1822	2236	657
56312	Laparoscopic lymphadenectomy	1961	2575	3161	838
56313	Laparoscopic lymphadenectomy	2281	2995	3676	1030
56315	Laparoscopic appendectomy	1106	1452	1782	552
56316	Laparoscopic hernia repair	1091	1432	1758	455
56317	Laparoscopic hernia repair	1202	1578	1937	555
56320	Laparoscopy, spermatic veins	917	1204	1478	433
56322	Laparoscopy, vagus nerves	1456	1911	2346	620
56323	Laparoscopy, vagus nerves	2113	2775	3406	745
56324	Laparoscopy, cholecystoenterostomy	2132	2799	3436	901
56340	Laparoscopic cholecystectomy	1979	2670	3330	800
56341	Laparoscopic cholecystectomy	2128	2822	3484	854
56342	Laparoscopic cholecystectomy	2249	2953	3625	986
56343	Laparoscopic salpingostomy	1178	1546	1898	763
56344	Laparoscopic fimbrioplasty	1190	1562	1918	728
56350	Hysteroscopy; diagnostic	517	679	833	189
56351	Hysteroscopy; biopsy	962	1263	1550	207
56352	Hysteroscopy; lysis	745	978	1200	307
56353	Hysteroscopy; resect septum	831	1091	1339	321
56354	Hysteroscopy; remove myoma	969	1273	1562	400
56355	Hysteroscopy; remove impact	731	960	1178	216
56356	Hysteroscopy; ablation	1458	1914	2349	370
56362	Laparoscopy with cholangiography	618	812	996	305
56363	Laparoscopy with biopsy	734	964	1183	374

MC = Medicare Fee

Code	Short Description	50th	75th	90th	MC

FEMALE GENITAL SYSTEM SURGERY

Vulva, Perineum and Introitus

Code	Short Description	50th	75th	90th	MC
56405	I & D of vulva/perineum	205	279	363	89
56420	Drainage of gland abscess	152	207	270	88
56440	Surgery for vulva lesion	490	670	870	234
56441	Lysis of labial lesion(s)	226	309	401	152
56501	Destruction, vulva lesion(s)	151	206	268	82
56515	Destruction, vulva lesion(s)	513	701	912	193
56605	Biopsy of vulva/perineum	150	205	266	75
56606	Biopsy of vulva/perineum	86	117	152	38
56620	Partial removal of vulva	1274	1740	2262	573
56625	Complete removal of vulva	1674	2287	2973	756
56630	Extensive vulva surgery	2063	2819	3665	1079
56631	Extensive vulva surgery	2757	3766	4896	1498
56632	Extensive vulva surgery	3205	4379	5693	1759
56633	Extensive vulva surgery	2417	3302	4293	1352
56634	Extensive vulva surgery	3071	4195	5454	1664
56637	Extensive vulva surgery	3382	4621	6007	1826
56640	Extensive vulva surgery	3445	4706	6118	1750
56700	Partial removal of hymen	371	507	659	180
56720	Incision of hymen	125	171	222	50
56740	Remove vagina gland lesion	548	749	974	275
56800	Repair vagina	569	777	1011	283
56805	Repair clitoris	1755	2398	3117	1213
56810	Repair perineum	590	807	1049	277

Vagina

Code	Short Description	50th	75th	90th	MC
57000	Exploration of vagina	478	653	849	207
57010	Drainage of pelvic abscess	633	865	1125	333
57020	Drainage of pelvic fluid	132	181	235	89
57061	Destruction vagina lesion(s)	160	218	284	86
57065	Destruction vagina lesion(s)	537	733	954	261
57100	Biopsy of vagina	124	170	221	67
57105	Biopsy of vagina	230	314	408	139
57108	Partial removal of vagina	1048	1432	1862	475
57110	Remove vagina	1676	2290	2977	901
57120	Closure of vagina	1332	1819	2365	601

SURGERY SERVICES

Code	Short Description	50th	75th	90th	MC
57130	Remove vagina lesion	524	715	930	220
57135	Remove vagina lesion	454	620	806	194
57150	Treat vagina infection	55	75	97	30
57160	Insertion of pessary/device	67	88	111	46
57170	Fitting of diaphragm/cap	95	130	169	50
57180	Treat vaginal bleeding	157	215	279	85
57200	Repair vagina	638	871	1133	274
57210	Repair vagina/perineum	738	1008	1311	338
57220	Revision of urethra	808	1103	1434	360
57230	Repair urethral lesion	782	1069	1389	374
57240	Repair bladder and vagina	1011	1381	1795	551
57250	Repair rectum and vagina	985	1346	1750	516
57260	Repair vagina	1370	1872	2433	716
57265	Extensive repair of vagina	1603	2190	2848	873
57268	Repair bowel bulge	1165	1592	2070	580
57270	Repair bowel pouch	1397	1908	2481	763
57280	Suspension of vagina	1625	2220	2887	955
57282	Repair vaginal prolapse	1535	2097	2726	737
57284	Repair paravaginal defect	1838	2511	3264	841
57288	Repair bladder defect	1888	2579	3353	958
57289	Repair bladder and vagina	1435	1961	2549	787
57291	Construction of vagina	1818	2484	3229	548
57292	Construct vagina with graft	2531	3458	4496	788
57300	Repair rectum-vagina fistula	1426	1948	2533	648
57305	Repair rectum-vagina fistula	1765	2411	3135	852
57307	Fistula repair and colostomy	1893	2587	3363	869
57310	Repair urethrovaginal lesion	1283	1753	2279	426
57311	Repair urethrovaginal lesion	1583	2162	2811	517
57320	Repair bladder-vagina lesion	1582	2161	2810	715
57330	Repair bladder-vagina lesion	1788	2442	3175	811
57335	Repair vagina	2322	3172	4124	992
57400	Dilation of vagina	168	229	298	101
57410	Pelvic examination	152	208	271	83
57415	Removal vaginal foreign body	175	238	310	96
57452	Examination of vagina	174	237	309	70
57454	Vagina examination and biopsy	247	338	439	108
57460	Cervix excision	509	696	905	208

MC = Medicare Fee

Code	Short Description	50th	75th	90th	MC
Cervix Uteri					
57500	Biopsy of cervix	134	176	219	65
57505	Endocervical curettage	138	181	225	72
57510	Cauterization of cervix	135	178	221	94
57511	Cryocautery of cervix	185	242	301	111
57513	Laser surgery of cervix	449	589	731	194
57520	Conization of cervix	755	991	1231	320
57522	Conization of cervix	585	767	953	294
57530	Remove cervix	693	909	1129	346
57540	Remove residual cervix	1380	1811	2250	771
57545	Remove cervix, repair pelvis	1501	1969	2446	692
57550	Remove residual cervix	1257	1649	2049	505
57555	Remove cervix, repair vagina	1727	2265	2814	808
57556	Remove cervix, repair bowel	1658	2175	2702	749
57700	Revision of cervix	742	973	1210	236
57720	Revision of cervix	603	790	982	279
57800	Dilation of cervical canal	101	133	165	53
57820	D & C of residual cervix	425	557	692	165
Corpus Uteri					
58100	Biopsy of uterus lining	140	184	228	59
58120	Dilation and curettage (D & C)	593	778	967	243
58140	Remove uterus lesion	1609	2110	2622	929
58145	Remove uterus lesion	1290	1691	2101	677
58150	Total hysterectomy	2147	2816	3499	1014
58152	Total hysterectomy	2570	3371	4188	1127
58180	Partial hysterectomy	1829	2398	2980	1023
58200	Extensive hysterectomy	2869	3763	4676	1410
58210	Extensive hysterectomy	4209	5520	6858	1919
58240	Remove pelvis contents	5473	7178	8919	2753
58260	Vaginal hysterectomy	2065	2708	3365	897
58262	Vaginal hysterectomy	2108	2764	3435	960
58263	Vaginal hysterectomy	2457	3223	4004	1050
58267	Hysterectomy and vagina repair	2489	3265	4057	1097
58270	Hysterectomy and vagina repair	2282	2993	3719	987
58275	Hysterectomy, revise vagina	2384	3127	3885	1072
58280	Hysterectomy, revise vagina	2409	3159	3925	1063
58285	Extensive hysterectomy	2766	3628	4508	1241

SURGERY SERVICES

Code	Short Description	50th	75th	90th	MC
58300	Insert intrauterine device	166	218	271	0
58301	Remove intrauterine device	86	112	139	69
58321	Artificial insemination	159	209	260	70
58322	Artificial insemination	196	258	320	77
58323	Sperm washing	49	64	79	17
58340	Inject for uterus/tube x-ray	134	176	219	60
58345	Reopen fallopian tube	686	900	1118	333
58350	Reopen fallopian tube	159	208	259	71
58400	Suspension of uterus	1261	1654	2056	491
58410	Suspension of uterus	1598	2096	2604	712
58520	Repair ruptured uterus	1193	1565	1944	632
58540	Revision of uterus	1759	2308	2867	834

Oviduct

Code	Short Description	50th	75th	90th	MC
58600	Division of fallopian tube	998	1331	1682	393
58605	Division of fallopian tube	796	1062	1342	337
58611	Ligate oviduct(s)	231	308	389	47
58615	Occlude fallopian tube(s)	944	1260	1592	278
58700	Remove fallopian tube	1199	1600	2021	535
58720	Remove ovary/tube(s)	1463	1952	2467	775
58740	Revise fallopian tube(s)	1456	1942	2454	552
58750	Repair oviduct	2015	2688	3396	854
58752	Revise ovarian tube(s)	1789	2387	3016	850
58760	Remove tubal obstruction	1603	2139	2702	728
58770	Create new tubal opening	1631	2176	2749	763

Ovary

Code	Short Description	50th	75th	90th	MC
58800	Drainage of ovarian cyst(s)	576	769	971	273
58805	Drainage of ovarian cyst(s)	1253	1671	2112	521
58820	Drainage of ovarian abscess	575	767	969	282
58822	Drainage of ovarian abscess	1073	1432	1809	519
58825	Transposition, ovary(s)	1240	1655	2091	415
58900	Biopsy of ovary(s)	1133	1512	1910	463
58920	Partial removal of ovary(s)	1254	1673	2114	571
58925	Remove ovarian cyst(s)	1316	1756	2218	726
58940	Remove ovary(s)	1286	1717	2169	566
58943	Remove ovary(s)	2556	3411	4309	1261
58950	Resect ovarian malignancy	2227	2971	3754	1087

MC = Medicare Fee

Code	Short Description	50th	75th	90th	MC
58951	Resect ovarian malignancy	3169	4228	5342	1676
58952	Resect ovarian malignancy	3604	4809	6076	1779
58960	Exploration of abdomen	2339	3122	3944	1166

In Vitro Fertilization

Code	Short Description	50th	75th	90th	MC
58970	Retrieval of oocyte	839	1119	1414	214
58974	Transfer of embryo	931	1243	1570	0
58976	Transfer of embryo	918	1225	1548	233

MATERNITY CARE AND DELIVERY

Fetal Testing or Monitoring

Code	Short Description	50th	75th	90th	MC
59000	Amniocentesis	176	253	334	96
59012	Fetal cord puncture, prenatal	457	656	864	250
59015	Chorion biopsy	297	426	561	136
59020	Fetal contract stress test	141	203	267	92
59025	Fetal non-stress test	107	154	202	50
59030	Fetal scalp blood sample	215	309	407	148
59050	Fetal monitor w/report	168	240	317	73
59051	Fetal monitor/interpret only	129	184	243	55
59100	Remove uterus lesion	1406	2017	2659	642
59120	Treat ectopic pregnancy	1503	2155	2841	785
59121	Treat ectopic pregnancy	1408	2020	2663	677
59130	Treat ectopic pregnancy	1423	2040	2690	779
59135	Treat ectopic pregnancy	1901	2726	3594	939
59136	Treat ectopic pregnancy	1802	2585	3408	783
59140	Treat ectopic pregnancy	1186	1702	2243	394
59150	Treat ectopic pregnancy	1097	1574	2075	467
59151	Treat ectopic pregnancy	1654	2372	3126	651
59160	D & C after delivery	487	699	922	241
59200	Insert cervical dilator	185	266	350	56
59300	Episiotomy or vaginal repair	271	388	512	135
59320	Revision of cervix	405	581	766	183
59325	Revision of cervix	636	913	1203	283
59350	Repair uterus	1204	1727	2276	365

SURGERY SERVICES

Code	Short Description	50th	75th	90th	MC
Vaginal Delivery, Antepartum and Postpartum Care					
59400	Obstetrical care	2359	3384	4461	1622
59409	Obstetrical care	1518	2178	2871	985
59410	Obstetrical care	1538	2207	2909	1075
59412	Antepartum manipulation	358	513	676	126
59414	Deliver placenta	296	424	559	119
59425	Antepartum care only	542	777	1025	326
59426	Antepartum care only	897	1287	1697	560
59430	Care after delivery	193	277	365	98
Cesarean Delivery					
59510	Cesarean delivery	2715	3894	5133	1838
59514	Cesarean delivery only	1894	2716	3581	1154
59515	Cesarean delivery	1914	2745	3619	1248
59525	Remove uterus after cesarean	1146	1644	2167	513
Vaginal Delivery After Previous Cesarean					
59610	VBAC delivery	2576	3695	4870	1681
59612	VBAC delivery only	1928	2765	3645	1044
59614	VBAC care after delivery	2116	3035	4001	1134
59618	Attempted VBAC delivery	2937	4212	5553	1896
59620	Attempted VBAC delivery only	2289	3283	4328	1213
59622	Attempted VBAC after care	2517	3611	4760	1307
Abortion					
59812	Treatment of miscarriage	566	811	1069	296
59820	Care of miscarriage	603	864	1139	325
59821	Treatment of miscarriage	604	866	1142	297
59830	Treat uterus infection	747	1072	1413	431
59840	Abortion	557	799	1053	269
59841	Abortion	603	865	1141	365
59850	Abortion	822	1179	1554	404
59851	Abortion	945	1356	1787	422
59852	Abortion	1279	1834	2417	567
59855	Abortion	858	1231	1623	427
59856	Abortion	1091	1564	2062	527

MC = Medicare Fee

Code	Short Description	50th	75th	90th	MC
59857	Abortion	1355	1944	2563	641
59866	Abortion	555	797	1050	294

Other Procedures Related to Pregnancy

59870	Evacuate mole of uterus	573	822	1083	300

ENDOCRINE SYSTEM SURGERY

Thyroid Gland

Code	Short Description	50th	75th	90th	MC
60000	Drain thyroid/tongue cyst	143	186	232	76
60001	Aspirate/inject thyroid cyst	162	211	263	70
60100	Biopsy of thyroid	172	225	280	70
60200	Remove thyroid lesion	1216	1585	1972	621
60210	Partial excision thyroid	1641	2139	2663	818
60212	Partial thyroid excision	2149	2801	3486	1023
60220	Partial removal of thyroid	1673	2180	2713	786
60225	Partial removal of thyroid	2128	2773	3451	1008
60240	Remove thyroid	2357	3071	3823	1102
60252	Remove thyroid	2925	3812	4744	1311
60254	Extensive thyroid surgery	3470	4522	5628	1758
60260	Repeat thyroid surgery	1791	2334	2905	687
60270	Remove thyroid	2759	3596	4476	1294
60271	Remove thyroid	2243	2923	3638	1121
60280	Remove thyroid duct lesion	1318	1718	2138	545
60281	Remove thyroid duct lesion	1336	1741	2167	546

Parathyroid, Thymus, Adrenal Glands, and Carotid Body

Code	Short Description	50th	75th	90th	MC
60500	Explore parathyroid glands	2154	2808	3495	1138
60502	Re-explore parathyroids	2430	3167	3942	1285
60505	Explore parathyroid glands	2801	3650	4543	1392
60512	Autotransplant, parathyroid	673	877	1092	284
60520	Remove thymus gland	2480	3232	4023	1250
60521	Removal thymus gland	2833	3693	4596	1324
60522	Remove thymus gland	3265	4256	5296	1473
60540	Explore adrenal gland	2382	3104	3864	1169
60545	Explore adrenal gland	2792	3639	4529	1376
60600	Remove carotid body lesion	2399	3126	3891	1152

SURGERY SERVICES

Code	Short Description	50th	75th	90th	MC
60605	Remove carotid body lesion	2801	3650	4543	1213

NERVOUS SYSTEM SURGERY

Skull, Meninges, and Brain

Code	Short Description	50th	75th	90th	MC
61000	Remove cranial cavity fluid	246	346	451	110
61001	Remove cranial cavity fluid	194	273	357	99
61020	Remove brain cavity fluid	256	360	469	117
61026	Injection into brain canal	337	475	619	129
61050	Remove brain canal fluid	260	366	477	94
61055	Injection into brain canal	375	527	687	135
61070	Brain canal shunt procedure	167	235	306	45
61105	Drill skull for examination	1302	1832	2388	514
61106	Drill skull for exam/surgery	1055	1484	1935	473
61107	Drill skull for implantation	1426	2006	2616	468
61108	Drill skull for drainage	2334	3284	4283	923
61120	Pierce skull for examination	1303	1833	2390	588
61130	Pierce skull, exam/surgery	978	1376	1794	481
61140	Pierce skull for biopsy	2752	3871	5048	1241
61150	Pierce skull for drainage	2841	3997	5213	1323
61151	Pierce skull for drainage	942	1326	1728	531
61154	Pierce skull, remove clot	2955	4158	5422	1364
61156	Pierce skull for drainage	3019	4247	5538	1360
61210	Pierce skull; implant device	1359	1911	2492	529
61215	Insert brain-fluid device	1531	2154	2809	586
61250	Pierce skull and explore	1795	2525	3292	741
61253	Pierce skull and explore	2704	3804	4960	887
61304	Open skull for exploration	4581	5913	7314	2037
61305	Open skull for exploration	4967	6412	7930	2330
61312	Open skull for drainage	4339	5601	6927	1991
61313	Open skull for drainage	4655	6009	7433	2009
61314	Open skull for drainage	5199	6712	8301	2097
61315	Open skull for drainage	5540	7151	8845	2156
61320	Open skull for drainage	4067	5250	6493	1803
61321	Open skull for drainage	4402	5683	7029	1959
61330	Decompress eye socket	3325	4293	5310	1391
61332	Explore/biopsy eye socket	4603	5942	7350	1941
61333	Explore orbit; remove lesion	4852	6264	7747	1976
61334	Explore orbit; remove object	4180	5396	6674	1316

MC = Medicare Fee

Code	Short Description	50th	75th	90th	MC
61340	Relieve cranial pressure	2708	3495	4323	1361
61343	Incise skull, pressure relief	5944	7673	9490	2494
61345	Relieve cranial pressure	3252	4198	5192	1879
61440	Incise skull for surgery	3727	4811	5951	1904
61450	Incise skull for surgery	4296	5545	6859	1890
61458	Incise skull for brain wound	5274	6808	8420	2292
61460	Incise skull for surgery	4851	6262	7745	2194
61470	Incise skull for surgery	4232	5464	6758	1595
61480	Incise skull for surgery	4134	5337	6601	1630
61490	Incise skull for surgery	2999	3871	4788	1477
61500	Remove skull lesion	4218	5445	6735	1605
61501	Remove infected skull bone	3800	4906	6067	1360
61510	Remove brain lesion	5135	6629	8199	2314
61512	Remove brain lining lesion	5166	6669	8248	2664
61514	Remove brain abscess	4756	6140	7594	2122
61516	Remove brain lesion	4752	6134	7587	2130
61518	Remove brain lesion	5867	7573	9367	2790
61519	Remove brain lining lesion	6533	8433	10431	3002
61520	Remove brain lesion	6935	8952	11072	3618
61521	Remove brain lesion	7915	10218	12638	3175
61522	Remove brain abscess	5058	6530	8076	2008
61524	Remove brain lesion	5317	6864	8490	2313
61526	Remove brain lesion	6459	8338	10313	3489
61530	Remove brain lesion	6562	8471	10478	3180
61531	Implant brain electrodes	4242	5476	6773	1172
61533	Implant brain electrodes	4543	5865	7254	1512
61534	Remove brain lesion	3691	4765	5893	1062
61535	Remove brain electrodes	2697	3481	4306	749
61536	Remove brain lesion	5097	6580	8138	2321
61538	Remove brain tissue	5580	7203	8909	2337
61539	Remove brain tissue	5325	6874	8502	2236
61541	Incision of brain tissue	6131	7914	9789	1978
61542	Remove brain tissue	5777	7458	9225	2066
61543	Remove brain tissue	4306	5559	6875	1834
61544	Remove and treat brain lesion	4751	6133	7585	2132
61545	Excision of brain tumor	7462	9633	11915	2816
61546	Remove pituitary gland	5353	6911	8547	2404
61548	Remove pituitary gland	5025	6487	8024	1937
61550	Release of skull seams	2820	3640	4502	1064
61552	Release of skull seams	3448	4451	5506	1391
61556	Incise skull/sutures	3565	4602	5692	1563

SURGERY SERVICES

Code	Short Description	50th	75th	90th	MC
61557	Incise skull/sutures	3885	5016	6203	1571
61558	Excision of skull/sutures	4594	5930	7335	1786
61559	Excision of skull/sutures	5437	7018	8680	2316
61563	Excision of skull tumor	4639	5988	7406	1893
61564	Excision of skull tumor	5909	7628	9435	2388
61570	Remove brain foreign body	4890	6312	7807	1661
61571	Incise skull for brain wound	5364	6925	8565	1804
61575	Skull base/brainstem surgery	4973	6419	7940	2772
61576	Skull base/brainstem surgery	5030	6493	8031	3197
61580	Craniofacial approach, skull	5044	6512	8054	2114
61581	Craniofacial approach, skull	5778	7459	9226	2399
61582	Craniofacial approach, skull	5236	6759	8360	2178
61583	Craniofacial approach, skull	5944	7673	9490	2485
61584	Orbitocranial approach/skull	5771	7450	9215	2406
61585	Orbitocranial approach/skull	6433	8304	10271	2692
61586	Resect nasopharynx, skull	3907	5044	6238	1857
61590	Infratemporal approach/skull	7070	9126	11288	2928
61591	Infratemporal approach/skull	7398	9550	11812	3071
61592	Orbitocranial approach/skull	6674	8616	10656	2785
61595	Transtemporal approach/skull	4931	6366	7874	2057
61596	Transcochlear approach/skull	5990	7732	9563	2500
61597	Transcondylar approach/skull	6336	8179	10116	2642
61598	Transpetrosal approach/skull	5590	7216	8925	2328
61600	Resect/excise cranial lesion	4301	5552	6868	1785
61601	Resect/excise cranial lesion	4615	5957	7368	1914
61605	Resect/excise cranial lesion	4870	6287	7776	2021
61606	Resect/excise cranial lesion	6517	8413	10406	2707
61607	Resect/excise cranial lesion	6081	7850	9709	2529
61608	Resect/excise cranial lesion	7085	9146	11313	2942
61609	Transect, artery, sinus	1707	2204	2726	723
61610	Transect, artery, sinus	5621	7256	8974	2170
61611	Transect, artery, sinus	1272	1642	2030	543
61612	Transect, artery, sinus	5279	6815	8429	2040
61613	Remove aneurysm, sinus	6954	8977	11104	2885
61615	Resect/excise lesion, skull	5365	6926	8566	2221
61616	Resect/excise lesion, skull	7274	9390	11614	3021
61618	Repair dura	2798	3612	4467	1143
61619	Repair dura	3502	4521	5592	1428
61624	Occlusion/embolization cath	3240	4330	5477	1203
61626	Occlusion/embolization cath	2658	3553	4493	992

MC = Medicare Fee

Code	Short Description	50th	75th	90th	MC
61680	Intracranial vessel surgery	6962	9305	11768	2604
61682	Intracranial vessel surgery	8234	11005	13917	3941
61684	Intracranial vessel surgery	7240	9677	12238	2797
61686	Intracranial vessel surgery	8623	11525	14575	3978
61690	Intracranial vessel surgery	6847	9152	11574	2336
61692	Intracranial vessel surgery	7795	10418	13175	3185
61700	Inner skull vessel surgery	6163	8237	10417	3344
61702	Inner skull vessel surgery	7271	9718	12290	3497
61703	Clamp neck artery	2503	3346	4231	1203
61705	Revise circulation to head	6453	8625	10907	2756
61708	Revise circulation to head	5161	6898	8724	2389
61710	Revise circulation to head	4373	5844	7391	1810
61711	Fusion of skull arteries	5830	7792	9855	2908
61712	Skull or spine microsurgery	1100	1470	1860	352
61720	Incise skull/brain surgery	4047	5409	6840	1595
61735	Incise skull/brain surgery	3759	5024	6354	1296
61750	Incise skull; brain biopsy	3545	4738	5992	1357
61751	Brain biopsy with cat scan	4304	5753	7275	1603
61760	Implant brain electrodes	4068	5437	6876	1474
61770	Incise skull for treatment	3214	4296	5433	1677
61790	Treat trigeminal nerve	2884	3854	4874	1052
61791	Treat trigeminal tract	2936	3924	4962	1055
61793	Focus radiation beam	5059	6761	8551	1582
61795	Brain surgery using computer	1138	1520	1923	430
61850	Implant neuroelectrodes	2909	3888	4916	1001
61855	Implant neuroelectrodes	2598	3473	4392	955
61860	Implant neuroelectrodes	2452	3278	4145	1135
61865	Implant neuroelectrodes	4033	5391	6817	1588
61870	Implant neuroelectrodes	1519	2030	2568	719
61875	Implant neuroelectrodes	2124	2839	3591	846
61880	Revise/remove neuroelectrode	1466	1959	2477	438
61885	Implant neuroreceiver	534	713	902	290
61888	Revise/remove neuroreceiver	747	998	1263	286
62000	Repair skull fracture	2048	2737	3461	697
62005	Repair skull fracture	2877	3846	4864	1092
62010	Treatment of head injury	3782	5055	6393	1618
62100	Repair brain fluid leakage	4249	5679	7182	1818
62115	Reduction of skull defect	3262	4360	5514	1480
62116	Reduction of skull defect	3595	4805	6077	1620
62117	Reduction of skull defect	4028	5384	6809	1832
62120	Repair skull cavity lesion	3406	4553	5758	1612

SURGERY SERVICES

Code	Short Description	50th	75th	90th	MC
62121	Incise skull repair	3988	5331	6742	1617
62140	Repair skull defect	2831	3783	4784	1122
62141	Repair skull defect	3533	4722	5971	1383
62142	Remove skull plate/flap	2509	3353	4240	1000
62143	Replace skull plate/flap	2895	3869	4893	898
62145	Repair skull and brain	3641	4866	6154	1297
62146	Repair skull with graft	3158	4221	5338	1106
62147	Repair skull with graft	3753	5017	6344	1326
62180	Establish brain cavity shunt	3169	4236	5357	1433
62190	Establish brain cavity shunt	2525	3375	4268	1043
62192	Establish brain cavity shunt	2659	3554	4495	1130
62194	Replace/irrigate catheter	649	868	1097	213
62200	Establish brain cavity shunt	3764	5030	6362	1472
62201	Establish brain cavity shunt	2416	3229	4083	939
62220	Establish brain cavity shunt	2946	3937	4980	1213
62223	Establish brain cavity shunt	3075	4110	5198	1245
62225	Replace/irrigate catheter	1004	1342	1697	397
62230	Replace/revise brain shunt	2170	2900	3668	842
62256	Remove brain cavity shunt	1345	1798	2274	531
62258	Replace brain cavity shunt	2877	3846	4864	1221

Spine and Spinal Cord

Code	Short Description	50th	75th	90th	MC
62268	Drain spinal cord cyst	1057	1483	1896	260
62269	Needle biopsy spinal cord	922	1294	1654	225
62270	Spinal fluid tap, diagnostic	176	238	298	61
62272	Drain spinal fluid	223	313	400	80
62273	Treat lumbar spine lesion	217	304	389	113
62274	Inject spinal anesthetic	181	254	324	86
62275	Inject spinal anesthetic	325	456	584	82
62276	Inject spinal anesthetic	257	361	461	113
62277	Inject spinal anesthetic	243	341	435	103
62278	Inject spinal anesthetic	263	366	467	89
62279	Inject spinal anesthetic	279	389	496	85
62280	Treat spinal cord lesion	340	478	611	109
62281	Treat spinal cord lesion	370	519	664	120
62282	Treat spinal canal lesion	444	622	796	142
62284	Injection for myelogram	372	498	621	153
62287	Percutaneous diskectomy	1690	2370	3031	673
62288	Injection into spinal canal	274	385	492	100

MC = Medicare Fee

Code	Short Description	50th	75th	90th	MC
62289	Injection into spinal canal	324	448	568	97
62290	Inject for spine disk x-ray	388	544	696	164
62291	Inject for spine disk x-ray	398	558	713	164
62292	Injection into disk lesion	1355	1901	2430	717
62294	Injection into spinal artery	955	1339	1712	678
62298	Injection into spinal canal	365	512	655	108
62350	Implant spinal catheter	1051	1474	1885	419
62351	Implant spinal catheter	1549	2173	2778	620
62355	Remove spinal canal catheter	853	1196	1530	351
62360	Insert spine infusion device	343	480	614	135
62361	Implant spine infusion pump	811	1137	1454	322
62362	Implant spine infusion pump	1054	1479	1891	422
62365	Remove spine infusion device	850	1192	1525	349
62367	Analyze spine infusion pump	82	115	147	0
62368	Analyze spine infusion pump	126	177	226	0
63001	Remove spinal lamina	3790	5317	6799	1445
63003	Remove spinal lamina	3896	5465	6989	1416
63005	Remove spinal lamina	3307	4638	5931	1358
63011	Remove spinal lamina	3170	4446	5686	989
63012	Remove spinal lamina	3735	5239	6699	1403
63015	Remove spinal lamina	4460	6256	8000	1708
63016	Remove spinal lamina	4390	6158	7874	1736
63017	Remove spinal lamina	4052	5684	7269	1555
63020	Neck spine disk surgery	3501	4911	6279	1313
63030	Low back disk surgery	3242	4548	5815	1167
63035	Added spinal disk surgery	893	1253	1603	315
63040	Neck spine disk surgery	4324	6065	7756	1756
63042	Low back disk surgery	3589	5034	6437	1707
63045	Remove spinal lamina	4110	5765	7372	1557
63046	Remove spinal lamina	4263	5979	7646	1502
63047	Remove spinal lamina	4042	5670	7250	1362
63048	Remove spinal lamina	1138	1642	2132	335
63055	Decompress spinal cord	4715	6613	8457	1920
63056	Decompress spinal cord	4302	6034	7717	1766
63057	Decompress spinal cord	952	1335	1707	390
63064	Decompress spinal cord	4638	6505	8319	2016
63066	Decompress spinal cord	843	1182	1511	242
63075	Neck spine disk surgery	3317	4653	5950	1546
63076	Neck spine disk surgery	1070	1501	1920	404
63077	Spine disk surgery, thorax	3783	5306	6785	1645
63078	Spine disk surgery, thorax	849	1191	1524	249

SURGERY SERVICES

Code	Short Description	50th	75th	90th	MC
63081	Remove vertebral body	4892	6861	8774	2089
63082	Remove vertebral body	1250	1754	2243	443
63085	Remove vertebral body	5214	7314	9352	2256
63086	Remove vertebral body	1171	1642	2100	331
63087	Remove vertebral body	5444	7636	9764	2629
63088	Remove vertebral body	1318	1848	2364	438
63090	Remove vertebral body	5271	7394	9455	2382
63091	Remove vertebral body	810	1136	1453	244
63170	Incise spinal cord tract(s)	4529	6353	8124	1591
63172	Drainage of spinal cyst	4024	5644	7217	1631
63173	Drainage of spinal cyst	3907	5480	7007	1474
63180	Revise spinal cord ligaments	4011	5626	7195	1189
63182	Revise spinal cord ligaments	4623	6485	8293	1474
63185	Incise spinal column/nerves	3627	5087	6505	1277
63190	Incise spinal column/nerves	4310	6046	7731	1623
63191	Incise spinal column/nerves	3822	5361	6855	1241
63194	Incise spinal column and cord	3831	5374	6871	1287
63195	Incise spinal column and cord	3851	5402	6907	1299
63196	Incise spinal column and cord	4113	5769	7377	1486
63197	Incise spinal column and cord	4047	5677	7259	1423
63198	Incise spinal column and cord	4684	6570	8401	1642
63199	Incise spinal column and cord	4909	6886	8806	1881
63200	Release of spinal cord	3903	5475	7001	1250
63250	Revise spinal cord vessels	5634	8623	11765	2813
63251	Revise spinal cord vessels	5402	8269	11281	2568
63252	Revise spinal cord vessels	6424	9832	13414	2842
63265	Excise intraspinal lesion	4503	6892	9403	1814
63266	Excise intraspinal lesion	4673	7153	9759	1971
63267	Excise intraspinal lesion	4163	6372	8693	1675
63268	Excise intraspinal lesion	3707	5673	7740	1264
63270	Excise intraspinal lesion	4657	7128	9725	1816
63271	Excise intraspinal lesion	5011	7670	10464	2223
63272	Excise intraspinal lesion	4564	6985	9530	2013
63273	Excise intraspinal lesion	4264	6526	8904	1698
63275	Biopsy/excise spinal tumor	4902	7503	10237	2176
63276	Biopsy/excise spinal tumor	4722	7227	9860	2043
63277	Biopsy/excise spinal tumor	4388	6715	9162	1880
63278	Biopsy/excise spinal tumor	4310	6596	8999	1856
63280	Biopsy/excise spinal tumor	5222	7993	10904	2358
63281	Biopsy/excise spinal tumor	5107	7817	10665	2329

MC = Medicare Fee

Code	Short Description	50th	75th	90th	MC
63282	Biopsy/excise spinal tumor	4840	7408	10107	2107
63283	Biopsy/excise spinal tumor	4328	6623	9036	1795
63285	Biopsy/excise spinal tumor	5890	9015	12300	2473
63286	Biopsy/excise spinal tumor	6047	9255	12626	2654
63287	Biopsy/excise spinal tumor	5975	9145	12477	2532
63290	Biopsy/excise spinal tumor	5250	8036	10963	2619
63300	Remove vertebral body	4453	6815	9298	1646
63301	Remove vertebral body	4934	7551	10302	1844
63302	Remove vertebral body	5053	7734	10552	1960
63303	Remove vertebral body	5063	7748	10571	1966
63304	Remove vertebral body	4848	7419	10122	2030
63305	Remove vertebral body	5279	8079	11023	2180
63306	Remove vertebral body	5258	8048	10980	2168
63307	Remove vertebral body	5307	8122	11082	2227
63308	Remove vertebral body	963	1473	2010	393
63600	Remove spinal cord lesion	2389	3657	4989	857
63610	Stimulation of spinal cord	1854	2838	3871	568
63615	Remove lesion of spinal cord	3137	4800	6549	1135
63650	Implant neuroelectrodes	1557	2383	3251	626
63655	Implant neuroelectrodes	2335	3574	4876	987
63660	Revise/remove neuroelectrode	1273	1949	2659	562
63685	Implant neuroreceiver	1269	1942	2650	599
63688	Revise/remove neuroreceiver	989	1514	2066	481
63690	Analysis of neuroreceiver	107	163	223	38
63691	Analysis of neuroreceiver	125	191	261	38
63700	Repair spinal herniation	2728	4175	5696	1143
63702	Repair spinal herniation	3014	4613	6294	1285
63704	Repair spinal herniation	3358	5140	7012	1428
63706	Repair spinal herniation	3679	5631	7683	1642
63707	Repair spinal fluid leakage	3001	4593	6266	1017
63709	Repair spinal fluid leakage	3414	5226	7129	1328
63710	Graft repair of spine defect	2848	4359	5947	953
63740	Install spinal shunt	2839	4345	5928	1059
63741	Install spinal shunt	2012	3079	4200	756
63744	Revision of spinal shunt	1521	2328	3176	678
63746	Remove spinal shunt	1166	1785	2435	481

SURGERY SERVICES

Code	Short Description	50th	75th	90th	MC

Extracranial Nerves, Peripheral Nerves, and Autonomic Nervous System

Code	Short Description	50th	75th	90th	MC
64400	Injection for nerve block	160	236	317	52
64402	Injection for nerve block	162	239	321	76
64405	Injection for nerve block	138	204	274	65
64408	Injection for nerve block	161	238	320	83
64410	Injection for nerve block	155	228	307	73
64412	Injection for nerve block	147	217	291	60
64413	Injection for nerve block	162	239	321	71
64415	Injection for nerve block	182	269	361	57
64417	Injection for nerve block	198	292	392	71
64418	Injection for nerve block	140	207	278	73
64420	Injection for nerve block	164	242	325	61
64421	Injection for nerve block	230	339	456	86
64425	Injection for nerve block	168	248	333	77
64430	Injection for nerve block	184	272	365	88
64435	Injection for nerve block	155	229	308	77
64440	Injection for nerve block	166	246	330	71
64441	Injection for nerve block	211	311	418	94
64442	Injection for nerve block	247	359	479	89
64443	Injection for nerve block	144	214	289	56
64445	Injection for nerve block	111	163	220	65
64450	Injection for nerve block	98	142	188	71
64505	Injection for nerve block	148	219	294	65
64508	Injection for nerve block	157	232	312	73
64510	Injection for nerve block	224	330	443	68
64520	Injection for nerve block	224	330	443	72
64530	Injection for nerve block	254	375	504	98
64550	Apply neurostimulator	65	92	121	22
64553	Implant neuroelectrodes	322	475	638	108
64555	Implant neuroelectrodes	227	335	450	87
64560	Implant neuroelectrodes	322	475	638	156
64565	Implant neuroelectrodes	199	294	395	82
64573	Implant neuroelectrodes	711	1049	1410	318
64575	Implant neuroelectrodes	614	905	1216	303
64577	Implant neuroelectrodes	610	900	1210	302
64580	Implant neuroelectrodes	587	867	1164	279
64585	Revise/remove neuroelectrode	375	553	743	119
64590	Implant neuroreceiver	475	700	941	178

MC = Medicare Fee

Code	Short Description	50th	75th	90th	MC
64595	Revise/remove neuroreceiver	314	463	622	118
64600	Injection treatment of nerve	356	486	617	168
64605	Injection treatment of nerve	552	753	955	237
64610	Injection treatment of nerve	917	1250	1586	512
64612	Destroy nerve, face muscle	237	323	410	138
64613	Destroy nerve, spine muscle	266	362	459	138
64620	Injection treatment of nerve	286	390	495	127
64622	Injection treatment of nerve	390	532	675	165
64623	Injection treatment of nerve	165	225	285	65
64630	Injection treatment of nerve	265	361	458	163
64640	Injection treatment of nerve	223	304	386	111
64680	Injection treatment of nerve	417	569	722	146
64702	Revise finger/toe nerve	686	936	1187	353
64704	Revise hand/foot nerve	927	1265	1605	417
64708	Revise arm/leg nerve	1311	1788	2268	566
64712	Revision of sciatic nerve	1779	2427	3078	715
64713	Revision of arm nerve(s)	1745	2381	3019	844
64714	Revise low back nerve(s)	1590	2169	2751	680
64716	Revision of cranial nerve	1452	1981	2513	443
64718	Revise ulnar nerve at elbow	1336	1823	2311	527
64719	Revise ulnar nerve at wrist	906	1236	1567	415
64721	Carpal tunnel surgery	1038	1381	1725	385
64722	Relieve pressure on nerve(s)	1125	1534	1946	447
64726	Release foot/toe nerve	526	717	910	181
64727	Internal nerve revision	640	872	1107	272
64732	Incision of brow nerve	855	1123	1405	362
64734	Incision of cheek nerve	877	1152	1442	385
64736	Incision of chin nerve	1006	1321	1653	365
64738	Incision of jaw nerve	1134	1490	1864	436
64740	Incision of tongue nerve	879	1154	1444	436
64742	Incision of facial nerve	1320	1734	2170	445
64744	Incise nerve, back of head	1000	1314	1644	478
64746	Incise diaphragm nerve	745	979	1225	397
64752	Incision of vagus nerve	1465	1925	2408	445
64755	Incision of stomach nerves	2522	3313	4145	1014
64760	Incision of vagus nerve	1560	2049	2563	579
64761	Incision of pelvis nerve	779	1024	1281	440
64763	Incise hip/thigh nerve	896	1177	1473	483
64766	Incise hip/thigh nerve	1320	1734	2170	634
64771	Sever cranial nerve	1271	1670	2089	555
64772	Incision of spinal nerve	1066	1401	1753	586

SURGERY SERVICES

Code	Short Description	50th	75th	90th	MC
64774	Remove skin nerve lesion	592	778	973	313
64776	Remove digit nerve lesion	597	785	982	313
64778	Added digit nerve surgery	379	498	623	246
64782	Remove limb nerve lesion	775	1018	1274	430
64783	Added limb nerve surgery	525	689	862	293
64784	Remove nerve lesion	1260	1656	2071	626
64786	Remove sciatic nerve lesion	1877	2466	3085	1173
64787	Implant nerve end	783	1028	1286	328
64788	Remove skin nerve lesion	781	1026	1284	331
64790	Remove nerve lesion	1465	1925	2408	752
64792	Remove nerve lesion	1791	2353	2944	977
64795	Biopsy of nerve	453	595	744	227
64802	Remove sympathetic nerves	1603	2105	2634	575
64804	Remove sympathetic nerves	2527	3320	4154	1136
64809	Remove sympathetic nerves	2394	3145	3935	996
64818	Remove sympathetic nerves	1537	2020	2526	775
64820	Remove sympathetic nerves	1741	2287	2861	732
64830	Microrepair of nerve	534	702	878	214
64831	Repair digit nerve	889	1168	1462	493
64832	Repair additional nerve	475	624	781	280
64834	Repair hand or foot nerve	1097	1441	1803	533
64835	Repair hand or foot nerve	1368	1798	2249	680
64836	Repair hand or foot nerve	1553	2040	2552	718
64837	Repair additional nerve	834	1095	1370	452
64840	Repair leg nerve	1705	2239	2802	913
64856	Repair/transpose nerve	1724	2264	2833	877
64857	Repair arm/leg nerve	1762	2315	2897	958
64858	Repair sciatic nerve	2096	2753	3445	1116
64859	Additional nerve surgery	710	933	1168	327
64861	Repair arm nerves	2216	2911	3641	1280
64862	Repair low back nerves	2535	3330	4166	1630
64864	Repair facial nerve	1692	2223	2781	815
64865	Repair facial nerve	1990	2614	3270	1119
64866	Fusion of facial/other nerve	2932	3852	4819	1095
64868	Fusion of facial/other nerve	3037	3990	4991	1020
64870	Fusion of facial/other nerve	3226	4238	5302	1210
64872	Subsequent repair of nerve	333	437	547	146
64874	Repair and revise nerve	505	663	830	218
64876	Repair nerve; shorten bone	476	626	783	204
64885	Nerve graft, head or neck	3078	4044	5058	1209

MC = Medicare Fee

DOES YOUR DOCTOR CHARGE TOO MUCH?

Code	Short Description	50th	75th	90th	MC
64886	Nerve graft, head or neck	3488	4583	5733	1442
64890	Nerve graft, hand or foot	2056	2701	3379	1128
64891	Nerve graft, hand or foot	2145	2818	3525	1069
64892	Nerve graft, arm or leg	1971	2590	3240	1042
64893	Nerve graft, arm or leg	2273	2986	3735	1212
64895	Nerve graft, hand or foot	2540	3336	4174	1334
64896	Nerve graft, hand or foot	2870	3771	4717	1524
64897	Nerve graft, arm or leg	2482	3260	4079	1271
64898	Nerve graft, arm or leg	2739	3598	4502	1377
64901	Additional nerve graft	1266	1663	2080	836
64902	Additional nerve graft	1461	1919	2401	973
64905	Nerve pedicle transfer	1451	1907	2386	910
64907	Nerve pedicle transfer	2033	2670	3341	1310

EYE AND OCULAR ADNEXA SURGERY

Eyeball

Code	Description	50th	75th	90th	MC
65091	Revise eye	1070	1341	1654	567
65093	Revise eye with implant	1241	1556	1919	603
65101	Remove eye	1219	1527	1884	606
65103	Remove eye/insert implant	1379	1729	2132	656
65105	Remove eye/attach implant	1664	2085	2572	726
65110	Remove eye	2193	2749	3390	1197
65112	Remove eye, revise socket	2268	2843	3506	1123
65114	Remove eye, revise socket	2539	3183	3926	1226
65125	Revise ocular implant	624	782	965	218
65130	Insert ocular implant	1180	1480	1825	628
65135	Insert ocular implant	1162	1456	1796	497
65140	Attach ocular implant	1350	1692	2087	548
65150	Revise ocular implant	1123	1408	1736	560
65155	Reinsert ocular implant	1419	1778	2193	775
65175	Remove ocular implant	921	1154	1424	546
65205	Remove foreign body from eye	62	78	96	43
65210	Remove foreign body from eye	76	96	118	52
65220	Remove foreign body from eye	78	98	120	41
65222	Remove foreign body from eye	99	124	153	60
65235	Remove foreign body from eye	1295	1623	2002	510
65260	Remove foreign body from eye	1727	2165	2670	761
65265	Remove foreign body from eye	1867	2340	2887	884

SURGERY SERVICES

Code	Short Description	50th	75th	90th	MC
65270	Repair eye wound	205	257	317	120
65272	Repair eye wound	343	430	531	205
65273	Repair eye wound	517	648	799	287
65275	Repair eye wound	628	787	971	218
65280	Repair eye wound	1477	1851	2283	659
65285	Repair eye wound	1739	2180	2689	981
65286	Repair eye wound	892	1118	1378	400
65290	Repair eye socket wound	911	1142	1408	459
65400	Remove eye lesion	895	1210	1572	490
65410	Biopsy of cornea	389	526	683	125
65420	Remove eye lesion	621	839	1090	334
65426	Remove eye lesion	917	1240	1610	470
65430	Corneal smear	97	132	171	79
65435	Curette/treat cornea	110	149	194	68
65436	Curette/treat cornea	312	422	548	216
65450	Treatment of corneal lesion	390	528	685	257
65600	Revision of cornea	584	789	1025	231
65710	Corneal transplant	2368	3202	4160	997
65730	Corneal transplant	2744	3711	4820	1180
65750	Corneal transplant	2887	3904	5071	1249
65755	Corneal transplant	2878	3891	5054	1252
65760	Revision of cornea	3202	4330	5624	0
65765	Revision of cornea	3507	4741	6159	0
65767	Corneal tissue transplant	2894	3913	5083	0
65770	Revise cornea with implant	2832	3830	4974	1217
65771	Radial keratotomy	1571	2125	2760	0
65772	Correction of astigmatism	1197	1618	2102	376
65775	Correction of astigmatism	1733	2343	3043	510
65800	Drainage of eye	302	408	530	146
65805	Drainage of eye	324	437	568	150
65810	Drainage of eye	920	1243	1615	407
65815	Drainage of eye	1072	1450	1883	372
65820	Relieve inner eye pressure	1214	1641	2132	697
65850	Incision of eye	1627	2199	2857	944
65855	Laser surgery of eye	1267	1670	2133	423
65860	Incise inner eye adhesions	731	988	1284	318
65865	Incise inner eye adhesions	1046	1415	1838	504
65870	Incise inner eye adhesions	932	1260	1637	475
65875	Incise inner eye adhesions	959	1297	1684	502
65880	Incise inner eye adhesions	1057	1429	1857	547

MC = Medicare Fee

Code	Short Description	50th	75th	90th	MC
65900	Remove eye lesion	1314	1777	2308	753
65920	Remove implant from eye	1537	2079	2700	657
65930	Remove blood clot from eye	1051	1421	1846	595
66020	Injection treatment of eye	313	423	549	145
66030	Injection treatment of eye	192	260	337	68
66130	Remove eye lesion	752	1004	1277	511
66150	Glaucoma surgery	1365	1822	2317	708
66155	Glaucoma surgery	1383	1847	2348	693
66160	Glaucoma surgery	1597	2132	2710	819
66165	Glaucoma surgery	1448	1932	2457	681
66170	Glaucoma surgery	1591	2131	2715	946
66172	Incision of eye	1983	2647	3365	1035
66180	Implant eye shunt	2143	2861	3637	1230
66185	Revise eye shunt	1253	1672	2126	716
66220	Repair eye lesion	1637	2185	2778	533
66225	Repair/graft eye lesion	2272	3033	3856	985
66250	Follow-up surgery of eye	1039	1387	1764	522
66500	Incision of iris	671	896	1139	333
66505	Incision of iris	639	853	1085	289
66600	Remove iris and lesion	1332	1779	2261	713
66605	Remove iris	2131	2845	3617	977
66625	Remove iris	968	1293	1644	465
66630	Remove iris	1060	1415	1799	541
66635	Remove iris	1009	1347	1712	551
66680	Repair iris and ciliary body	1055	1408	1791	470
66682	Repair iris and ciliary body	1182	1579	2007	536
66700	Destruction, ciliary body	887	1184	1505	424
66710	Destruction, ciliary body	1035	1382	1757	426
66720	Destruction, ciliary body	892	1191	1514	425
66740	Destruction, ciliary body	936	1249	1588	426
66761	Revision of iris	1091	1432	1800	370
66762	Revision of iris	896	1196	1520	428
66770	Remove inner eye lesion	844	1127	1433	457
66820	Incision, secondary cataract	681	898	1086	350
66821	After cataract laser surgery	852	1118	1349	252
66825	Reposition intraocular lens	1209	1594	1928	606
66830	Remove lens lesion	1359	1792	2167	624
66840	Remove lens material	1532	2020	2443	698
66850	Remove lens material	2076	2738	3311	808
66852	Remove lens material	1803	2377	2874	894
66920	Extraction of lens	1933	2549	3082	786

SURGERY SERVICES

Code	Short Description	50th	75th	90th	MC
66930	Extraction of lens	2207	2910	3519	818
66940	Extraction of lens	1787	2357	2849	788
66983	Remove cataract, insert lens	2224	2933	3546	808
66984	Remove cataract, insert lens	2514	3420	4204	929
66985	Insert lens prosthesis	1879	2479	2997	736
66986	Exchange lens prosthesis	1987	2621	3169	968

Posterior Segment

Code	Short Description	50th	75th	90th	MC
67005	Partial removal of eye fluid	1732	2291	2914	674
67010	Partial removal of eye fluid	2044	2703	3438	702
67015	Release of eye fluid	1083	1432	1822	530
67025	Replace eye fluid	1035	1369	1741	533
67028	Injection eye drug	648	857	1090	234
67030	Incise inner eye strands	1246	1648	2096	423
67031	Laser surgery, eye strands	1325	1752	2229	411
67036	Remove inner eye fluid	3320	4391	5585	1128
67038	Strip retinal membrane	4184	5535	7040	1891
67039	Laser treatment of retina	3013	3986	5070	1326
67040	Laser treatment of retina	3871	5120	6513	1535
67101	Repair, detached retina	1826	2415	3072	659
67105	Repair, detached retina	1780	2355	2995	672
67107	Repair detached retina	2834	3748	4767	1304
67108	Repair detached retina	4480	5926	7537	1863
67110	Repair detached retina	1780	2355	2995	780
67112	Re-repair detached retina	2660	3518	4475	1318
67115	Release, encircling material	904	1196	1521	435
67120	Remove eye implant material	950	1256	1598	520
67121	Remove eye implant material	1375	1819	2313	788
67141	Treatment of retina	1094	1447	1840	461
67145	Treatment of retina	1214	1606	2043	477
67208	Treatment of retinal lesion	1313	1736	2208	597
67210	Treatment of retinal lesion	1318	1673	2068	745
67218	Treatment of retinal lesion	2134	2823	3590	1052
67227	Treatment of retinal lesion	1276	1688	2147	586
67228	Treatment of retinal lesion	1408	1800	2237	870
67250	Reinforce eye wall	1744	2307	2934	617
67255	Reinforce/graft eye wall	2144	2836	3608	790

MC = Medicare Fee

Code	Short Description	50th	75th	90th	MC
Ocular Adnexa					
67311	Revise eye muscle	1231	1699	2228	586
67312	Revise two eye muscles	1473	2033	2666	725
67314	Revise eye muscle	1385	1911	2507	665
67316	Revise two eye muscles	1690	2332	3058	796
67318	Revise eye muscle(s)	1358	1874	2458	548
67320	Revise eye muscle(s)	1665	2298	3013	771
67331	Eye surgery follow-up	1406	1940	2545	717
67332	Re-revise eye muscles	1713	2364	3100	797
67334	Revise eye muscle w/suture	1297	1789	2346	556
67335	Eye suture during surgery	572	790	1036	270
67340	Revise eye muscle	1623	2240	2937	695
67343	Release eye tissue	1225	1691	2217	514
67345	Destroy nerve of eye muscle	337	465	610	211
67350	Biopsy eye muscle	629	868	1139	211
67400	Explore/biopsy eye socket	1433	1977	2592	818
67405	Explore/drain eye socket	1318	1818	2384	695
67412	Explore/treat eye socket	1793	2473	3243	850
67413	Explore/treat eye socket	1655	2283	2994	721
67414	Explore/decompress eye socket	1810	2498	3275	740
67415	Aspiration orbital contents	306	422	553	154
67420	Explore/treat eye socket	2336	3223	4227	1446
67430	Explore/treat eye socket	2002	2763	3623	939
67440	Explore/drain eye socket	2065	2849	3736	1158
67445	Explore/decompress eye socket	2027	2797	3668	981
67450	Explore/biopsy eye socket	2091	2885	3783	1143
67500	Inject/treat eye socket	116	160	210	62
67505	Inject/treat eye socket	157	217	285	76
67515	Inject/treat eye socket	85	117	153	47
67550	Insert eye socket implant	1326	1830	2400	787
67560	Revise eye socket implant	1184	1634	2142	739
67570	Decompress optic nerve	1178	1625	2131	796
67599	Orbit surgery procedure	0	0	0	0
67700	Drainage of eyelid abscess	108	145	186	70
67710	Incision of eyelid	120	162	207	80
67715	Incision of eyelid fold	174	235	301	109
67800	Remove eyelid lesion	137	184	237	91
67801	Remove eyelid lesions	196	263	338	130
67805	Remove eyelid lesions	220	297	381	141

SURGERY SERVICES

Code	Short Description	50th	75th	90th	MC
67808	Remove eyelid lesion(s)	366	494	633	226
67810	Biopsy of eyelid	127	171	220	91
67820	Revise eyelashes	55	73	92	50
67825	Revise eyelashes	143	192	247	89
67830	Revise eyelashes	265	357	459	156
67835	Revise eyelashes	1121	1510	1937	505
67840	Remove eyelid lesion	198	266	341	128
67850	Treat eyelid lesion	145	196	251	97
67875	Closure of eyelid by suture	248	335	429	126
67880	Revision of eyelid	543	732	939	304
67882	Revision of eyelid	761	1025	1315	444
67900	Repair brow defect	759	1022	1312	382
67901	Repair eyelid defect	1245	1678	2153	640
67902	Repair eyelid defect	1446	1949	2501	649
67903	Repair eyelid defect	1436	1935	2483	590
67904	Repair eyelid defect	1507	2031	2606	566
67906	Repair eyelid defect	1340	1805	2316	488
67908	Repair eyelid defect	1124	1514	1943	468
67909	Revise eyelid defect	1094	1474	1891	490
67911	Revise eyelid defect	1420	1914	2456	493
67914	Repair eyelid defect	664	894	1147	340
67915	Repair eyelid defect	244	329	423	171
67916	Repair eyelid defect	892	1201	1542	474
67917	Repair eyelid defect	1084	1461	1874	545
67921	Repair eyelid defect	551	742	952	289
67922	Repair eyelid defect	226	305	391	164
67923	Repair eyelid defect	893	1203	1544	511
67924	Repair eyelid defect	1036	1396	1791	525
67930	Repair eyelid wound	426	574	737	189
67935	Repair eyelid wound	730	984	1262	393
67938	Remove eyelid foreign body	89	119	153	71
67950	Revision of eyelid	1148	1547	1985	526
67961	Revision of eyelid	1134	1527	1960	516
67966	Revision of eyelid	1325	1786	2291	602
67971	Reconstruction of eyelid	1553	2093	2686	823
67973	Reconstruction of eyelid	1856	2501	3210	1065
67974	Reconstruction of eyelid	1984	2673	3429	1084
67975	Reconstruction of eyelid	817	1101	1413	514

MC = Medicare Fee

Code	Short Description	50th	75th	90th	MC

Conjunctiva

Code	Short Description	50th	75th	90th	MC
68020	Incise/drain eyelid lining	85	117	154	72
68040	Treatment of eyelid lesions	84	116	153	51
68100	Biopsy of eyelid lining	164	226	299	94
68110	Remove eyelid lining lesion	204	281	371	118
68115	Remove eyelid lining lesion	353	487	642	170
68130	Remove eyelid lining lesion	638	878	1159	355
68135	Remove eyelid lining lesion	175	241	318	99
68200	Treat eyelid by injection	83	115	152	41
68320	Revise/graft eyelid lining	1092	1503	1984	465
68325	Revise/graft eyelid lining	1321	1819	2401	652
68326	Revise/graft eyelid lining	1282	1766	2330	627
68328	Revise/graft eyelid lining	1497	2061	2720	734
68330	Revise eyelid lining	887	1221	1612	422
68335	Revise/graft eyelid lining	1279	1762	2325	639
68340	Separate eyelid adhesions	514	708	934	283
68360	Revise eyelid lining	682	939	1240	385
68362	Revise eyelid lining	1078	1484	1959	606
68400	Incise/drain tear gland	201	278	366	105
68420	Incise/drain tear sac	194	267	352	129
68440	Incise tear duct opening	118	163	215	66
68500	Remove tear gland	1292	1779	2348	736
68505	Partial removal tear gland	1292	1780	2349	766
68510	Biopsy of tear gland	417	574	757	336
68520	Remove tear sac	1277	1759	2322	661
68525	Biopsy of tear sac	411	567	748	327
68530	Clearance of tear duct	734	1011	1334	259
68540	Remove tear gland lesion	1448	1995	2632	740
68550	Remove tear gland lesion	1786	2460	3246	970
68700	Repair tear ducts	968	1333	1759	349
68705	Revise tear duct opening	170	234	309	119
68720	Create tear sac drain	1658	2283	3012	755
68745	Create tear duct drain	1406	1936	2555	596
68750	Create tear duct drain	1630	2244	2962	772
68760	Close tear duct opening	162	224	295	102
68761	Close tear duct opening	140	193	255	89
68770	Close tear system fistula	741	1021	1347	432
68801	Dilate tear duct opening	83	115	152	51
68810	Probe nasolacrimal duct	116	160	211	71

SURGERY SERVICES

Code	Short Description	50th	75th	90th	MC
68811	Probe nasolacrimal duct	240	330	436	149
68815	Probe nasolacrimal duct	316	435	574	196
68840	Explore/irrigate tear ducts	88	121	160	67
68850	Injection for tear sac x-ray	75	103	136	53

AUDITORY SYSTEM SURGERY

External Ear

Code	Short Description	50th	75th	90th	MC
69000	Drain external ear lesion	95	124	150	68
69005	Drain external ear lesion	290	378	460	130
69020	Drain outer ear canal lesion	116	152	185	74
69090	Pierce earlobes	81	106	129	0
69100	Biopsy of external ear	93	122	148	60
69105	Biopsy of external ear canal	137	179	218	68
69110	Partial removal external ear	538	703	854	248
69120	Remove external ear	627	818	995	183
69140	Remove ear canal lesion(s)	1264	1649	2006	652
69145	Remove ear canal lesion(s)	375	489	594	210
69150	Extensive ear canal surgery	1710	2232	2714	968
69155	Extensive ear/neck surgery	2503	3267	3972	1435
69200	Clear outer ear canal	81	105	128	39
69205	Clear outer ear canal	209	273	332	92
69210	Remove impacted ear wax	50	64	78	27
69220	Clean out mastoid cavity	77	101	123	54
69222	Clean out mastoid cavity	168	219	267	84
69300	Revise external ear	1109	1448	1761	467
69310	Rebuild outer ear canal	1966	2566	3120	845
69320	Rebuild outer ear canal	2228	2908	3536	1292

Middle Ear

Code	Short Description	50th	75th	90th	MC
69400	Inflate middle ear canal	61	79	98	52
69401	Inflate middle ear canal	45	59	73	35
69405	Catheterize middle ear canal	139	182	225	118
69410	Inset middle ear baffle	48	62	77	40
69420	Incision of eardrum	149	195	241	80
69421	Incision of eardrum	246	322	398	115
69424	Remove ventilating tube	121	159	196	59
69433	Create eardrum opening	254	332	411	116

MC = Medicare Fee

Code	Short Description	50th	75th	90th	MC
69436	Create eardrum opening	424	553	685	168
69440	Exploration of middle ear	1270	1659	2052	669
69450	Eardrum revision	1331	1739	2152	537
69501	Mastoidectomy	1397	1825	2257	825
69502	Mastoidectomy	1801	2352	2910	1056
69505	Remove mastoid structures	2445	3193	3950	1205
69511	Extensive mastoid surgery	2563	3348	4142	1254
69530	Extensive mastoid surgery	3009	3930	4862	1432
69535	Remove part of temporal bone	3845	5023	6213	2448
69540	Remove ear lesion	158	206	255	101
69550	Remove ear lesion	2160	2821	3490	1045
69552	Remove ear lesion	3060	3997	4945	1469
69554	Remove ear lesion	4123	5386	6663	2219
69601	Mastoid surgery revision	1869	2441	3020	1118
69602	Mastoid surgery revision	2165	2828	3499	1232
69603	Mastoid surgery revision	2488	3249	4020	1298
69604	Mastoid surgery revision	2490	3253	4024	1335
69605	Mastoid surgery revision	2691	3515	4348	1366
69610	Repair eardrum	246	322	398	207
69620	Repair eardrum	1540	2012	2489	564
69631	Repair eardrum structures	2187	2857	3534	925
69632	Rebuild eardrum structures	2529	3303	4086	1187
69633	Rebuild eardrum structures	2632	3438	4254	1131
69635	Repair eardrum structures	2585	3377	4178	1249
69636	Rebuild eardrum structures	2750	3593	4444	1426
69637	Rebuild eardrum structures	2841	3711	4591	1420
69641	Revise middle ear and mastoid	2926	3822	4729	1183
69642	Revise middle ear and mastoid	3233	4223	5225	1550
69643	Revise middle ear and mastoid	3123	4080	5047	1435
69644	Revise middle ear and mastoid	3168	4139	5120	1592
69645	Revise middle ear and mastoid	3033	3961	4901	1525
69646	Revise middle ear and mastoid	3233	4223	5225	1650
69650	Release middle ear bone	1535	2005	2480	900
69660	Revise middle ear bone	2479	3238	4006	1122
69661	Revise middle ear bone	2631	3437	4251	1410
69662	Revise middle ear bone	2691	3515	4348	1382
69666	Repair middle ear structures	2033	2655	3285	916
69667	Repair middle ear structures	2023	2643	3269	913
69670	Remove mastoid air cells	2001	2613	3233	876
69676	Remove middle ear nerve	1756	2294	2838	731
69700	Close mastoid fistula	945	1234	1527	656

SURGERY SERVICES

Code	Short Description	50th	75th	90th	MC
69710	Implant/replace hearing aid	1092	1426	1765	0
69711	Remove/repair hearing aid	1021	1334	1650	744
69720	Release facial nerve	2724	3559	4402	1335
69725	Release facial nerve	3848	5027	6219	1564
69740	Repair facial nerve	2871	3750	4639	1132
69745	Repair facial nerve	3626	4737	5860	1321

Inner Ear

Code	Short Description	50th	75th	90th	MC
69801	Incise inner ear	1995	2606	3224	812
69802	Incise inner ear	2621	3423	4235	978
69805	Explore inner ear	2504	3271	4046	1115
69806	Explore inner ear	2756	3601	4454	1168
69820	Establish inner ear window	2239	2924	3618	784
69840	Revise inner ear window	1625	2123	2627	747
69905	Remove inner ear	2313	3021	3738	1048
69910	Remove inner ear and mastoid	2832	3699	4577	1275
69915	Incise inner ear nerve	3844	5021	6211	1555
69930	Implant cochlear device	3343	4367	5402	1503

Temporal Bone, Middle Fossa Approach

Code	Short Description	50th	75th	90th	MC
69950	Incise inner ear nerve	3927	5130	6346	1741
69955	Release facial nerve	4065	5309	6568	1882
69960	Release inner ear canal	3762	4914	6079	1769
69970	Remove inner ear lesion	4580	5982	7401	1971

MC = Medicare Fee

Code	Short Description	50th	75th	90th	MC

RADIOLOGY SERVICES

Radiology services include diagnostic x-rays, diagnostic ultrasound, radiation therapy, and nuclear medicine. Diagnostic services may be provided in the doctor's office, hospital or emergency department. Therapeutic x-rays and nuclear medicine are provided in the hospital radiology department. Radiology services may be performed by a radiologist, other medical specialists, or by radiology technicians working under the supervision of a doctor.

Interventional radiologic procedures or diagnostic studies involving injection of contrast media include necessary local anesthesia, placement of needle or catheter, injection of contrast media, supervision of the study, and interpretation of results. When one of these procedures is performed in full by a single doctor, it is designated as a "complete procedure."

You may receive two separate bills for radiology services performed in the hospital or emergency department. It is common for radiology services provided in the hospital or emergency department to be split into what are called *technical* and *professional* components.

The technical component, billed by the hospital and identified with a -TC after the service code, covers the process of taking the x-ray, and includes supplies and the radiology technician's services. The professional component, billed by the radiologist and identified with a -26 after the service code, is for the reading of the x-ray and reporting the results.

Code	Short Description	50th	75th	90th	MC

DIAGNOSTIC RADIOLOGY

Head and Neck X-ray

70010	Contrast x-ray of brain	341	426	511	206
70015	Contrast x-ray of brain	267	334	400	104
70030	X-ray eye for foreign body	70	88	105	23
70100	X-ray exam of jaw	71	88	106	27

MC = Medicare Fee

DOES YOUR DOCTOR CHARGE TOO MUCH?

Code	Short Description	50th	75th	90th	MC
70110	X-ray exam of jaw	94	118	141	34
70120	X-ray exam of mastoids	69	87	104	30
70130	X-ray exam of mastoids	104	130	155	44
70134	X-ray exam of middle ear	93	116	139	42
70140	X-ray exam of facial bones	81	101	121	31
70150	X-ray exam of facial bones	102	128	153	40
70160	X-ray exam of nasal bones	75	94	113	26
70170	X-ray exam of tear duct	95	119	142	47
70190	X-ray exam of eye sockets	71	88	106	32
70200	X-ray exam of eye sockets	100	126	150	41
70210	X-ray exam of sinuses	70	87	104	30
70220	X-ray exam of sinuses	98	121	145	40
70240	X-ray exam pituitary saddle	57	72	86	24
70250	X-ray exam of skull	82	103	123	33
70260	X-ray exam of skull	115	143	172	47
70300	X-ray exam of teeth	28	35	42	14
70310	X-ray exam of teeth	45	56	67	22
70320	Full mouth x-ray of teeth	79	99	118	38
70328	X-ray exam of jaw joint	62	78	93	26
70330	X-ray exam of jaw joints	99	123	148	41
70332	X-ray exam of jaw joint	203	253	304	99
70336	Magnetic image jaw joint	1122	1401	1680	447
70350	X-ray head for orthodontia	53	66	79	21
70355	Panoramic x-ray of jaws	88	110	131	29
70360	X-ray exam of neck	60	75	90	23
70370	Throat x-ray and fluoroscopy	138	173	207	60
70371	Speech evaluation, complex	254	317	380	113
70373	Contrast x-ray of larynx	178	223	267	83
70380	X-ray exam of salivary gland	67	84	101	31
70390	X-ray exam of salivary duct	172	215	258	80
70450	CAT scan of head or brain	583	730	880	203
70460	Contrast CAT scan of head	650	804	963	249
70470	Contrast CAT scans of head	759	942	1129	304
70480	CAT scan of skull	512	634	758	224
70481	Contrast CAT scan of skull	594	736	881	261
70482	Contrast CAT scans of skull	707	875	1048	313
70486	CAT scan of face, jaw	519	643	769	217
70487	Contrast CAT scan, face/jaw	597	739	885	257
70488	Contrast CAT scans face/jaw	724	897	1074	311
70490	CAT scan of neck tissue	565	699	837	224
70491	Contrast CAT of neck tissue	647	801	959	261

RADIOLOGY SERVICES

Code	Short Description	50th	75th	90th	MC
70492	Contrast CAT of neck tissue	742	919	1100	313
70540	Magnetic image, face, neck	1298	1607	1924	456
70541	Magnetic image, head (MRA)	1040	1288	1541	466
70551	Magnetic image, brain (MRI)	1196	1456	1722	456
70552	Magnetic image, brain (MRI)	1304	1615	1933	547
70553	Magnetic image, brain	1809	2162	2523	968

Chest X-ray

Code	Short Description	50th	75th	90th	MC
71010	Chest x-ray	58	74	89	25
71015	X-ray exam of chest	63	80	95	28
71020	Chest x-ray	74	93	110	32
71021	Chest x-ray	91	116	139	39
71022	Chest x-ray	93	118	141	40
71023	Chest x-ray and fluoroscopy	112	142	170	46
71030	Chest x-ray	100	127	151	42
71034	Chest x-ray and fluoroscopy	154	196	234	72
71035	Chest x-ray	73	93	111	27
71036	X-ray guidance for biopsy	198	251	300	81
71038	X-ray guidance for biopsy	189	240	287	84
71040	Contrast x-ray of bronchi	166	211	252	79
71060	Contrast x-ray of bronchi	234	298	356	112
71090	X-ray and pacemaker insertion	212	270	323	84
71100	X-ray exam of ribs	77	98	117	31
71101	X-ray exam of ribs/chest	93	118	141	36
71110	X-ray exam of ribs	101	129	154	41
71111	X-ray exam of ribs/chest	118	150	179	46
71120	X-ray exam of breastbone	75	96	114	32
71130	X-ray exam of breastbone	75	95	114	35
71250	Cat scan of chest	635	808	964	259
71260	Contrast CAT scan of chest	734	926	1100	302
71270	Contrast CAT scans of chest	832	1059	1265	369
71550	Magnetic image, chest	1157	1472	1758	462
71555	Magnetic imaging/chest (MRA)	985	1253	1497	0

Spine and Pelvis X-ray

Code	Short Description	50th	75th	90th	MC
72010	X-ray exam of spine	146	182	219	57
72020	X-ray exam of spine	55	70	85	22
72040	X-ray exam of neck spine	82	104	126	31

MC = Medicare Fee

Code	Short Description	50th	75th	90th	MC
72050	X-ray exam of neck spine	115	144	172	46
72052	X-ray exam of neck spine	140	175	209	57
72069	X-ray exam of trunk spine	72	91	109	27
72070	X-ray exam of thorax spine	84	105	126	33
72072	X-ray exam of thoracic spine	96	120	144	36
72074	X-ray exam of thoracic spine	118	148	178	42
72080	X-ray exam of trunk spine	85	107	128	34
72090	X-ray exam of trunk spine	92	115	138	37
72100	X-ray exam of lower spine	87	110	132	34
72110	X-ray exam of lower spine	122	152	183	47
72114	X-ray exam of lower spine	149	186	224	58
72120	X-ray exam of lower spine	108	136	163	41
72125	CAT scan of neck spine	657	814	974	259
72126	Contrast CAT scan of neck	779	966	1156	301
72127	Contrast CAT scans of neck	851	1055	1262	364
72128	CAT scan of thorax spine	633	785	939	259
72129	Contrast CAT scan of thorax	709	878	1051	301
72130	Contrast CAT scans of thorax	811	1005	1203	364
72131	CAT scan of lower spine	654	810	969	259
72132	Contrast CAT of lower spine	737	913	1093	301
72133	Contrast CAT scans, low spine	814	1009	1207	364
72141	Magnetic image, neck spine	1201	1489	1781	462
72142	Magnetic image, neck spine	1261	1563	1870	554
72146	Magnetic image, chest spine	1193	1478	1769	504
72147	Magnetic image, chest spine	1257	1558	1864	554
72148	Magnetic image, lumbar spine	1232	1493	1759	498
72149	Magnetic image, lumbar spine	1285	1593	1906	547
72156	Magnetic image, neck spine	1804	2235	2675	978
72157	Magnetic image, chest spine	1826	2263	2707	978
72158	Magnetic image, lumbar spine	1806	2238	2678	968
72159	Magnetic imaging/spine (MRA)	1077	1335	1598	0
72170	X-ray exam of pelvis	71	88	105	26
72190	X-ray exam of pelvis	92	114	136	33
72192	CAT scan of pelvis	624	773	925	255
72193	Contrast CAT scan of pelvis	713	899	1089	291
72194	Contrast CAT scans of pelvis	809	1003	1200	349
72196	Magnetic image, pelvis	1251	1550	1855	462
72198	Magnetic imaging/pelvis (MRA)	1014	1256	1503	0
72200	X-ray exam sacroiliac joints	70	87	104	26
72202	X-ray exam sacroiliac joints	83	103	123	31
72220	X-ray exam of tailbone	75	93	111	28

RADIOLOGY SERVICES

Code	Short Description	50th	75th	90th	MC
72240	Contrast x-ray of neck spine	421	522	624	207
72255	Contrast x-ray thorax spine	343	425	508	193
72265	Contrast x-ray lower spine	352	436	522	180
72270	Contrast x-ray of spine	489	606	726	273
72285	X-ray of neck spine disk	656	813	973	328
72295	X-ray of lower spine disk	663	822	983	310

Upper Extremities X-ray

Code	Short Description	50th	75th	90th	MC
73000	X-ray exam of collarbone	65	81	96	26
73010	X-ray exam of shoulder blade	69	87	103	26
73020	X-ray exam of shoulder	59	74	88	24
73030	X-ray exam of shoulder	74	93	111	28
73040	Contrast x-ray of shoulder	212	265	316	99
73050	X-ray exam of shoulders	76	95	113	33
73060	X-ray exam of humerus	70	87	104	28
73070	X-ray exam of elbow	67	84	100	25
73080	X-ray exam of elbow	73	91	109	28
73085	Contrast x-ray of elbow	210	263	314	99
73090	X-ray exam of forearm	65	81	97	26
73092	X-ray exam of arm, infant	55	69	82	25
73100	X-ray exam of wrist	63	78	92	25
73110	X-ray exam of wrist	69	87	104	27
73115	Contrast x-ray of wrist	165	206	246	81
73120	X-ray exam of hand	62	78	93	25
73130	X-ray exam of hand	71	90	107	27
73140	X-ray exam of finger(s)	57	71	84	21
73200	CAT scan of arm	530	663	791	223
73201	Contrast CAT scan of arm	614	768	917	259
73202	Contrast CAT scans of arm	699	874	1044	313
73220	Magnetic image, arm, hand	1090	1362	1627	456
73221	Magnetic image, joint of arm	1247	1559	1861	447
73225	Magnetic imaging/upper (MRA)	995	1244	1485	0

Lower Extremities X-ray

Code	Short Description	50th	75th	90th	MC
73500	X-ray exam of hip	61	77	92	25
73510	X-ray exam of hip	81	101	121	30
73520	X-ray exam of hips	104	133	162	36
73525	Contrast x-ray of hip	213	268	322	99

MC = Medicare Fee

DOES YOUR DOCTOR CHARGE TOO MUCH?

Code	Short Description	50th	75th	90th	MC
73530	X-ray exam of hip	84	106	127	32
73540	X-ray exam of pelvis and hips	74	93	112	30
73550	X-ray exam of thigh	74	93	112	28
73560	X-ray exam of knee	67	84	101	26
73562	X-ray exam of knee	77	97	116	29
73564	X-ray exam of knee	86	108	130	32
73565	X-ray exam of knee	81	105	129	25
73580	Contrast x-ray of knee joint	237	297	358	117
73590	X-ray exam of lower leg	69	87	105	26
73592	X-ray exam of leg, infant	57	72	86	25
73600	X-ray exam of ankle	63	79	95	25
73610	X-ray exam of ankle	73	92	110	27
73615	Contrast x-ray of ankle	182	229	276	99
73620	X-ray exam of foot	61	76	91	25
73630	X-ray exam of foot	71	89	107	27
73650	X-ray exam of heel	60	76	91	24
73660	X-ray exam of toe(s)	55	69	84	21
73700	CAT scan of leg	574	691	818	223
73701	Contrast CAT scan of leg	628	756	894	259
73702	Contrast CAT scans of leg	723	871	1030	313
73720	Magnetic image, leg, foot	1197	1443	1706	456
73721	Magnetic image, joint of leg	1243	1498	1772	447
73725	Magnetic imaging/lower (MRA)	1016	1224	1447	0

Abdomen X-ray

Code	Short Description	50th	75th	90th	MC
74000	X-ray exam of abdomen	67	84	99	27
74010	X-ray exam of abdomen	76	95	112	31
74020	X-ray exam of abdomen	89	113	134	35
74022	X-ray exam series, abdomen	114	143	169	41
74150	CAT scan of abdomen	633	779	931	252
74160	Contrast CAT scan of abdomen	737	916	1101	296
74170	Contrast CAT scans, abdomen	872	1073	1281	359
74181	Magnetic image, abdomen (MRI)	1317	1621	1936	462
74185	Magnetic image/abdomen (MRA)	1018	1253	1497	0
74190	X-ray exam of peritoneum	206	254	303	65

Gastrointestinal Tract X-ray

Code	Short Description	50th	75th	90th	MC
74210	Contrast x-ray exam of throat	133	166	200	58

RADIOLOGY SERVICES

Code	Short Description	50th	75th	90th	MC
74220	Contrast x-ray exam, esophagus	137	170	203	63
74230	Cinema x-ray throat/esophagus	171	214	257	71
74235	Remove esophagus obstruction	350	437	526	148
74240	X-ray exam upper GI tract	178	223	268	84
74241	X-ray exam upper GI tract	197	246	297	85
74245	X-ray exam upper GI tract	273	341	411	126
74246	Contrast x-ray upper GI tract	202	252	303	90
74247	Contrast x-ray upper GI tract	224	280	338	92
74249	Contrast x-ray upper GI tract	298	373	449	132
74250	X-ray exam of small bowel	151	188	227	67
74251	X-ray exam of small bowel	186	233	280	74
74260	X-ray exam of small bowel	165	206	248	75
74270	Contrast x-ray exam of colon	196	243	291	92
74280	Contrast x-ray exam of colon	260	323	387	125
74283	Contrast x-ray exam of colon	303	378	455	186
74290	Contrast x-ray exam gallbladder	99	123	148	41
74291	Contrast x-rays, gallbladder	59	74	89	24
74300	X-ray bile ducts, pancreas	99	124	149	0
74301	Additional x-rays at surgery	51	64	77	0
74305	X-ray bile ducts, pancreas	121	151	182	48
74320	Contrast x-ray of bile ducts	351	438	528	135
74327	X-ray for bile stone removal	310	387	466	95
74328	X-ray for bile duct endoscopy	336	420	506	142
74329	X-ray for pancreas endoscopy	308	384	462	142
74330	X-ray, bile/pancreas endoscopy	341	426	513	148
74340	X-ray guide for GI tube	284	355	428	117
74350	X-ray guide, stomach tube	301	375	452	145
74355	X-ray guide, intestinal tube	283	354	426	127
74360	X-ray guide, GI dilation	324	404	487	135
74363	X-ray, bile duct dilation	647	808	973	252

Urinary Tract X-ray

Code	Short Description	50th	75th	90th	MC
74400	Contrast x-ray urinary tract	190	247	305	82
74405	Contrast x-ray urinary tract	215	279	345	92
74410	Contrast x-ray urinary tract	207	268	332	91
74415	Contrast x-ray urinary tract	251	321	392	96
74420	Contrast x-ray urinary tract	229	297	368	108
74425	Contrast x-ray urinary tract	159	207	256	62
74430	Contrast x-ray of bladder	127	164	203	52

MC = Medicare Fee

Code	Short Description	50th	75th	90th	MC
74440	X-ray exam male genital tract	124	161	199	57
74445	X-ray exam of penis	197	256	316	94
74450	X-ray exam urethra/bladder	174	226	280	66
74455	X-ray exam urethra/bladder	189	245	304	70
74470	X-ray exam of kidney lesion	151	196	243	70
74475	X-ray control catheter insert	490	636	787	166
74480	X-ray control catheter insert	499	649	802	166
74485	X-ray guide, GU dilation	334	434	537	135

Gynecological and Obstetrical X-ray

Code	Short Description	50th	75th	90th	MC
74710	X-ray measurement of pelvis	109	142	176	53
74740	X-ray female genital tract	138	179	221	63
74742	X-ray fallopian tube	274	356	440	137
74775	X-ray exam of perineum	173	225	278	81

Heart X-ray

Code	Short Description	50th	75th	90th	MC
75552	Magnetic image, myocardium	1016	1244	1492	462
75553	Magnetic image, myocardium	987	1210	1451	474
75554	Cardiac MRI/function	1003	1228	1473	469
75555	Cardiac MRI/limited study	875	1072	1286	466
75556	Cardiac MRI/flow mapping	889	1089	1306	0

Aorta and Arteries X-ray

Code	Short Description	50th	75th	90th	MC
75600	Contrast x-ray of aorta, thoracic	894	1188	1497	456
75605	Contrast x-ray of aorta, thoracic	785	1043	1314	487
75625	Contrast x-ray of aorta, abdominal	815	1082	1364	487
75630	Contrast x-ray of aorta, abdominal	869	1154	1454	528
75650	Artery x-rays, head and neck	790	1050	1323	504
75658	Artery x-rays, arm	815	1083	1365	495
75660	Artery x-rays, head and neck	773	1027	1295	495
75662	Artery x-rays, head and neck	985	1309	1650	512
75665	Artery x-rays, head and neck	903	1199	1512	495
75671	Artery x-rays, head and neck	868	1153	1453	512
75676	Artery x-rays, neck	786	1044	1316	495
75680	Artery x-rays, neck	937	1244	1569	512
75685	Artery x-rays, spine	762	1012	1275	495
75705	Artery x-rays, spine	970	1289	1624	538

RADIOLOGY SERVICES

Code	Short Description	50th	75th	90th	MC
75710	Artery x-rays, arm/leg	740	984	1240	487
75716	Artery x-rays, arms/legs	803	1067	1344	495
75722	Artery x-rays, kidney	786	1045	1317	487
75724	Artery x-rays, kidneys	967	1285	1620	504
75726	Artery x-rays, abdomen	853	1133	1428	487
75731	Artery x-rays, adrenal gland	689	915	1153	487
75733	Artery x-rays, adrenal glands	790	1050	1323	495
75736	Artery x-rays, pelvis	905	1203	1516	487
75741	Artery x-rays, lung	751	997	1257	495
75743	Artery x-rays, lungs	839	1114	1404	512
75746	Artery x-rays, lung	598	794	1001	487
75756	Artery x-rays, chest	741	985	1242	487
75774	Artery x-ray, each vessel	993	1320	1663	449
75790	Visualize A-V shunt	427	567	715	136

Veins and Lymphatics X-ray

Code	Short Description	50th	75th	90th	MC
75801	Lymph vessel x-ray, arm/leg	392	543	707	225
75803	Lymph vessel x-ray, arms/legs	441	611	796	242
75805	Lymph vessel x-ray, trunk	431	597	778	249
75807	Lymph vessel x-ray, trunk	476	659	859	265
75809	Nonvascular shunt, x-ray	126	175	228	49
75810	Vein x-ray, spleen/liver	604	837	1091	487
75820	Vein x-ray, arm/leg	202	279	364	67
75822	Vein x-ray, arms/legs	300	416	542	102
75825	Vein x-ray, trunk	865	1199	1563	487
75827	Vein x-ray, chest	894	1239	1615	487
75831	Vein x-ray, kidney	675	935	1219	487
75833	Vein x-ray, kidneys	692	959	1251	504
75840	Vein x-ray, adrenal gland	631	874	1140	487
75842	Vein x-ray, adrenal glands	674	935	1218	504
75860	Vein x-ray, neck	676	937	1222	487
75870	Vein x-ray, skull	637	882	1150	487
75872	Vein x-ray, skull	661	916	1194	487
75880	Vein x-ray, eye socket	219	304	396	67
75885	Vein x-ray, liver	689	955	1245	502
75887	Vein x-ray, liver	678	939	1224	502
75889	Vein x-ray, liver	749	1037	1352	487
75891	Vein x-ray, liver	675	935	1218	487
75893	Venous sampling by catheter	1022	1416	1845	458

MC = Medicare Fee

Code	Short Description	50th	75th	90th	MC
75894	X-rays, transcatheter therapy	1317	1846	2428	891
75896	X-rays, transcatheter therapy	1209	1695	2229	783
75898	Follow-up angiogram	275	386	507	116
75900	Arterial catheter exchange	1142	1602	2107	743
75940	X-ray placement, vein filter	1029	1443	1898	458
75945	Intravascular ultrasound	294	413	543	174
75946	Intravascular ultrasound	163	228	300	96
75960	Transcatheter introduction of stent	1066	1494	1965	550
75961	Retrieval, broken catheter	972	1362	1792	565
75962	Repair arterial blockage	1302	1826	2401	566
75964	Repair artery blockage, each	729	1022	1344	305
75966	Repair arterial blockage	1023	1434	1886	603
75968	Repair artery blockage, each	630	884	1163	305
75970	Vascular biopsy	598	839	1103	436
75978	Repair venous blockage	1048	1470	1933	574
75980	Contrast x-ray exam bile duct	459	643	846	256
75982	Contrast x-ray exam bile duct	527	739	972	279
75984	X-ray control catheter change	230	322	424	102
75989	Abscess drainage under x-ray	420	589	775	165
75992	Atherectomy, x-ray exam	1085	1521	2000	566
75993	Atherectomy, x-ray exam	614	860	1132	305
75994	Atherectomy, x-ray exam	1204	1688	2221	603
75995	Atherectomy, x-ray exam	1211	1698	2233	603
75996	Atherectomy, x-ray exam	617	865	1138	305
76000	Fluoroscope examination	190	259	323	53
76001	Fluoroscope exam, extensive	283	385	479	123
76003	Needle localization by x-ray	184	250	312	71
76010	X-ray, nose to rectum	61	84	104	27
76020	X-rays, bone age	76	104	129	27
76040	X-rays, bone evaluation	112	153	190	41
76061	X-rays, bone survey	153	208	259	56
76062	X-rays, bone survey	203	276	344	76
76065	X-rays, bone evaluation	84	114	142	39
76066	Joint(s) survey, single film	105	144	179	53
76070	CAT scan, bone density study	360	490	611	114
76075	Dual energy x-ray study	314	411	501	120
76080	X-ray exam of fistula	143	194	242	63
76086	X-ray of mammary duct	216	294	365	108
76088	X-ray of mammary ducts	281	382	476	147
76090	Mammogram, one breast	102	133	162	59
76091	Mammogram, both breasts	133	173	209	73

RADIOLOGY SERVICES

Code	Short Description	50th	75th	90th	MC
76092	Mammogram, screening	102	132	160	0
76093	Magnetic image, breast	1201	1634	2035	683
76094	Magnetic image, both breasts	1632	2222	2766	898
76095	Stereotactic breast biopsy	597	812	1012	323
76096	X-ray of needle wire, breast	240	327	407	72
76098	X-ray exam, breast specimen	66	89	111	22
76100	X-ray exam of body section	148	201	251	71
76101	Complex body section x-ray	174	237	295	77
76102	Complex body section x-rays	216	294	365	88
76120	Cinematic x-rays	158	215	268	55
76125	Cinematic x-rays	83	113	140	40
76140	X-ray consultation	45	62	77	0
76150	X-ray exam, dry process	34	47	58	15
76350	Special x-ray contrast study	36	49	61	0
76355	CAT scan for localization	808	1100	1369	341
76360	CAT scan for needle biopsy	727	989	1231	339
76365	CAT scan for cyst aspiration	796	1083	1348	339
76370	CAT scan for therapy guide	367	499	622	142
76375	CAT scans, other planes	696	948	1180	129
76380	CAT scan follow-up study	327	446	555	168
76400	Magnetic image, bone marrow	1045	1422	1770	462

DIAGNOSTIC ULTRASOUND

Head and Neck Ultrasound

Code	Short Description	50th	75th	90th	MC
76506	Echo exam of head	197	266	330	79
76511	Echo exam of eye	189	254	316	82
76512	Echo exam of eye	273	366	452	85
76513	Echo exam of eye, water bath	211	285	354	85
76516	Echo exam of eye	204	272	334	70
76519	Echo exam of eye	197	262	323	70
76529	Echo exam of eye	187	253	314	75
76536	Echo exam of head and neck	201	271	337	76

Chest Ultrasound

Code	Short Description	50th	75th	90th	MC
76604	Echo exam of chest	196	247	297	72
76645	Echo exam of breast	161	209	257	63

MC = Medicare Fee

Code	Short Description	50th	75th	90th	MC

Abdomen and Retroperitoneum Ultrasound

76700	Echo exam of abdomen	264	334	403	107
76705	Echo exam of abdomen	187	238	290	78
76770	Echo exam abdomen back wall	253	316	380	104
76775	Echo exam abdomen back wall	194	245	296	77
76778	Echo exam kidney transplant	291	365	440	104

Spinal Canal Ultrasound

76800	Echo exam spinal canal	243	310	377	103

Pelvis Ultrasound

76805	Echo exam of pregnant uterus	260	332	404	120
76810	Echo exam of pregnant uterus	509	652	791	239
76815	Echo exam of pregnant uterus	195	249	303	80
76816	Echo exam follow-up or repeat	159	203	246	66
76818	Fetal biophysical profile	241	308	374	93
76825	Echo exam of fetal heart	242	309	375	133
76826	Echo exam of fetal heart	178	228	277	75
76827	Echo exam of fetal heart	221	283	344	103
76828	Echo exam of fetal heart	147	188	228	66
76830	Echo exam, transvaginal	223	286	347	86
76856	Echo exam of pelvis	221	284	344	86
76857	Echo exam of pelvis	159	207	255	55

Genitalia Ultrasound

76870	Echo exam of scrotum	216	281	343	83
76872	Echo exam, transrectal	272	357	439	86

Extremities Ultrasound

76880	Echo exam of extremity	236	306	374	78

Ultrasonic Guidance Procedures

76930	Echo guide for heart sac tap	191	261	335	85
76932	Echo guide for heart biopsy	205	280	358	85

RADIOLOGY SERVICES

Code	Short Description	50th	75th	90th	MC
76934	Echo guide for chest tap	202	277	354	85
76936	Echo guide for artery repair	463	633	810	323
76938	Echo exam for drainage	215	294	377	85
76941	Echo guide for transfusion	227	310	397	118
76942	Echo guide for biopsy	225	306	389	85
76945	Echo guide, villus sampling	208	285	364	97
76946	Echo guide for amniocentesis	159	218	279	71
76948	Echo guide, ova aspiration	159	218	279	71
76950	Echo guidance radiotherapy	166	227	291	73
76960	Echo guidance radiotherapy	204	279	356	73
76965	Echo guidance radiotherapy	466	637	815	309
76970	Ultrasound exam follow-up	118	162	207	56
76975	GI endoscopic ultrasound	246	337	431	91
76986	Echo exam at surgery	413	565	723	148

RADIATION ONCOLOGY

Clinical Treatment Planning

77261	Radiation therapy planning	243	335	432	67
77262	Radiation therapy planning	367	506	653	102
77263	Radiation therapy planning	496	689	892	152
77280	Set radiation therapy field	377	521	672	153
77285	Set radiation therapy field	571	788	1017	242
77290	Set radiation therapy field	690	910	1142	299
77295	Set radiation therapy field	2325	3206	4138	1178

Medical Radiation Physics, Dosimetry, Treatment Devices, and Special Services

77300	Radiation therapy dose plan	199	265	332	76
77305	Radiation therapy dose plan	255	341	431	98
77310	Radiation therapy dose plan	300	403	508	131
77315	Radiation therapy dose plan	411	538	669	167
77321	Radiation therapy port plan	502	674	850	184
77326	Radiation therapy dose plan	298	399	503	126
77327	Radiation therapy dose plan	439	589	744	186
77328	Radiation therapy dose plan	623	836	1054	271
77331	Special radiation dosimetry	160	222	287	59
77332	Radiation treatment aid(s)	176	236	298	73

MC = Medicare Fee

Code	Short Description	50th	75th	90th	MC
77333	Radiation treatment aid(s)	257	344	435	106
77334	Radiation treatment aid(s)	429	568	711	171
77336	Radiation physics consult	178	232	288	102
77370	Radiation physics consult	205	275	347	120

Radiation Treatment Delivery

Code	Short Description	50th	75th	90th	MC
77401	Radiation treatment delivery	107	145	185	61
77402	Radiation treatment delivery	124	161	201	61
77403	Radiation treatment delivery	133	170	209	61
77404	Radiation treatment delivery	140	182	227	61
77406	Radiation treatment delivery	138	179	223	61
77407	Radiation treatment delivery	160	208	259	72
77408	Radiation treatment delivery	160	207	257	72
77409	Radiation treatment delivery	155	201	251	72
77411	Radiation treatment delivery	103	134	167	72
77412	Radiation treatment delivery	188	242	300	80
77413	Radiation treatment delivery	193	254	319	80
77414	Radiation treatment delivery	214	279	350	80
77416	Radiation treatment delivery	209	278	352	80
77417	Radiology port film(s)	53	72	92	20

Clinical Treatment Management

Code	Short Description	50th	75th	90th	MC
77419	Weekly radiation therapy	367	566	707	174
77420	Weekly radiation therapy	244	377	471	78
77425	Weekly radiation therapy	366	565	707	119
77430	Weekly radiation therapy	504	778	973	174
77431	Radiation therapy management	168	259	324	88
77432	Stereotactic radiation treatment	968	1494	1869	427
77470	Special radiation treatment	882	1362	1703	483
77600	Hyperthermia treatment	539	831	1040	180
77605	Hyperthermia treatment	570	880	1101	241
77610	Hyperthermia treatment	431	665	832	180
77615	Hyperthermia treatment	570	879	1100	241
77620	Hyperthermia treatment	432	666	833	180
77750	Infuse radioactive materials	575	787	995	268
77761	Radioelement application	578	790	999	258
77762	Radioelement application	872	1192	1507	383
77763	Radioelement application	1232	1685	2131	541

RADIOLOGY SERVICES

Code	Short Description	50th	75th	90th	MC
77776	Radioelement application	711	973	1230	301
77777	Radioelement application	1183	1617	2045	484
77778	Radioelement application	1814	2480	3136	682
77781	High intensity brachytherapy	1786	2442	3088	771
77782	High intensity brachytherapy	2068	2827	3576	809
77783	High intensity brachytherapy	2256	3085	3901	864
77784	High intensity brachytherapy	2493	3408	4310	950
77789	Radioelement application	160	219	277	66
77790	Radioelement handling	207	283	358	68

NUCLEAR MEDICINE

Diagnostic Nuclear Medicine

Code	Short Description	50th	75th	90th	MC
78000	Thyroid, single uptake	113	146	180	42
78001	Thyroid, multiple uptakes	142	184	226	57
78003	Thyroid suppress/stimulation	111	144	177	49
78006	Thyroid imaging with uptake	280	363	446	106
78007	Thyroid imaging with uptakes	315	407	501	113
78010	Thyroid imaging	214	276	340	81
78011	Thyroid imaging with flow	260	336	413	105
78015	Thyroid metastases imaging	275	355	437	121
78016	Thyroid metastases imaging/studies	330	426	524	160
78017	Thyroid metastases imaging, multiple	358	463	569	170
78018	Thyroid metastases imaging, body	534	690	848	232
78070	Parathyroid nuclear imaging	213	276	339	97
78075	Adrenal nuclear imaging	449	580	713	222
78102	Bone marrow imaging, limited	210	311	411	97
78103	Bone marrow imaging, multiple	302	448	592	145
78104	Bone marrow imaging, body	372	553	730	179
78110	Plasma volume, single	95	140	185	42
78111	Plasma volume, multiple	203	301	398	99
78120	Red cell mass, single	155	230	304	71
78121	Red cell mass, multiple	253	375	496	115
78122	Blood volume	383	568	750	180
78130	Red cell survival study	260	386	510	128
78135	Red cell survival kinetics	412	611	808	198
78140	Red cell sequestration	332	492	650	165
78160	Plasma iron turnover	300	445	588	142
78162	Iron absorption exam	264	391	517	131

MC = Medicare Fee

Code	Short Description	50th	75th	90th	MC
78170	Red cell iron utilization	387	575	760	202
78172	Total body iron estimation	149	222	293	0
78185	Spleen imaging	246	365	482	101
78190	Platelet survival, kinetics	507	753	995	249
78191	Platelet survival	566	840	1109	281
78195	Lymph system imaging	338	502	663	190
78201	Liver imaging	259	341	407	102
78202	Liver imaging with flow	323	426	508	124
78205	Liver imaging (3D)	538	708	845	238
78215	Liver and spleen imaging	362	476	568	124
78216	Liver and spleen image, flow	379	498	594	147
78220	Liver function study	400	527	628	151
78223	Hepatobiliary imaging	378	497	593	167
78230	Salivary gland imaging	220	289	345	97
78231	Serial salivary imaging	287	377	450	134
78232	Salivary gland function exam	300	394	470	144
78258	Esophageal motility study	275	362	431	135
78261	Gastric mucosa imaging	340	448	534	175
78262	Gastroesophageal reflux exam	380	500	597	179
78264	Gastric emptying study	407	535	638	180
78270	Vitamin B-12 absorption exam	153	201	240	63
78271	Vitamin B-12 absorption exam	201	265	316	66
78272	Vitamin B-12 absorption, combined	224	294	351	93
78278	Acute GI blood loss imaging	470	619	738	216
78282	GI protein loss exam	157	206	246	0
78290	Meckel's diverticulum exam	309	407	485	138
78291	Leveen/shunt patency exam	307	404	482	147
78300	Bone imaging, limited area	284	361	442	116
78305	Bone imaging, multiple areas	380	484	592	166
78306	Bone imaging, whole body	464	581	703	188
78315	Bone imaging, 3 phase	520	662	809	213
78320	Bone imaging (3D)	627	798	975	253
78350	Bone mineral, single photon	159	203	248	37
78351	Bone mineral, dual photon	240	306	374	0
78414	Non-imaging heart function	516	681	843	0
78428	Cardiac shunt imaging	249	328	406	116
78445	Vascular flow imaging	250	329	408	88
78455	Venous thrombosis study	348	459	569	172
78457	Venous thrombosis imaging	287	378	468	129
78458	Venous thrombosis images, bilateral	407	537	665	181
78459	Heart muscle imaging (PET)	233	307	381	0

RADIOLOGY SERVICES

Code	Short Description	50th	75th	90th	MC
78460	Heart muscle blood single	346	456	565	123
78461	Heart muscle blood multiple	667	879	1089	221
78464	Heart image (3D) single	674	889	1101	295
78465	Heart image (3D) multiple	1163	1468	1771	475
78466	Heart infarct image	286	377	467	124
78468	Heart infarct image	375	494	612	164
78469	Heart infarct image (3D)	500	659	817	224
78472	Gated heart, resting	585	771	955	237
78473	Gated heart, multiple	774	1020	1263	354
78478	Heart wall motion (add-on)	198	260	321	84
78480	Heart function, (add-on)	181	239	296	84
78481	Heart first pass single	505	666	825	227
78483	Heart first pass multiple	870	1147	1421	341
78580	Lung perfusion imaging	336	435	535	154
78584	Lung V/Q image single breath	371	480	590	158
78585	Lung V/Q imaging	579	750	921	246
78586	Aerosol lung image, single	290	375	461	109
78587	Aerosol lung image, multiple	353	457	562	120
78591	Ventilation image, single projection	310	401	493	117
78593	Ventilation image, single projection	381	493	606	142
78594	Ventilation image, multiple projection	533	690	848	197
78596	Lung differential function	534	690	849	304
78600	Brain imaging, limited static	264	346	426	120
78601	Brain imaging, limited, vascular flow	305	399	491	142
78605	Brain imaging, complete	360	471	580	143
78606	Brain imaging, complete, vascular flow	397	519	640	164
78607	Brain imaging (3D)	701	918	1130	284
78608	Brain imaging (PET)	342	448	552	0
78609	Brain imaging (PET)	343	449	553	0
78610	Brain flow imaging only	192	251	309	69
78615	Cerebral blood flow imaging	397	520	641	152
78630	Cerebrospinal fluid scan	499	653	804	206
78635	CSF ventriculography	259	339	417	117
78645	CSF shunt evaluation	327	428	528	146
78647	Cerebrospinal fluid scan	466	609	751	247
78650	CSF leakage imaging	391	512	630	189
78660	Nuclear exam of tear flow	204	268	330	99
78700	Kidney imaging, static	298	393	496	126
78701	Kidney imaging with flow	427	564	711	146
78704	Imaging renogram	419	553	698	172

MC = Medicare Fee

Code	Short Description	50th	75th	90th	MC
78707	Kidney flow and function image	512	676	853	199
78710	Kidney imaging (3D)	523	691	872	235
78715	Renal vascular flow exam	201	266	336	69
78725	Kidney function study	263	348	439	80
78726	Kidney function w/intervention	349	460	581	144
78727	Kidney transplant evaluation	443	585	739	185
78730	Urinary bladder retention	140	185	233	67
78740	Ureteral reflux study	234	309	390	101
78760	Testicular imaging	257	339	428	124
78761	Testicular imaging and flow	331	437	551	145
78800	Tumor imaging, limited area	352	485	620	148
78801	Tumor imaging, multiple areas	443	611	780	184
78802	Tumor imaging, whole body	579	799	1021	232
78803	Tumor imaging (3D)	638	880	1124	277
78805	Abscess imaging, limited area	349	481	614	152
78806	Abscess imaging, whole body	629	868	1108	262
78807	Nuclear localization/abscess	558	769	983	277
78810	Tumor imaging (PET)	239	330	421	0
78890	Nuclear medicine data, simple	448	619	790	0
78891	Nuclear medicine data, complex	520	718	916	0
78990	Provide diagnostic radionuclide(s)	110	152	194	0

Therapeutic

Code	Short Description	50th	75th	90th	MC
79000	Initial hyperthyroid therapy	443	589	733	178
79001	Repeat hyperthyroid therapy	210	279	347	95
79020	Thyroid ablation	391	521	648	178
79030	Thyroid ablation, carcinoma	458	609	758	192
79035	Thyroid metastatic therapy	474	630	784	213
79100	Hematopoietic nuclear therapy	335	446	554	154
79200	Intracavitary nuclear treatment	393	522	650	187
79300	Interstitial nuclear therapy	638	848	1056	0
79400	Non-hematologic nuclear therapy	447	594	739	185
79420	Intravascular nuclear therapy	421	560	698	0
79440	Nuclear joint therapy	425	565	703	187

LABORATORY SERVICES

Laboratory services may be provided your doctor's office, a hospital laboratory, or an independent laboratory. Most laboratory services are performed by laboratory technicians working under the supervision of a doctor.

Many doctors have office laboratories, staffed by qualified technicians, where most commonly ordered laboratory tests are performed. Doctors who do not have office laboratories will either refer you to a hospital or independent laboratory, or will collect blood, urine, PAP smears or other samples and send them to an independent laboratory for analysis and reporting.

Laboratory services are billed in addition to any visit services, surgery services, or other procedures. You will be billed by the doctor for laboratory tests performed in the office laboratory. For services performed in an independent laboratory you may be billed by the laboratory or the doctor's office.

It is common for several laboratory tests to be performed at the same time by using automated multichannel equipment. It is less expensive to perform laboratory tests in this manner, even when the doctor is interested in only a few tests.

Code	Short Description	50th	75th	90th	MC
AUTOMATED LABORATORY PANELS					
80002	1-2 clinical chemistry tests	22	32	42	0
80003	3 clinical chemistry tests	31	44	58	0
80004	4 clinical chemistry tests	31	43	56	0
80005	5 clinical chemistry tests	35	49	64	0
80006	6 clinical chemistry tests	36	52	68	0
80007	7 clinical chemistry tests	35	49	64	0
80008	8 clinical chemistry tests	38	55	73	0
80009	9 clinical chemistry tests	38	54	72	0
80010	10 clinical chemistry tests	38	54	70	0
80011	11 clinical chemistry tests	39	56	73	0
80012	12 clinical chemistry tests	39	54	71	0

MC = Medicare Fee

Code	Short Description	50th	75th	90th	MC
80016	13-16 blood/urine tests	39	55	72	0
80018	17-18 blood/urine tests	43	59	77	0
80019	19 blood/urine tests	44	62	80	0

ORGAN OR DISEASE ORIENTED PANELS

Code	Short Description	50th	75th	90th	MC
80050	General health panel	91	116	137	0
80055	Obstetric panel	78	102	123	0
80058	Hepatic function panel	36	48	59	0
80059	Hepatitis panel	162	211	254	0
80061	Lipid panel	49	63	75	0
80072	Arthritis panel	66	87	104	0
80090	Torch antibody panel	109	142	170	0
80091	Thyroid panel	38	48	57	0
80092	Thyroid panel with TSH	85	107	126	0

DRUG TESTING

Code	Short Description	50th	75th	90th	MC
80100	Drug screen	46	64	79	0
80101	Drug screen	39	51	62	0
80102	Drug confirmation	69	90	108	0
80103	Drug analysis, tissue prep	17	22	26	0

THERAPEUTIC DRUG ASSAYS

Code	Short Description	50th	75th	90th	MC
80150	Assay amikacin	67	87	104	0
80152	Assay amitriptyline	62	81	98	0
80154	Assay benzodiazepines	74	96	115	0
80156	Assay carbamazepine	57	73	87	0
80158	Assay cyclosporine	87	114	137	0
80160	Assay desipramine	73	95	114	0
80162	Assay digoxin	51	65	77	0
80164	Assay dipropylacetic acid	61	77	92	0
80166	Assay doxepin	60	78	94	0
80168	Assay ethosuximide	65	85	102	0
80170	Assay gentamicin	69	89	107	0
80172	Assay gold	62	81	98	0
80174	Assay imipramine	69	90	108	0
80176	Assay lidocaine	46	60	72	0
80178	Assay lithium	29	37	44	0

LABORATORY SERVICES

Code	Short Description	50th	75th	90th	MC
80182	Assay nortriptyline	72	94	113	0
80184	Assay phenobarbital	53	68	82	0
80185	Assay phenytoin	54	70	83	0
80186	Assay phenytoin, free	63	82	99	0
80188	Assay primidone	56	73	87	0
80190	Assay procainamide	53	69	83	0
80192	Assay procainamide	72	93	112	0
80194	Assay quinidine	59	77	91	0
80196	Assay salicylate	38	50	60	0
80197	Assay tacrolimus	0	0	0	0
80198	Assay theophylline	50	65	77	0
80200	Assay tobramycin	78	102	122	0
80202	Assay vancomycin	74	94	112	0

EVOCATIVE/SUPPRESSION TESTING

Code	Short Description	50th	75th	90th	MC
80400	ACTH stimulation panel	86	112	134	0
80402	ACTH stimulation panel	170	221	266	0
80406	ACTH stimulation panel	168	219	263	0
80408	Aldosterone suppression evaluation	252	329	395	0
80410	Calcitonin stimulation panel	108	141	169	0
80412	CRH stimulation panel	596	777	933	0
80414	Testosterone response	151	196	235	0
80415	Estradiol response panel	156	204	245	0
80416	Renin stimulation panel	305	397	477	0
80417	Renin stimulation panel	303	395	474	0
80418	Pituitary evaluation panel	1181	1538	1847	0
80420	Dexamethasone panel	132	172	206	0
80422	Glucagon tolerance panel	78	102	122	0
80424	Glucagon tolerance panel	115	150	181	0
80426	Gonadotropin hormone panel	340	442	531	0
80428	Growth hormone panel	114	149	179	0
80430	Growth hormone panel	123	161	193	0
80432	Insulin suppression panel	296	386	463	0
80434	Insulin tolerance panel	196	256	307	0
80435	Insulin tolerance panel	205	267	320	0
80436	Metyrapone panel	149	194	232	0
80438	TRH stimulation panel	88	115	138	0
80439	TRH stimulation panel	203	265	318	0
80440	TRH stimulation panel	181	236	283	0

MC = Medicare Fee

Code	Short Description	50th	75th	90th	MC

CONSULTATIONS (CLINICAL PATHOLOGY)

80500	Lab pathology consultation	48	66	86	19
80502	Lab pathology consultation	118	169	224	53

URINALYSIS

81000	Urinalysis, non-auto with scope	13	17	22	0
81001	Urinalysis, auto, w/scope	18	25	32	0
81002	Urinalysis, non-auto without scope	10	13	17	0
81003	Urinalysis, auto, w/o scope	11	16	21	0
81005	Urinalysis	9	12	16	0
81007	Urine screen for bacteria	10	14	18	0
81015	Microscopic exam of urine	9	13	16	0
81020	Urinalysis, glass test	15	20	26	0
81025	Urine pregnancy test	16	21	28	0
81050	Urinalysis, volume measure	14	20	26	0

CHEMISTRY

82000	Assay blood acetaldehyde	37	50	64	0
82003	Assay acetaminophen	54	72	92	0
82009	Test for acetone/ketones	12	17	21	0
82010	Assay acetone/ketones	27	37	47	0
82013	Assay acetylcholinesterase	37	50	63	0
82024	Assay ACTH	116	156	198	0
82030	Assay ADP & AMP	67	90	114	0
82040	Assay serum albumin	17	22	28	0
82042	Assay urine albumin	21	29	36	0
82043	Microalbumin, quantitative	23	30	38	0
82044	Microalbumin, semiquantitative	21	28	36	0
82055	Assay ethanol	42	56	71	0
82075	Assay breath ethanol	42	57	72	0
82085	Assay aldolase	41	55	70	0
82088	Aldosterone	117	158	200	0
82101	Assay urine alkaloids	88	119	151	0
82103	Alpha-1-antitrypsin, total	41	55	70	0
82104	Alpha-1-antitrypsin, pheno	56	76	96	0
82105	Alpha-fetoprotein, serum	69	93	118	0
82106	Alpha-fetoprotein, amniotic	50	68	86	0

LABORATORY SERVICES

Code	Short Description	50th	75th	90th	MC
82108	Assay aluminum	89	114	139	0
82128	Test for amino acids	30	40	51	0
82130	Assay amino acids, urine/plasma	130	175	222	0
82131	Assay amino acids, quantitation	89	120	152	0
82135	Assay aminolevulinic acid	56	76	96	0
82140	Assay ammonia	57	77	98	0
82143	Amniotic fluid scan	41	55	70	0
82145	Assay amphetamines	44	59	74	0
82150	Assay amylase	22	30	38	0
82157	Assay androstenedione	96	129	164	0
82160	Assay androsterone	89	120	152	0
82163	Assay angiotensin II	55	74	94	0
82164	Assay angiotensin I	69	93	119	0
82172	Assay apolipoprotein	42	56	70	0
82175	Assay arsenic	62	83	106	0
82180	Assay ascorbic acid	30	41	52	0
82190	Atomic absorption	45	61	77	0
82205	Assay barbiturates	50	67	85	0
82232	Assay beta-2 protein	66	87	110	0
82239	Assay bile acids, total	54	73	92	0
82240	Assay bile acids, cholylglycine	69	93	118	0
82250	Assay bilirubin	17	23	29	0
82251	Assay bilirubin	24	32	41	0
82252	Test for bilirubin, feces	15	20	25	0
82270	Test for blood, feces	10	14	19	0
82273	Test for blood, other source	12	16	21	0
82286	Assay bradykinin	19	25	32	0
82300	Assay cadmium	68	92	117	0
82306	Assay vitamin D	149	200	254	0
82307	Assay vitamin D	109	147	186	0
82308	Assay calcitonin	99	134	170	0
82310	Assay calcium	17	23	28	0
82330	Assay calcium	45	60	74	0
82331	Calcium infusion test	24	32	41	0
82340	Assay calcium in urine	25	34	43	0
82355	Calculus (stone) analysis	46	61	78	0
82360	Calculus (stone) assay	38	51	65	0
82365	Calculus (stone) assay	52	69	88	0
82370	X-ray assay, calculus (stone)	40	53	68	0
82374	Assay blood carbon dioxide	16	21	27	0

MC = Medicare Fee

Code	Short Description	50th	75th	90th	MC
82375	Assay blood carbon monoxide	35	47	59	0
82376	Test for carbon monoxide	13	17	22	0
82378	Assay carcinoembryonic antigen	69	90	112	0
82380	Assay carotene	33	45	57	0
82382	Assay urine catecholamines	68	91	116	0
82383	Assay blood catecholamines	88	118	150	0
82384	Assay three catecholamines	111	149	190	0
82387	Assay cathepsin-D	61	82	104	0
82390	Assay ceruloplasmin	42	56	71	0
82397	Chemiluminescent assay	51	68	87	0
82415	Assay chloramphenicol	41	55	70	0
82435	Assay blood chloride	14	19	24	0
82436	Assay urine chloride	18	25	31	0
82438	Assay other fluid chlorides	18	24	31	0
82441	Test for chlorohydrocarbons	23	30	38	0
82465	Assay serum cholesterol	15	20	24	0
82480	Assay serum cholinesterase	33	45	57	0
82482	Assay RBC cholinesterase	37	50	64	0
82485	Assay chondroitin sulfate	52	70	89	0
82486	Gas/liquid chromatography	58	78	98	0
82487	Paper chromatography	60	80	102	0
82488	Paper chromatography	84	113	143	0
82489	Thin layer chromatography	60	81	103	0
82491	Chromatography, quantitative	63	84	107	0
82495	Assay chromium	56	76	96	0
82507	Assay citrate	96	130	164	0
82520	Assay cocaine	38	51	65	0
82525	Assay copper	43	58	73	0
82528	Assay corticosterone	55	74	94	0
82530	Assay cortisol, free	64	86	109	0
82533	Assay cortisol, total	66	86	107	0
82540	Assay creatine	17	23	29	0
82550	Assay CK/CPK, total	22	29	37	0
82552	Assay CK/CPK, isoenzymes	48	64	80	0
82553	Assay CK/CPK, MB fraction	36	48	61	0
82554	Assay CK/CPK, isoforms	36	48	61	0
82565	Assay creatinine, blood	17	23	29	0
82570	Assay creatinine, other	21	28	36	0
82575	Assay creatinine, clearance	35	47	59	0
82585	Assay cryofibrinogen	28	38	48	0
82595	Assay cryoglobulin	36	49	62	0

LABORATORY SERVICES

Code	Short Description	50th	75th	90th	MC
82600	Assay cyanide	58	78	99	0
82607	Assay vitamin B-12	54	70	87	0
82608	Assay B-12 binding capacity	48	65	83	0
82615	Test for urine cystines	38	51	64	0
82626	Assay dehydroepiandrosterone	122	162	203	0
82627	Assay dehydroepiandrosterone	92	122	153	0
82633	Assay desoxycorticosterone	117	155	194	0
82634	Assay deoxycortisol	112	150	187	0
82638	Assay dibucaine number	34	46	57	0
82646	Assay dihydrocodeinone	53	70	88	0
82649	Assay dihydromorphinone	67	89	112	0
82651	Assay dihydrotestosterone	70	93	116	0
82652	Assay dihydroxyvitamin D	135	179	224	0
82654	Assay dimethadione	58	77	97	0
82664	Electrophoretic test	70	94	117	0
82666	Assay epiandrosterone	90	120	150	0
82668	Assay erythropoietin	90	120	150	0
82670	Assay estradiol	91	122	152	0
82671	Assay estrogens assay	89	118	148	0
82672	Assay estrogen assay	102	136	170	0
82677	Assay estriol	74	99	124	0
82679	Assay estrone	102	135	169	0
82690	Assay ethchlorvynol	75	100	125	0
82693	Assay ethylene glycol	46	61	77	0
82696	Assay etiocholanolone	84	112	140	0
82705	Test for fats/lipids, feces	26	35	43	0
82710	Assay fats/lipids, feces	57	76	95	0
82715	Assay fecal fat	45	60	75	0
82725	Assay blood fatty acids	33	44	55	0
82728	Assay ferritin	41	54	67	0
82735	Assay fluoride	61	81	101	0
82742	Assay flurazepam	60	79	99	0
82746	Assay folic acid, serum	52	67	82	0
82747	Assay folic acid, RBC	65	87	109	0
82757	Assay semen fructose	43	58	72	0
82759	Assay RBC galactokinase	51	68	85	0
82760	Assay galactose	36	48	60	0
82775	Assay galactose transferase	67	89	111	0
82776	Test for galactose transferase	20	27	33	0
82784	Assay gammaglobulin IgM	30	39	49	0

MC = Medicare Fee

Code	Short Description	50th	75th	90th	MC
82785	Assay gammaglobulin IgE	58	76	94	0
82787	Assay gammaglobulin IgG1, 2, 3, 4	82	109	136	0
82800	Blood gases, pH only	25	34	43	0
82803	Blood gases; pH, pO_2 & pCO_2	64	86	108	0
82805	Blood gases with O_2 saturation	55	73	92	0
82810	Blood gases, O_2 saturation only	25	33	42	0
82820	Hemoglobin-oxygen affinity	25	33	42	0
82926	Assay gastric acid	26	35	44	0
82928	Assay gastric acid	16	21	27	0
82938	Assay gastrin	70	93	117	0
82941	Assay gastrin	64	85	107	0
82943	Assay glucagon	53	70	88	0
82946	Glucagon tolerance test	37	49	61	0
82947	Assay quantitative, glucose	15	19	24	0
82948	Reagent strip/blood glucose	11	15	18	0
82950	Glucose test	17	22	27	0
82951	Glucose tolerance test (GTT)	37	49	62	0
82952	GTT-added samples	15	20	25	0
82953	Glucose-tolbutamide test	52	69	87	0
82955	Assay G6PD enzyme	33	44	55	0
82960	Assay G6PD enzyme	22	29	36	0
82962	Glucose blood test	11	15	18	0
82963	Glucosidase assay	75	100	125	0
82965	Assay GDH enzyme	25	34	43	0
82975	Assay glutamine	42	56	70	0
82977	Assay GGT	20	27	33	0
82978	Glutathione assay	40	53	66	0
82979	Assay RBC glutathione enzyme	24	32	40	0
82980	Assay glutethimide	53	70	88	0
82985	Assay glycated protein	41	54	68	0
83001	Assay gonadotropin (FSH)	70	91	112	0
83002	Assay gonadotropin (LH)	70	90	111	0
83003	Assay growth hormone (HGH)	56	74	93	0
83008	Assay guanosine	48	64	80	0
83010	Assay haptoglobin, quantitative	45	60	75	0
83012	Assay haptoglobin, phenotypes	57	75	94	0
83015	Assay heavy metal, screen	75	100	125	0
83018	Assay heavy metal, quantitative	98	131	164	0
83020	Assay hemoglobin	42	58	74	0
83026	Assay hemoglobin, copper sulfate	9	12	15	0
83030	Assay fetal hemoglobin	31	41	51	0

LABORATORY SERVICES

Code	Short Description	50th	75th	90th	MC
83033	Test for fetal fecal hemoglobin	21	28	36	0
83036	Assay glycated hemoglobin	35	46	57	0
83045	Test for methemoglobin	15	20	26	0
83050	Assay methemoglobin	26	35	44	0
83051	Assay plasma hemoglobin	22	30	37	0
83055	Test for sulfhemoglobin	18	25	31	0
83060	Assay sulfhemoglobin	32	43	53	0
83065	Assay hemoglobin heat	26	34	43	0
83068	Assay hemoglobin stability screen	26	35	43	0
83069	Assay urine hemoglobin	13	18	22	0
83070	Test for hemosiderin	21	27	34	0
83071	Assay hemosiderin	27	36	45	0
83088	Assay histamine	89	118	148	0
83150	Assay HVA	65	87	109	0
83491	Assay corticosteroids	64	85	107	0
83497	Assay 5-HIAA	59	78	98	0
83498	Assay progesterone	90	120	150	0
83499	Assay progesterone	73	97	122	0
83500	Assay free hydroxyproline	78	103	130	0
83505	Assay total hydroxyproline	126	167	209	0
83516	Immunoassay, non antibody	46	62	82	0
83518	Immunoassay, dipstick	43	58	76	0
83519	Immunoassay, non-antibody	66	89	117	0
83520	Immunoassay, RIA	53	74	99	0
83525	Assay insulin	45	60	79	0
83527	Assay insulin	49	66	87	0
83528	Assay intrinsic factor	60	81	107	0
83540	Assay iron	18	24	31	0
83550	Assay iron binding capacity	23	30	39	0
83570	Assay IDH enzyme	34	46	60	0
83582	Assay ketogenic steroids	47	63	83	0
83586	Assay ketosteroids total	54	72	95	0
83593	Assay ketosteroids, fractionation	86	115	152	0
83605	Assay lactic acid assay	34	46	60	0
83615	Assay lactate (LD)(LDH) enzyme	21	28	37	0
83625	Assay LDH enzymes	41	56	73	0
83632	Assay placental lactogen	66	89	117	0
83633	Test for lactose, urine	26	35	46	0
83634	Assay lactose, urine	43	58	76	0
83655	Assay lead	45	60	79	0

MC = Medicare Fee

Code	Short Description	50th	75th	90th	MC
83661	Assay L/S ratio	33	45	59	0
83662	Assay L/S ratio, foam stability	53	71	93	0
83670	Assay LAP enzyme	29	40	52	0
83690	Assay lipase	27	37	49	0
83715	Assay lipoprotein, blood	37	48	63	0
83717	Assay lipoprotein, blood	63	85	112	0
83718	Assay lipoprotein, cholesterol (HDL)	25	32	42	0
83719	Assay lipoprotein, cholesterol	39	52	67	0
83721	Assay lipoprotein, cholesterol (LDL)	25	34	44	0
83727	Assay LRH hormone	58	79	103	0
83735	Assay magnesium	19	26	34	0
83775	Assay malate dehydrogenase	24	33	43	0
83785	Assay manganese	72	98	128	0
83805	Assay meprobamate	62	84	110	0
83825	Assay mercury	54	73	95	0
83835	Assay metanephrines	93	125	165	0
83840	Assay methadone	18	24	31	0
83857	Assay methemalbumin	38	51	67	0
83858	Assay methsuximide	53	71	94	0
83864	Assay mucopolysaccharides	44	59	77	0
83866	Assay mucopolysaccharides, screen	36	49	64	0
83872	Assay mucin, synovial fluid	20	28	36	0
83873	Assay myelin basic protein	71	95	125	0
83874	Assay myoglobin	44	59	78	0
83883	Nephelometry, not specified	35	46	57	0
83885	Assay nickel	62	81	101	0
83887	Assay nicotine	83	109	135	0
83890	Molecular diagnostics	24	32	39	0
83892	Molecular diagnostics	28	37	46	0
83894	Molecular diagnostics	24	31	39	0
83896	Molecular diagnostics	32	42	53	0
83898	Molecular diagnostics	69	91	113	0
83912	Molecular diagnostics	48	63	78	0
83915	Assay nucleotidase	36	47	59	0
83916	Assay oligoclonal bands	69	91	113	0
83918	Assay organic acids	77	101	126	0
83925	Assay opiates	32	42	52	0
83930	Assay blood osmolality	20	27	34	0
83935	Assay urine osmolality	31	40	50	0
83937	Assay osteocalcin	51	67	83	0
83945	Assay oxalate	52	68	85	0

LABORATORY SERVICES

Code	Short Description	50th	75th	90th	MC
83970	Assay parathormone	145	179	213	0
83986	Assay body fluid acidity	13	17	22	0
83992	Assay phencyclidine	44	58	73	0
84022	Assay phenothiazine	72	94	117	0
84030	Assay blood PKU	14	19	23	0
84035	Test for phenylketones	16	21	26	0
84060	Assay acid phosphatase, total	34	45	56	0
84061	Assay acid phosphatase, forensic	25	33	41	0
84066	Assay prostate phosphatase	37	47	58	0
84075	Assay alkaline phosphatase	18	24	30	0
84078	Assay alkaline phosphatase	31	41	51	0
84080	Assay alkaline phosphatases	55	72	89	0
84081	Assay phosphatidylglycerol	65	86	107	0
84085	Assay phosphogluconate enzyme	21	28	35	0
84087	Assay phosphohexose enzymes	35	47	58	0
84100	Assay phosphorus inorganic	16	21	26	0
84105	Assay phosphorus, urine	21	28	34	0
84106	Test for porphobilinogen	14	18	23	0
84110	Assay porphobilinogen	30	40	50	0
84119	Test for porphyrins, urine	30	40	50	0
84120	Assay porphyrins, urine	68	89	110	0
84126	Assay porphyrins, feces	72	95	118	0
84127	Test for porphyrins, feces	31	40	50	0
84132	Assay potassium, serum	17	21	26	0
84133	Assay potassium, urine	21	28	34	0
84134	Assay prealbumin	45	57	69	0
84135	Assay pregnanediol	78	103	128	0
84138	Assay pregnanetriol	75	99	123	0
84140	Assay pregnenolone	58	77	95	0
84143	Assay/17-hydroxypregnenolone	87	115	143	0
84144	Assay progesterone	65	86	106	0
84146	Assay prolactin	92	119	146	0
84150	Assay prostaglandin	84	110	137	0
84153	Assay prostate specific antigen	66	85	103	0
84155	Assay protein	21	28	35	0
84160	Assay serum protein	17	22	28	0
84165	Assay serum proteins	41	53	66	0
84181	Assay protein, Western blot test	55	72	90	0
84182	Assay protein, Western blot test	91	119	148	0
84202	Assay protoporphyrin, RBC	41	54	67	0

MC = Medicare Fee

DOES YOUR DOCTOR CHARGE TOO MUCH?

Code	Short Description	50th	75th	90th	MC
84203	Test for protoporphyrin, RBC	23	30	37	0
84206	Assay proinsulin	49	65	80	0
84207	Assay vitamin B-6	74	97	121	0
84210	Assay pyruvate	36	48	60	0
84220	Assay pyruvate kinase	36	47	59	0
84228	Assay quinine	47	62	78	0
84233	Assay estrogen	145	191	238	0
84234	Assay progesterone	143	189	235	0
84235	Assay endocrine hormone	161	213	264	0
84238	Assay non-endocrine receptor	125	165	205	0
84244	Assay renin	86	113	140	0
84252	Assay vitamin B-2	62	82	102	0
84255	Assay selenium	67	89	112	0
84260	Assay serotonin	120	160	201	0
84270	Assay sex hormone globulin (SHBG)	67	89	112	0
84275	Assay sialic acid	72	96	121	0
84285	Assay silica	89	119	149	0
84295	Assay serum sodium	15	20	25	0
84300	Assay urine sodium	20	27	34	0
84305	Assay somatomedin	101	134	168	0
84307	Assay somatostatin	53	70	88	0
84311	Spectrophotometry	32	43	54	0
84315	Specific gravity, body fluid	9	12	15	0
84375	Assay sugars, chromatogram	47	62	78	0
84392	Assay urine sulfate	25	33	42	0
84402	Assay testosterone, free	90	120	150	0
84403	Assay testosterone, total	101	131	161	0
84425	Assay vitamin B-1	52	70	88	0
84430	Assay thiocyanate	45	60	76	0
84432	Assay thyroglobulin	73	98	123	0
84436	Assay total thyroxine	22	29	36	0
84437	Assay neonatal thyroxine	18	24	31	0
84439	Assay free thyroxine	37	51	65	0
84442	Assay thyroid activity (TBG)	43	57	71	0
84443	Assay thyroid stimulation hormone	56	74	92	0
84445	Assay thyroid immunoglobulins (TSI)	165	221	277	0
84446	Assay vitamin E	42	56	71	0
84449	Assay transcortin	57	76	95	0
84450	Assay transferase (AST)(SGOT)	17	23	29	0
84460	Assay alanine amino (ALT)(SGPT)	19	25	31	0
84466	Assay transferrin	44	59	73	0

LABORATORY SERVICES

Code	Short Description	50th	75th	90th	MC
84478	Assay triglycerides	17	23	29	0
84479	Assay thyroid (T-3 or T-4)	21	27	34	0
84480	Assay triiodothyronine T-3, total	49	66	82	0
84481	Assay triiodothyronine T-3, free	62	82	103	0
84482	Assay triiodothyronine T-3, reverse	74	99	124	0
84485	Assay duodenal fluid trypsin	22	30	37	0
84488	Test feces for trypsin	20	27	33	0
84490	Assay feces for trypsin	22	29	37	0
84510	Assay tyrosine	36	49	61	0
84520	Assay urea nitrogen	16	21	26	0
84525	Assay urea nitrogen, semi	12	16	20	0
84540	Assay urea nitrogen, urine	23	31	39	0
84545	Assay urea nitrogen, clearance	22	29	37	0
84550	Assay blood uric acid	17	22	27	0
84560	Assay urine uric acid	20	27	34	0
84577	Assay feces urobilinogen	46	61	76	0
84578	Test for urine urobilinogen	12	16	20	0
84580	Assay urine urobilinogen	25	33	41	0
84583	Assay urine urobilinogen	15	20	25	0
84585	Assay urine VMA	67	90	113	0
84586	Assay VIP	54	72	90	0
84588	Assay vasopressin	80	107	135	0
84590	Assay vitamin-A	42	56	71	0
84597	Assay vitamin-K	50	67	84	0
84600	Assay volatiles	49	65	82	0
84620	Xylose tolerance test	49	66	82	0
84630	Assay zinc	42	55	70	0
84681	Assay C-peptide	81	108	135	0
84702	Test for chorionic gonadotropin	57	76	95	0
84703	Assay chorionic gonadotropin	38	50	63	0
84830	Ovulation tests	35	47	59	0

HEMATOLOGY AND COAGULATION

Code	Short Description	50th	75th	90th	MC
85002	Bleeding time test	21	28	35	0
85007	Differential WBC count	12	16	21	0
85008	Non-differential WBC count	10	14	18	0
85009	Differential WBC count	12	16	20	0
85013	Hematocrit	10	13	17	0
85014	Hematocrit	10	14	17	0

MC = Medicare Fee

Code	Short Description	50th	75th	90th	MC
85018	Hemoglobin	11	14	18	0
85021	Automated hemogram	18	23	28	0
85022	Automated hemogram	21	28	35	0
85023	Automated hemogram	26	34	42	0
85024	Automated hemogram	24	31	39	0
85025	Automated hemogram	25	32	40	0
85027	Automated hemogram	23	30	37	0
85029	Automated hemogram	14	19	24	0
85030	Automated hemogram	14	20	25	0
85031	Manual hemogram, complete CBC	20	26	33	0
85041	Red blood cell (RBC) count	11	15	18	0
85044	Reticulocyte count	17	23	30	0
85045	Reticulocyte count	15	19	24	0
85048	White blood cell (WBC) count	12	16	20	0
85060	Blood smear interpretation	43	57	71	22
85095	Bone marrow aspiration	115	150	187	58
85097	Bone marrow interpretation	98	129	163	47
85102	Bone marrow biopsy	145	190	239	71
85130	Chromogenic substrate assay	42	63	84	0
85170	Blood clot retraction	16	24	32	0
85175	Blood clot lysis time	16	24	32	0
85210	Blood clot factor II test	39	58	78	0
85220	Blood clot factor V test	67	100	133	0
85230	Blood clot factor VII test	67	100	134	0
85240	Blood clot factor VIII test	82	123	164	0
85244	Blood clot factor VIII test	83	124	165	0
85245	Blood clot factor VIII test	79	117	157	0
85246	Blood clot factor VIII test	84	125	167	0
85247	Blood clot factor VIII test	89	133	178	0
85250	Blood clot factor IX test	69	103	138	0
85260	Blood clot factor X test	69	103	138	0
85270	Blood clot factor XI test	69	103	138	0
85280	Blood clot factor XII test	69	103	138	0
85290	Blood clot factor XIII test	64	95	127	0
85291	Blood clot factor XIII test	32	47	63	0
85292	Blood clot factor assay	72	108	144	0
85293	Blood clot factor assay	72	108	144	0
85300	Antithrombin III test	49	73	97	0
85301	Antithrombin III test	48	72	96	0
85302	Blood clot inhibitor antigen	73	109	146	0
85303	Blood clot inhibitor test	50	75	101	0

LABORATORY SERVICES

Code	Short Description	50th	75th	90th	MC
85305	Blood clot inhibitor assay	66	99	132	0
85306	Blood clot inhibitor test	55	81	109	0
85335	Factor inhibitor test	35	52	70	0
85337	Thrombomodulin	33	49	66	0
85345	Coagulation time	18	27	36	0
85347	Coagulation time	12	18	24	0
85348	Coagulation time	15	22	29	0
85360	Euglobulin lysis	23	34	46	0
85362	Fibrin degradation products	30	45	61	0
85366	Fibrinogen test	24	36	48	0
85370	Fibrinogen test	35	52	69	0
85378	Fibrin degradation	29	44	59	0
85379	Fibrin degradation	34	51	68	0
85384	Fibrinogen	27	41	54	0
85385	Fibrinogen	31	46	61	0
85390	Fibrinolysins screen	23	34	45	0
85400	Fibrinolytic plasmin	19	28	38	0
85410	Fibrinolytic antiplasmin	19	29	39	0
85415	Fibrinolytic plasminogen	54	81	108	0
85420	Fibrinolytic plasminogen	27	40	53	0
85421	Fibrinolytic plasminogen	62	92	123	0
85441	Heinz bodies; direct	11	15	18	0
85445	Heinz bodies; induced	23	31	38	0
85460	Hemoglobin, fetal	23	31	38	0
85461	Hemoglobin, fetal	19	26	31	0
85475	Hemolysin	28	38	47	0
85520	Heparin assay	37	50	61	0
85525	Heparin	38	51	63	0
85530	Heparin-protamine tolerance	45	60	74	0
85535	Iron stain, blood cells	27	37	45	0
85540	WBC alkaline phosphatase	37	49	60	0
85547	RBC mechanical fragility	34	46	56	0
85549	Muramidase	63	84	103	0
85555	RBC osmotic fragility	25	33	40	0
85557	RBC osmotic fragility	51	69	84	0
85576	Blood platelet aggregation	20	27	33	0
85585	Blood platelet estimation	10	14	17	0
85590	Platelet count, manual	15	21	25	0
85595	Platelet count, automated	15	20	24	0
85597	Platelet neutralization	56	75	93	0

MC = Medicare Fee

Code	Short Description	50th	75th	90th	MC
85610	Prothrombin time	16	22	26	0
85611	Prothrombin test	15	20	25	0
85612	Viper venom prothrombin time	28	37	46	0
85613	Russell viper venom, diluted	34	46	56	0
85635	Reptilase test	38	51	63	0
85651	RBC sedimentation rate, non-auto	15	19	24	0
85652	RBC sedimentation rate, auto	22	29	36	0
85660	RBC sickle cell test	19	26	32	0
85670	Thrombin time, plasma	21	28	34	0
85675	Thrombin time, titer	20	27	34	0
85705	Thromboplastin inhibition	29	39	48	0
85730	Thromboplastin time, partial	23	30	36	0
85732	Thromboplastin time, partial	24	32	39	0
85810	Blood viscosity examination	44	59	72	0

IMMUNOLOGY

Code	Short Description	50th	75th	90th	MC
86000	Agglutinins; febrile	20	27	35	0
86003	Allergen specific IgE	37	49	65	0
86005	Allergen specific IgE	27	36	47	0
86021	WBC antibody identification	73	97	129	0
86022	Platelet antibodies	105	140	186	0
86023	Immunoglobulin assay	56	75	100	0
86038	Antinuclear antibodies	43	57	74	0
86039	Antinuclear antibodies (ANA)	36	48	63	0
86060	Antistreptolysin O titer	25	33	44	0
86063	Antistreptolysin O screen	25	33	43	0
86077	Physician blood bank service	88	118	156	40
86078	Physician blood bank service	104	140	185	41
86079	Physician blood bank service	85	114	151	41
86140	C-reactive protein	22	30	41	0
86147	Cardiolipin antibody	71	95	126	0
86155	Chemotaxis assay	42	56	75	0
86156	Cold agglutinin screen	25	34	45	0
86157	Cold agglutinin, titer	26	35	47	0
86160	Complement, antigen	46	63	85	0
86161	Complement/function activity	38	51	68	0
86162	Complement, total (CH50)	87	116	154	0
86171	Complement fixation, each	44	59	79	0
86185	Counterimmunoelectrophoresis	30	40	53	0

LABORATORY SERVICES

Code	Short Description	50th	75th	90th	MC
86215	Deoxyribonuclease, antibody	50	67	89	0
86225	DNA antibody	48	65	86	0
86226	DNA antibody, single strand	56	74	99	0
86235	Nuclear antigen antibody	45	62	83	0
86243	Fc receptor	75	100	132	0
86255	Fluorescent antibody; screen	45	60	79	0
86256	Fluorescent antibody; titer	45	62	85	0
86277	Growth hormone antibody	57	77	102	0
86280	Hemagglutination inhibition	33	44	58	0
86287	Hepatitis B (HBsAg)	40	51	66	0
86289	Hepatitis BC antibody test	49	65	86	0
86290	Hepatitis BC antibody test	47	58	73	0
86291	Hepatitis BS antibody test	40	51	65	0
86293	Hepatitis Be antibody test	44	59	78	0
86295	Hepatitis Be antibody test	44	59	78	0
86296	Hepatitis A antibody test	50	65	85	0
86299	Hepatitis A antibody test	45	59	76	0
86302	Hepatitis C antibody	54	69	90	0
86303	Hepatitis C antibody	48	64	85	0
86306	Hepatitis, delta agent	51	68	90	0
86308	Heterophile antibodies	23	31	41	0
86309	Heterophile antibodies	28	38	50	0
86310	Heterophile antibodies	30	40	52	0
86311	HIV antigen test	65	87	116	0
86313	Immunoassay, infectious agent	60	80	106	0
86315	Immunoassay, infectious agent	46	61	81	0
86316	Immunoassay, tumor antigen	67	87	113	0
86317	Immunoassay, infectious agent	43	59	80	0
86318	Immunoassay, infectious agent	40	54	71	0
86320	Serum immunoelectrophoresis	74	99	131	0
86325	Other immunoelectrophoresis	82	110	145	0
86327	Immunoelectrophoresis assay	84	113	150	0
86329	Immunodiffusion	46	61	81	0
86331	Immunodiffusion ouchterlony	40	53	71	0
86332	Immune complex assay	77	103	137	0
86334	Immunofixation procedure	80	107	141	0
86337	Insulin antibodies	76	102	136	0
86340	Intrinsic factor antibody	68	90	120	0
86341	Islet cell antibody	66	89	118	0
86343	Leukocyte histamine release	51	68	90	0

MC = Medicare Fee

DOES YOUR DOCTOR CHARGE TOO MUCH?

Code	Short Description	50th	75th	90th	MC
86344	Leukocyte phagocytosis	40	54	71	0
86353	Lymphocyte transformation	104	139	185	0
86359	T cells, total count	86	115	153	0
86360	T cell ratio	145	194	257	0
86376	Microsomal antibody	52	70	92	0
86378	Migration inhibitory factor	74	99	131	0
86382	Neutralization test, viral	74	99	131	0
86384	Nitroblue tetrazolium dye	38	51	68	0
86403	Particle agglutination test	29	41	56	0
86406	Particle agglutination test	38	51	68	0
86430	Rheumatoid factor test	20	27	37	0
86431	Rheumatoid factor, quantitative	25	33	43	0
86485	Skin test, candida	25	33	44	0
86490	Coccidioidomycosis skin test	21	29	38	10
86510	Histoplasmosis skin test	18	25	32	11
86580	TB intradermal test	16	21	27	9
86585	TB tine test	14	19	25	7
86588	Streptococcus, direct screen	23	31	41	0
86590	Streptokinase, antibody	24	33	43	0
86592	Blood serology, qualitative	14	19	26	0
86593	Blood serology, quantitative	15	21	27	0
86602	Actinomyces antibody	34	46	56	0
86603	Adenovirus, antibody	40	54	66	0
86606	Aspergillus antibody	44	59	73	0
86609	Bacterium, antibody	44	60	75	0
86612	Blastomyces, antibody	46	62	77	0
86615	Bordetella antibody	46	63	77	0
86617	Lyme disease antibody	56	75	93	0
86618	Lyme disease antibody	76	99	121	0
86619	Borrelia antibody	40	54	66	0
86622	Brucella, antibody	27	37	46	0
86625	Campylobacter, antibody	64	87	108	0
86628	Candida, antibody	36	49	61	0
86631	Chlamydia, antibody	49	66	82	0
86632	Chlamydia, IgM, antibody	40	54	66	0
86635	Coccidioides, antibody	40	55	68	0
86638	Q fever antibody	46	63	78	0
86641	Cryptococcus antibody	50	68	83	0
86644	CMV antibody	62	84	103	0
86645	CMV antibody, IgM	68	93	115	0
86648	Diphtheria antibody	49	66	82	0

LABORATORY SERVICES

Code	Short Description	50th	75th	90th	MC
86651	Encephalitis antibody	41	56	69	0
86652	Encephalitis antibody	41	56	69	0
86653	Encephalitis antibody	41	56	69	0
86654	Encephalitis antibody	41	56	69	0
86658	Enterovirus antibody	39	53	65	0
86663	Epstein-barr antibody	44	60	74	0
86664	Epstein-barr antibody	50	68	83	0
86665	Epstein-barr antibody	58	79	98	0
86668	Francisella tularensis	31	42	52	0
86671	Fungus, antibody	43	58	72	0
86674	Giardia lamblia	50	68	84	0
86677	Helicobacter pylori	66	89	109	0
86682	Helminth, antibody	41	56	69	0
86684	Hemophilus influenza	49	66	82	0
86687	HTLV I	33	45	55	0
86688	HTLV-II	41	56	69	0
86689	HTLV/HIV confirmatory test	63	86	106	0
86692	Hepatitis, delta agent	60	82	101	0
86694	Herpes simplex test	58	78	97	0
86695	Herpes simplex test	54	74	91	0
86698	Histoplasma	45	61	76	0
86701	HIV-1	58	77	94	0
86702	HIV-2	43	59	72	0
86703	HIV-1/HIV-2, single assay	42	57	71	0
86710	Influenza virus	48	65	80	0
86713	Legionella	54	73	90	0
86717	Leishmania	39	53	65	0
86720	Leptospira	39	53	65	0
86723	Listeria monocytogenes	41	56	69	0
86727	Lymph choriomeningitis	39	53	65	0
86729	Lymphogranuloma venereum	38	52	64	0
86732	Mucormycosis	41	56	69	0
86735	Mumps	30	41	50	0
86738	Mycoplasma	62	84	104	0
86741	Neisseria meningitidis	41	56	69	0
86744	Nocardia	41	56	69	0
86747	Parvovirus	46	63	77	0
86750	Malaria	50	68	84	0
86753	Protozoa, not elsewhere	45	61	75	0
86756	Respiratory virus	39	53	66	0

MC = Medicare Fee

Code	Short Description	50th	75th	90th	MC
86759	Rotavirus	42	57	70	0
86762	Rubella	38	52	64	0
86765	Rubeola	53	72	88	0
86768	Salmonella	41	56	69	0
86771	Shigella	41	56	69	0
86774	Tetanus	52	71	88	0
86777	Toxoplasma	56	76	94	0
86778	Toxoplasma, IgM	59	80	99	0
86781	Treponema pallidum confirm	47	64	79	0
86784	Trichinella	41	56	69	0
86787	Varicella-zoster	55	75	92	0
86790	Virus, not specified	59	80	99	0
86793	Yersinia	43	58	72	0
86800	Thyroglobulin antibody	59	80	99	0
86805	Lymphocytotoxicity assay	140	190	235	0
86806	Lymphocytotoxicity assay	117	159	197	0
86807	Cytotoxic antibody screening	105	142	176	0
86808	Cytotoxic antibody screening	75	103	127	0
86812	HLA typing, A, B, or C	144	196	242	0
86813	HLA typing, A, B, or C	150	204	252	0
86816	HLA typing, DR/DQ	106	144	178	0
86817	HLA typing, DR/DQ	209	284	351	0
86821	Lymphocyte culture, mixed	179	244	301	0
86822	Lymphocyte culture, primed	131	179	221	0

TRANSFUSION MEDICINE

Code	Short Description	50th	75th	90th	MC
86850	RBC antibody screen	34	46	58	0
86860	RBC antibody elution	61	81	102	0
86870	RBC antibody identification	41	55	69	0
86880	Coombs test	23	31	38	0
86885	Coombs test	24	32	40	0
86886	Coombs test	22	29	37	0
86890	Autologous blood process	63	85	106	0
86891	Autologous blood, op salvage	129	173	217	0
86900	Blood typing, ABO	14	18	23	0
86901	Blood typing, Rh (D)	18	23	30	0
86903	Blood typing, antigen screen	29	39	48	0
86904	Blood typing, patient serum	27	36	45	0
86905	Blood typing, RBC antigens	15	20	25	0

LABORATORY SERVICES

Code	Short Description	50th	75th	90th	MC
86906	Blood typing, Rh phenotype	21	29	36	0
86910	Blood typing, paternity test	113	151	190	0
86911	Blood typing, antigen system	33	44	55	0
86915	Bone marrow	62	83	104	0
86920	Compatibility test	46	61	77	0
86921	Compatibility test	34	45	56	0
86922	Compatibility test	33	45	56	0
86927	Plasma, fresh frozen	36	47	60	0
86930	Frozen blood prep	209	279	351	0
86931	Frozen blood thaw	210	280	352	0
86932	Frozen blood, freeze/thaw	217	290	364	0
86940	Hemolysins/agglutinins auto	27	36	46	0
86941	Hemolysins/agglutinins	42	56	71	0
86945	Blood product/irradiation	49	65	82	0
86950	Leukocyte transfusion	134	179	225	0
86965	Pooling blood platelets	36	48	60	0
86970	RBC pretreatment	57	75	95	0
86971	RBC pretreatment	29	38	48	0
86972	RBC pretreatment	29	39	49	0
86975	RBC pretreatment, serum	73	98	123	0
86976	RBC pretreatment, serum	73	98	123	0
86977	RBC pretreatment, serum	73	98	123	0
86978	RBC pretreatment, serum	88	118	148	0
86985	Split blood or products	46	61	77	0

MICROBIOLOGY

Code	Short Description	50th	75th	90th	MC
87001	Small animal inoculation	49	66	82	0
87003	Small animal inoculation	58	78	97	0
87015	Specimen concentration	24	32	40	0
87040	Blood culture for bacteria	44	59	74	0
87045	Stool culture for bacteria	38	51	64	0
87060	Nose/throat culture, bacteria	28	37	47	0
87070	Culture specimen, bacteria	34	45	56	0
87072	Culture of specimen by kit	22	29	36	0
87075	Culture specimen, bacteria	37	51	64	0
87076	Bacteria identification	38	52	64	0
87081	Bacteria culture screen	22	30	37	0
87082	Culture of specimen by kit	22	30	38	0
87083	Culture of specimen by kit	23	31	39	0

MC = Medicare Fee

DOES YOUR DOCTOR CHARGE TOO MUCH?

Code	Short Description	50th	75th	90th	MC
87084	Culture of specimen by kit	27	35	42	0
87085	Culture of specimen by kit	28	35	43	0
87086	Urine culture, colony count	30	40	49	0
87087	Urine bacteria culture	23	30	38	0
87088	Urine bacteria culture	25	33	41	0
87101	Skin fungus culture	25	34	42	0
87102	Fungus isolation culture	31	40	50	0
87103	Blood fungus culture	39	52	65	0
87106	Fungus identification	32	41	49	0
87109	Mycoplasma culture	45	61	76	0
87110	Culture, chlamydia	52	70	87	0
87116	Mycobacteria culture	39	52	65	0
87117	Mycobacteria culture	48	64	80	0
87118	Mycobacteria identification	35	47	59	0
87140	Culture typing, fluorescent	29	39	49	0
87143	Culture typing, GLC method	50	67	84	0
87145	Culture typing, phage method	28	37	47	0
87147	Culture typing, serologic	21	28	35	0
87151	Culture typing, serologic	20	27	33	0
87155	Culture typing, precipitin	15	21	26	0
87158	Culture typing, added method	15	20	25	0
87163	Special microbiology culture	37	47	57	0
87164	Dark field examination	44	59	73	0
87166	Dark field examination	35	47	59	0
87174	Endotoxin, bacterial	54	73	91	0
87175	Assay, endotoxin, bacterial	41	55	68	0
87176	Endotoxin, bacterial	27	37	46	0
87177	Ova and parasites smears	33	46	58	0
87178	Microbe identification	47	61	75	0
87179	Microbe identification	57	77	96	0
87181	Antibiotic sensitivity, each	15	20	25	0
87184	Antibiotic sensitivity, each	22	29	36	0
87186	Antibiotic sensitivity, MIC	29	38	47	0
87187	Antibiotic sensitivity, MBC	27	36	45	0
87188	Antibiotic sensitivity, each	18	24	30	0
87190	TB antibiotic sensitivity	15	20	25	0
87192	Antibiotic sensitivity, each	28	38	47	0
87197	Bactericidal level, serum	42	56	70	0
87205	Smear, stain and interpret	16	22	27	0
87206	Smear, stain and interpret	23	30	36	0
87207	Smear, stain and interpret	21	28	35	0

LABORATORY SERVICES

Code	Short Description	50th	75th	90th	MC
87208	Smear, stain and interpret	19	26	32	0
87210	Smear, stain and interpret	15	20	24	0
87211	Smear, stain and interpret	18	24	30	0
87220	Tissue exam for fungi	18	24	30	0
87230	Assay, toxin or antitoxin	66	89	110	0
87250	Virus inoculation for test	68	92	114	0
87252	Virus inoculation for test	82	110	138	0
87253	Virus inoculation for test	57	77	96	0

ANATOMIC PATHOLOGY

Code	Short Description	50th	75th	90th	MC
88000	Autopsy (necropsy), gross	678	882	1081	0
88005	Autopsy (necropsy), gross	782	1018	1248	0
88007	Autopsy (necropsy), gross	882	1147	1406	0
88012	Autopsy (necropsy), gross	719	935	1147	0
88014	Autopsy (necropsy), gross	719	935	1147	0
88016	Autopsy (necropsy), gross	678	882	1081	0
88020	Autopsy (necropsy), complete	905	1178	1444	0
88025	Autopsy (necropsy), complete	972	1263	1550	0
88027	Autopsy (necropsy), complete	1067	1388	1702	0
88028	Autopsy (necropsy), complete	890	1157	1419	0
88029	Autopsy (necropsy), complete	890	1157	1419	0
88036	Limited autopsy	736	957	1174	0
88037	Limited autopsy	590	767	941	0
88040	Forensic autopsy (necropsy)	2207	2870	3520	0
88104	Microscopic exam of cells	59	77	94	34
88106	Microscopic exam of cells	56	73	89	31
88107	Microscopic exam of cells	83	108	133	41
88108	Cytopathology	84	109	133	35
88125	Forensic cytopathology	52	67	82	12
88130	Sex chromatin identification	40	51	63	0
88140	Sex chromatin identification	27	35	43	0
88150	Cytopathology, pap smear	22	28	35	0
88151	Cytopathology interpretation	23	29	35	0
88155	Cytopathology, pap smear	23	30	36	0
88156	TBS smear (Bethesda system)	27	33	40	0
88157	TBS smear (Bethesda system)	26	34	41	0
88160	Cytopathology	50	65	80	28
88161	Cytopathology	57	74	91	30
88162	Cytopathology, extensive	86	112	137	52

MC = Medicare Fee

Code	Short Description	50th	75th	90th	MC
88170	Fine needle aspiration	124	162	198	76
88171	Fine needle aspiration	140	183	224	88
88172	Evaluation of smear	83	108	133	44
88173	Interpretation of smear	107	139	171	74
88180	Cell marker study	80	108	135	23
88182	Cell marker study	144	188	230	56
88230	Tissue culture, lymphocyte	247	321	394	0
88233	Tissue culture, skin/biopsy	296	385	473	0
88235	Tissue culture, placenta	337	438	537	0
88237	Tissue culture, bone marrow	294	382	469	0
88239	Tissue culture, other	334	435	533	0
88245	Chromosome analysis	311	405	496	0
88248	Chromosome analysis	310	404	495	0
88250	Chromosome analysis	355	462	567	0
88260	Chromosome analysis: 5 cells	260	338	414	0
88261	Chromosome analysis: 5 cells	354	460	564	0
88262	Chromosome analysis: 15-20 cells	403	524	642	0
88263	Chromosome analysis: 45 cells	374	486	596	0
88267	Chromosome analysis: placenta	645	839	1029	0
88269	Chromosome analysis: amniotic	396	515	632	0
88280	Chromosome karyotype study	76	99	121	0
88283	Chromosome banding study	146	190	233	0
88285	Chromosome count: additional	33	43	53	0
88289	Chromosome study: additional	77	100	122	0

SURGICAL PATHOLOGY

Code	Short Description	50th	75th	90th	MC
88300	Surgical pathology, gross	33	44	54	10
88302	Tissue exam by pathologist	62	83	103	19
88304	Tissue exam by pathologist	80	106	131	29
88305	Tissue exam by pathologist	121	159	196	61
88307	Tissue exam by pathologist	211	283	352	105
88309	Tissue exam by pathologist	304	405	503	140
88311	Decalcify tissue	33	44	55	15
88312	Special stains	41	55	68	26
88313	Special stains	37	50	63	15
88314	Histochemical stain	53	71	88	36
88318	Chemical histochemistry	60	79	98	21
88319	Enzyme histochemistry	61	81	101	34
88321	Microslide consultation	106	138	169	55

LABORATORY SERVICES

Code	Short Description	50th	75th	90th	MC
88323	Microslide consultation	91	121	151	68
88325	Comprehensive review of data	146	195	242	86
88329	Pathology consult in surgery	89	115	141	34
88331	Pathology consult in surgery	140	182	223	77
88332	Pathology consult in surgery	75	100	124	39
88342	Immunocytochemistry	94	123	150	49
88346	Immunofluorescent study	102	135	168	48
88347	Immunofluorescent study	106	142	176	42
88348	Electron microscopy	333	443	551	129
88349	Scanning electron microscopy	265	352	438	80
88355	Analysis, skeletal muscle	205	273	339	121
88356	Analysis, nerve	270	359	446	190
88358	Analysis, tumor	239	318	395	171
88362	Nerve teasing preparations	244	325	403	138
88365	Tissue hybridization	89	119	148	56
88371	Protein, western blot tissue	51	67	84	0
88372	Protein analysis w/probe	55	73	90	0

OTHER LABORATORY PROCEDURES

Code	Short Description	50th	75th	90th	MC
89050	Body fluid cell count	18	25	32	0
89051	Body fluid cell count	22	30	38	0
89060	Exam, synovial fluid crystals	28	39	50	0
89100	Sample intestinal contents	79	109	139	34
89105	Sample intestinal contents	80	111	142	30
89125	Specimen fat stain	21	30	38	0
89130	Sample stomach contents	63	87	111	29
89132	Sample stomach contents	38	52	66	13
89135	Sample stomach contents	82	113	145	46
89136	Sample stomach contents	58	80	102	15
89140	Sample stomach contents	111	154	196	59
89141	Sample stomach contents	115	159	203	53
89160	Exam feces for meat fibers	12	17	22	0
89190	Nasal smear for eosinophils	17	24	30	0
89250	Fertilization of oocyte	804	1111	1418	0
89300	Semen analysis	35	49	62	0
89310	Semen analysis	33	45	58	0
89320	Semen analysis	44	60	77	0
89325	Sperm antibody test	41	57	73	0
89329	Sperm evaluation test	127	175	223	0

MC = Medicare Fee

Code	Short Description	50th	75th	90th	MC
89330	Evaluation, cervical mucus	40	55	70	0
89350	Sputum specimen collection	28	39	50	14
89355	Exam feces for starch	15	21	27	0
89360	Collect sweat for test	35	48	62	16
89365	Water load test	39	53	68	0

APPENDIX

GEOGRAPHIC VARIABILITY AND ADJUSTMENT

In order to more accurately determine the percentile doctors fees in the area where you live, we have included this appendix of geographic adjustment factors. A *geographic adjustment factor* (GAF) is a multiplier used to determine the correct fee for a specific location of medical practice. This appendix includes a list of geographic adjustment factors for cities, counties, areas, regions and states which can be used to "fine tune" the doctors fees listed in this book. The geographic adjustment factors listed below are based upon the Medicare Fee Schedule.

The percentile fees presented in this book are based on national fee data. However, doctors fees vary substantially by geographic area. In rural areas and smaller towns and cities, doctors fees may be significantly lower than the percentiles presented in this book. Likewise, in larger cities, doctors fees may be significantly higher than the fees presented. There are two primary reasons for the geographic variation in doctors fees; namely, the cost of running a medical practice and the cost of medical malpractice insurance.

The cost of practice includes rent, employee costs, and other overhead costs, but not medical malpractice costs. According to the cost of practice indexes published in the *Medicare Fee Schedule*, New York City has the highest cost of practice and small eastern cities of Missouri have the lowest cost of practice. The cost of running a medical practice in New York City is almost 68% higher than running a medical practice in a small eastern city of Missouri.

The second reason for the geographic variation in doctors fees is the cost of medical malpractice insurance. According to the malpractice expense indexes published in the Medicare Fee Schedule, New York City has the highest cost of medical malpractice insurance and South Dakota has the lowest cost of medical malpractice insurance. Medical malpractice insurance costs are just over 248% higher in New York City than they are in South Dakota.

These differences in the cost of practice and medical malpractice insurance are reflected in the wide range of fees charged by doctors for identical services provided in different geographic locations.

MC = Medicare Fee

CITY, COUNTY, STATE OR AREA

This is the geographic region included in the geographic adjustment factor. The specific geographic regions listed below are taken directly from the Medicare Fee Schedule. As is common with government programs, there is no uniformity in what the areas are called or how they are assigned. You will note that most geographic adjustment factors correspond to entire states or specific cities. But others correspond to specific counties, or terms such as urban, metropolitan, rural, large, small, north west, south west, etc.

GAF

The geographic adjustment factor (GAF) for the city, county, area, region or state listed. Multiplying the GAF times the doctor's fee listed in this book results in a fee that has been adjusted to a particular geographic area.

HOW TO ADJUST FEES FOR YOUR LOCATION

To use the geographic adjustment factor, first look up the CPT codes in the book that you want to compare to your doctor's fees or health insurance carrier allowances. Write down the 50th, 75th and 90th percentile fees for each CPT code. Then look up the geographic adjustment factor for your city, county, area, region or state in this appendix. Finally, multiply the percentile fees times the geographic adjustment factor to determine the adjusted fee.

In order to clearly illustrate let's look at two medical services provided in Phoenix, New York City, or anywhere in South Dakota. We first look up and write down the percentile fees for each service. Then, looking up these locations in this appendix, we find that the GAF for Phoenix is 1.007, the GAF for New York City is 1.246 and the GAF for South Dakota is .866. Finally, we multiply the percentile fees times the GAF for each location to determine the adjusted fee.

Code	Short Description		50th	75th	90th	MC
99205	Office visit, new patient; xx minutes		158	192	227	121
	Phoenix	(multiply by 1.007)	159	193	229	122
	New York City	(multiply by 1.246)	197	239	285	151
	South Dakota	(multiply by .866)	137	166	197	105

Code	Short Description		50th	75th	90th	MC
33513	CABG, vein, four		5644	7876	9664	2972
	Phoenix	(multiply by 1.007)	5684	7931	9732	2993
	New York City	(multiply by 1.246)	7032	9814	12041	3703
	South Dakota	(multiply by .866)	4888	6821	8369	2574

As these examples clearly illustrate, medical fees in Phoenix are very close to the national average, medical fees in New York are almost 25% higher than the national average and medical fees in South Dakota are a little over 13% lower than the national average. As previously explained, these variations are due to the cost of practice and cost of medical malpractice insurance.

GEOGRAPHIC ADJUSTMENT FACTORS BY STATE

STATE/LOCALITY	GAF
ALABAMA	
Birmingham	0.952
Mobile	0.919
North Central	0.914
Northwest	0.932
Southeast	0.916
Rest of State	0.895
ALASKA	
Entire State	1.143
ARIZONA	
Flagstaff	0.979
Phoenix	1.007
Prescott	0.968
Tucson	0.985
Yuma	0.980
Rest of State	0.993
ARKANSAS	
Entire State	0.872
CALIFORNIA	
Anaheim/Santa Ana	1.094

MC = Medicare Fee

STATE/LOCALITY	GAF
CALIFORNIA (continued)	
Bakersfield	0.986
Fresno/Madera	0.962
Kings/Tulare	0.945
Los Angeles	1.104
Marin/Napa/Solano	1.061
Merced/Surrounding Counties	0.968
Monterey/Santa Cruz	1.041
North Coastal Counties	1.015
Northeast Rural	0.942
Oakland/Berkeley	1.090
Riverside	1.009
Sacramento/Surrounding Counties	1.013
San Bernardino/East Central Counties	1.015
San Diego/Imperial	1.017
San Francisco	1.154
San Mateo	1.132
Santa Barbara	1.040
Santa Clara	1.134
Stockton/Surrounding Counties	0.991
Ventura	1.079
COLORADO	
Entire State	0.961
CONNECTICUT	
Eastern	1.076
Northwest and North Central	1.096
South Central	1.129
CONNECTICUT (continued)	
Southwest	1.151
DELAWARE	
Entire State	1.010
DISTRICT OF COLUMBIA	
Washington, D.C. and Suburbs	1.110

APPENDIX

STATE/LOCALITY	GAF
FLORIDA	
Fort Lauderdale	1.075
Miami	1.147
North/North Central Cities	0.996
Rest of State	0.976
GEORGIA	
Atlanta	1.010
Small Cities	0.946
Rest of State	0.911
HAWAII AND GUAM	
Entire State and territory	1.094
IDAHO	
North	0.889
South	0.903
ILLINOIS	
Champaign-Urbana	0.925
Chicago	1.076
De Kalb	0.905
Decatur	0.912
East St. Louis	0.976
Kankakee	0.920
Normal	0.918
Northwest	0.886
Peoria	0.929
Quincy	0.876
Rock Island	0.904
Rockford	0.950
South East	0.871
Southern	0.881
Springfield	0.958
Suburban Chicago	1.056
INDIANA	
Metropolitan	0.922
Urban	0.895
Rest of State	0.884

STATE/LOCALITY	GAF
IOWA	
Entire State	0.903
KANSAS	
Kansas City	0.985
Suburban Kansas City	0.985
Rest of State	0.937
KENTUCKY	
Lexington & Louisville	0.939
Small Cities	0.900
Rest of State	0.886
LOUISIANA	
Alexandria	0.912
Baton Rouge	0.938
Lafayette	0.915
Lake Charles	0.936
Monroe	0.913
New Orleans	0.975
Shreveport	0.930
Rest of State	0.909
MAINE	
Central	0.933
Northern	0.930
Southern	0.989
MARYLAND	
Baltimore/Surrounding Counties	1.034
South & East Shore	0.971
Western	0.950
MASSACHUSETTS	
Suburbs/Rural Cities	1.051
Urban	1.089
MICHIGAN	
Detroit	1.178
Rest of State	1.027

STATE/LOCALITY	GAF
MINNESOTA	
Entire State	0.951
MISSISSIPPI	
Urban	0.904
Rest of State	0.872
MISSOURI	
Kansas City (Jackson County)	0.986
North Kansas City (Clay/Platte)	0.985
Rural North West Counties	0.912
Small Eastern Cities	0.895
St. Joseph	0.920
St. Louis/Large Eastern Cities	0.969
Rest of State	0.898
MONTANA	
Entire State	0.899
NEBRASKA	
Entire State	0.880
NEVADA	
Elko & Ely	0.978
Las Vegas	1.008
Reno	1.013
Rest of State	0.997
NEW HAMPSHIRE	
Entire State	1.004
NEW JERSEY	
Middle	1.061
Northern	1.109
Southern	1.032
NEW MEXICO	
Entire State	0.930

STATE/LOCALITY	GAF
NEW YORK	
Buffalo/Surrounding Counties	0.960
Manhattan	1.246
North Central Cities	0.975
New York City Suburbs/Long Island	1.191
Poughkpsie/N. New York City Suburbs	1.057
Queens	1.184
Rochester/Surrounding Counties	0.990
Rest of State	0.954
NORTH CAROLINA	
Entire State	0.910
NORTH DAKOTA	
Entire State	0.887
OHIO	
Entire State	0.972
OKLAHOMA	
Entire State	0.896
OREGON	
Eugene	0.927
Portland	0.974
Salem	0.926
South West Cities	0.938
Rest of State	0.915
PENNSYLVANIA	
Large Cities	0.999
Philadelphia/Pittsburgh	1.046
Small Cities	0.936
Rest of State	0.922
PUERTO RICO	
Entire Territory	0.775
RHODE ISLAND	
Entire State	1.082

APPENDIX

STATE/LOCALITY	GAF
SOUTH CAROLINA	
Entire State	0.899
SOUTH DAKOTA	
Entire State	0.866
TENNESSEE	
Entire State	0.910
TEXAS	
Abilene	0.901
Amarillo	0.923
Austin	0.975
Beaumont	0.977
Brazoria	1.010
Brownsville	0.898
Corpus Christi	0.934
Dallas	1.004
Denton	0.951
El Paso	0.931
Fort Worth	0.975
Galveston	1.009
Grayson	0.911
Houston	1.042
Laredo	0.900
Longview	0.913
Lubbock	0.918
McAllen	0.895
Midland	0.938
Northeast Rural	0.904
Odessa	0.938
Orange	0.936
San Angelo	0.892
San Antonio	0.944
Southeast Rural	0.917
Temple	0.920
Texarkana	0.908
Tyler	0.926
Victoria	0.920
Waco	0.916

STATE/LOCALITY	GAF
TEXAS (continued)	
Western Texas	0.884
Wichita Falls	0.899
UTAH	
Entire State	0.916
VERMONT	
Entire State	0.945
VIRGIN ISLANDS	
Entire territory	0.975
VIRGINIA	
Richmond & Charlottesville	0.964
Small Town/Industrial	0.908
Tidewater & North Counties	0.947
Rest of State	0.898
WASHINGTON	
East Central & Northeast	0.950
Seattle (King County)	1.020
West & Southeast (excluding Seattle)	0.960
WEST VIRGINIA	
Charleston	0.937
Eastern Valley	0.935
Ohio River Valley	0.905
Southern Valley	0.893
Wheeling	0.907
WISCONSIN	
Central	0.923
Green Bay (Northeast)	0.951
Janesville (South Central)	0.947
La Crosse (West Central)	0.943
Madison (Dane County)	1.006
Milwaukee Suburbs (Southeast)	0.987
Milwaukee	1.001
Northwest	0.924
Oshkosh (East Central)	0.946

STATE/LOCALITY	GAF
WISCONSIN	
Southwest	0.923
Wausau (North Central)	0.932
WYOMING	
Entire State	0.918

THE AUTHOR

James B. Davis has been in the health care field for over 30 years working closely with doctors, hospitals and insurance carriers. He is currently President of Practice Management Information Corporation, the nation's leading publisher of medical business books.

A nationally known expert on the subject of medical billing, he has given seminars to hundreds of doctors and is the author of several books on the subject. He is also the founder of Kid Care Los Angeles, a non-profit organization which meals-on-wheels to hundreds of pre-school aged children in the Los Angeles area. He resides in Los Angeles, California with his two young sons.

INDEX

A

abdomen 155, 171-173
abdomen x-ray 220
abortion 191, 192
accident and health insurance 5, 32
addictive disorders 22
adenoids 160
adjusting fees 39, 40
adrenal glands 192, 223
allergy and immunology 80
allergy testing 80
anatomic pathology 255
ankle joint 124-127
anus 168, 169
aorta and arteries x-ray 222
appendix 166
application of casts 132
arthroscopy 133, 134
assignment of benefits 17, 26, 34
audiologic function tests 73
auditory system surgery 211
automated laboratory panels 233
autonomic nervous system 201

B

back and flank 103
basic medical plans 17, 18
beneficiaries 15-17
benefit period limitation 22
biliary tract 170
biofeedback 69
bladder 176-180
Blue Cross 17-19
Blue Shield 17-19
brain 193-197, 215-217, 231
breast 96, 97, 224, 225
bronchi 138, 217

C

capitation 28, 42
cardiac catheterization 76
cardiography 74
cardiovascular services 74
cardiovascular system surgery 141
care plan oversight services 65
carrier 16
case management services 64
central nervous system 82
cerebrovascular arterial studies 78
cervix uteri 188
cesarean delivery 191
CHAMPUS 19
chemistry 233, 236
chemotherapy administration 83
chest ultrasound 225
chest x-ray 37, 217
chiropractic treatment 85
co-insurance 23, 27, 28, 57
co-payment 18, 19, 23, 50
coding errors 38, 52-54
commercial carriers 17
comprehensive medical plans 18
conjunctiva 210
consultations 62
consultations (pathology) 236
contact lens service 71
coordination of benefits 23, 24
corpus uteri 188
CPT 36
critical care services 63
custodial services 64

D

deductible 23
deductible carryover 23

271

dentoalveolar structures 158
dependents 17, 19
dermatology procedures 83
destruction of lesions 95
determining eligibility 24
diagnosis coding 37
diagnostic nuclear medicine 229
diagnostic radiology 215
diagnostic ultrasound 215, 225
diaphragm 155
digestive system surgery 156
discount business 41, 50, 87
doctor billing 33-38
doctor fees 39-42
doctor visits 61-65
drug testing 234
dual coverage 23, 24

E

ear, nose and throat services 72
echocardiography 75
electroencephalograph 82
emergency department services 63
endocrine system surgery 192
enrollee 17
EOB 49, 50
epididymis 183
esophagus 70, 160-163, 221
evocative/suppression testing 235
exclusions 17, 21
explanation of benefits 37, 45, 49-51, 53
external ear 74, 146, 168, 211
extracranial nerves 201
extremity arterial studies 78
extremity arterial-venous studies 78
extremity ultrasound 226
extremity venous studies 78
eye surgery 204
eye examinations 70
eye glasses 71, 72

eye prosthesis 71, 72
eyeball 204

F

fee-for-service 26
female genital system surgery 186
femur (thigh) and knee joint 121
fetal testing 190
fibula 98, 124-126
fingers 114
foot and toes 127, 129
forearm and wrist 110
forms and documents 33, 35

G

gastroenterology services 70
gastrointestinal tract x-ray 220
genitalia ultrasound 226
geographic adjustment factor 52, 58, 59, 259, 260
geographic variability and adjustment 58, 259
government plans 24
government programs 16, 28, 260
group plans 16, 23
group policies 16

H

hand and fingers 114
HCFA 19, 37
HCFA1500 45, 47, 48, 50, 57
head 81, 92, 98, 99, 106, 108, 109, 120, 196, 202-204, 215-217, 222, 225
head and neck ultrasound 215, 222, 225
health insurance claim form 45, 47-50, 52, 57

health insurance company 19, 26, 35, 47, 53, 57
health insurance fraud 30-32
health insurance plan 15, 17, 24, 25, 27, 28, 33-35, 38-40, 45, 47, 49, 50, 52-54, 58
health insurance policy 16, 17, 22, 23, 34
health maintenance organizations 17, 19, 21
heart and pericardium 141
heart x-ray 222
hematology and coagulation 245
HMO 26, 42
home services 64
hospital inpatient services 62
humerus (upper arm) and elbow 108
hysteroscopy 185

I-J

ICD-9-CM 36
immunization injections 67
immunology 80, 248
in vitro fertilization 190
increased operating costs 41
indemnity schedule 28
individual plans 23
individual policies 16
individual/family deductible 23
infusion therapy 68
inner ear 213
insured 16, 17, 23-25, 28, 47, 50, 52
insurer 16, 32
integumentary system 87
intestines 164
intracardiac electrophysiologic procedures 76
introitus 186
IPA 42

K

kidney 174-176, 179, 222, 223, 226, 231, 232
kidney dialysis services 69
knee joint 121-124, 220

L

laboratory services 233
laparoscopy and hysteroscopy 185
larynx 137, 138, 216
leg 92, 121-127, 132, 133
leg and ankle joint 124
limitation of benefits 50, 52
limitation of insurance coverage 21
lips 156
liver 170, 171
lower extremities x-ray 219
lungs and pleura 139
lymph nodes 154

M

major medical insurance 10
major medical plans 18
male genital system surgery 181
managed care 32, 34, 49
maternity care and delivery 190
maximum coverage amounts 22
maximum fee schedule 28
Meckel's diverticulum 166
mediastinum and diaphragm 155
Medicaid 20
medical coding systems 33, 36
medical radiation physics 227
Medicare 19
medicine services 67-85
mental and addictive disorders 22
mesentery 166
microbiology 253, 254
middle ear 211, 212, 216

musculoskeletal system surgery 97

N

nails 90
neck (soft tissues) and thorax 103
neonatal intensive care 63, 244
nervous system surgery 193
neurology procedures 81, 82
neuromuscular testing 81
new patient 61
newborn care 65
non-invasive vascular diagnostic studies 78
nose 72, 80, 101, 134, 135
nuclear medicine 229
nursing facility services 63

O

office services 62
omentum 172
ophthalmology services 70
osteopathic treatment 85
outpatient services 62
ovary 189
oviduct 189

P-Q

palate and uvula 158
pancreas 162, 171, 172
parathyroid 192
pelvis and hip joint 118
pelvis ultrasound 226
penile vascular studies 78
penis 154, 181, 182
pericardium 141
perineum 186, 187
peripheral nerves 201
peritoneum 172
pharynx, adenoids and tonsils 160
physical therapy 83
pleura 139
policy holder 17
posterior segment 207
postpartum care 191
PPO 42
pre-authorization 24, 25, 50
pre-determination 25
pre-existing conditions 21
premium 18, 19, 23
prenatal care 191
preventive medicine services 65
primary carrier 24
procedure coding 36
prolonged services 64
prostate 179, 184
provider 16, 17, 27, 35
psychiatry services 68
pulmonary services 79

R

radiation oncology 227
radiation treatment 227, 228
radiology services 215-232
reasonable charge 26
rectum 164, 166-168
rehabilitation 83
relative value scale 28-30, 39, 41
respiratory system surgery 134
rest home services 64

S

salivary gland and ducts 159
schedule of allowances 28-30
scrotum 183, 226
secondary carrier 12
seminal vesicles 184
shoulder 105-107, 132, 133, 219
sinuses 136, 216

skin, subcutaneous and
        accessory structures 87
skull 101, 104, 193-197, 216, 223
sleep testing 81
special services and reports 85
specialty differential 60
spermatic cord 184
spinal canal ultrasound 226
spinal cord 197-200
spine and pelvis x-ray 217
spine and spinal cord 197
spleen and lymphatic systems 154
stomach 162-164, 202, 221
subscriber 17, 19, 47
superbill 45, 46, 50
surgery services 87-213
surgical pathology 256

T

table of allowances 28
testis 182, 183
therapeutic drug assays 234
therapeutic injections 68
thorax 103, 104, 151 219
thymus 192
thyroid gland 192
tibia 124-126, 128
toes 127, 129, 133
tongue and floor of mouth 157
tonsils 160
trachea and bronchi 138
transfusion medicine 252
tunica vaginalis 183

U

ultrasonic guidance procedures 226
underwriter 16
upper extremities x-ray 219
ureter 174-178
urethra 178-182, 187
urinalysis 236
urinary system surgery 174
urinary tract x-ray 221
usual, customary, and reasonable 26

V

vagina 178, 186-188
vaginal delivery 191
veins and lymphatics x-ray 223
verifying benefits 24
vertebral column 103
vestibular function tests 72
vestibule of mouth 156
visit services 61-65
vulva, perineum and introitus 186

W-X-Y-Z

workers' compensation 20
wound repair 90
wrist 110-114, 132-134, 219